Yoga Biomechanics

Jules Mitchell

Stretching Redefined

Yoga Biomechanics

Jules Mitchell

Stretching Redefined

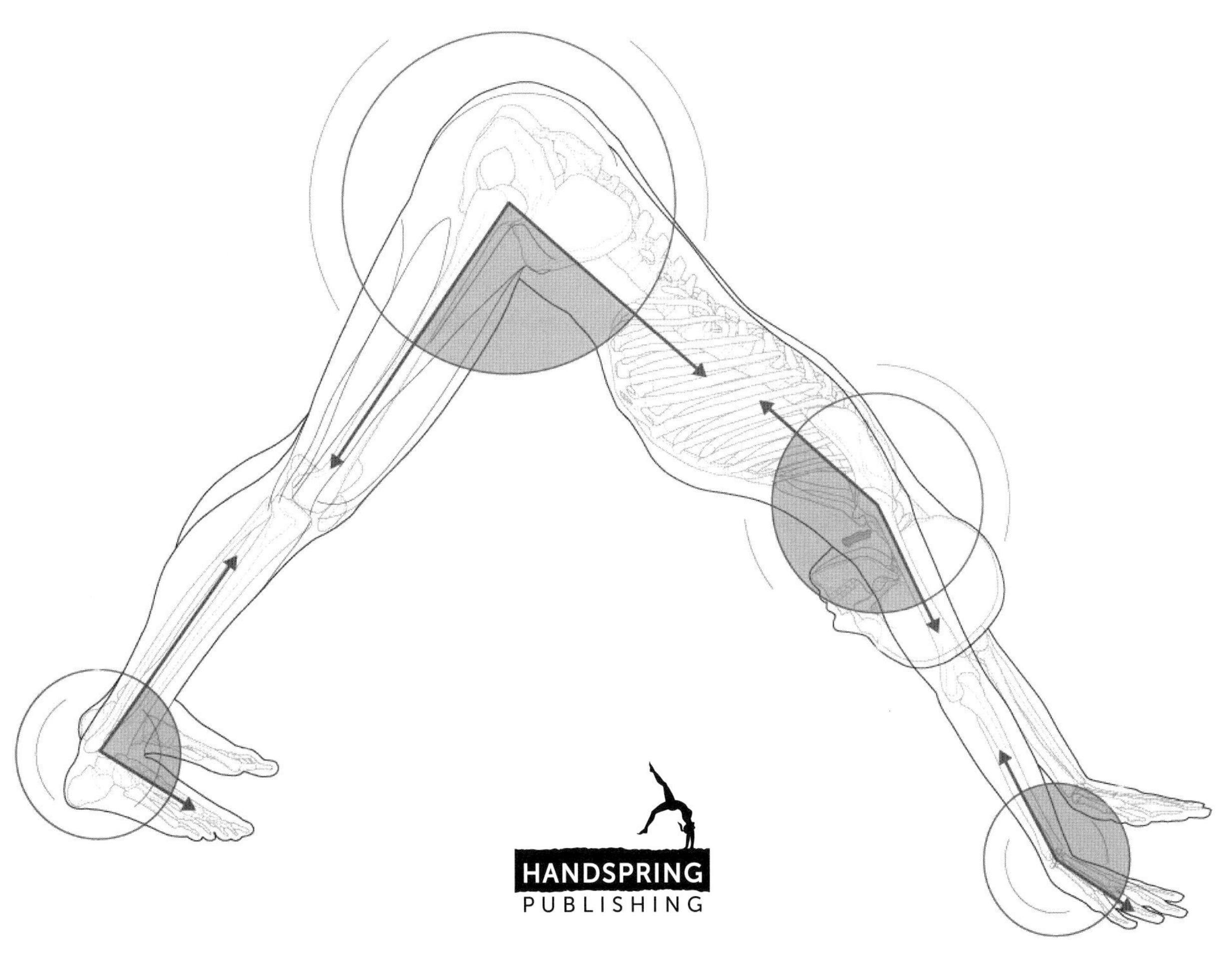

HANDSPRING
PUBLISHING

HANDSPRING PUBLISHING LIMITED
The Old Manse, Fountainhall,
Pencaitland, East Lothian
EH34 5EY, Scotland
Tel: +44 1875 341 859
Website: www.handspringpublishing.com

First published 2019 in the United Kingdom by Handspring Publishing
Reprinted 2019, 2020

ISBN 978-1-909141-61-2
ISBN (Kindle eBook) 978-1-909141-62-9

British Library Cataloguing in Publication Data
A catalogue record for this book is available from the British Library

Library of Congress Cataloguing in Publication Data
A catalog record for this book is available from the Library of Congress

Commissioning Editor Sarena Wolfaard
Project Manager Morven Dean
Copy-editor Barbara McAviney
Designer Kirsteen Wright
Cover design Bruce Hogarth
Indexer Aptara, India
Typesetter DSM Soft, India
Printed by Replika, India

The Publisher's policy is to use paper manufactured from sustainable forests

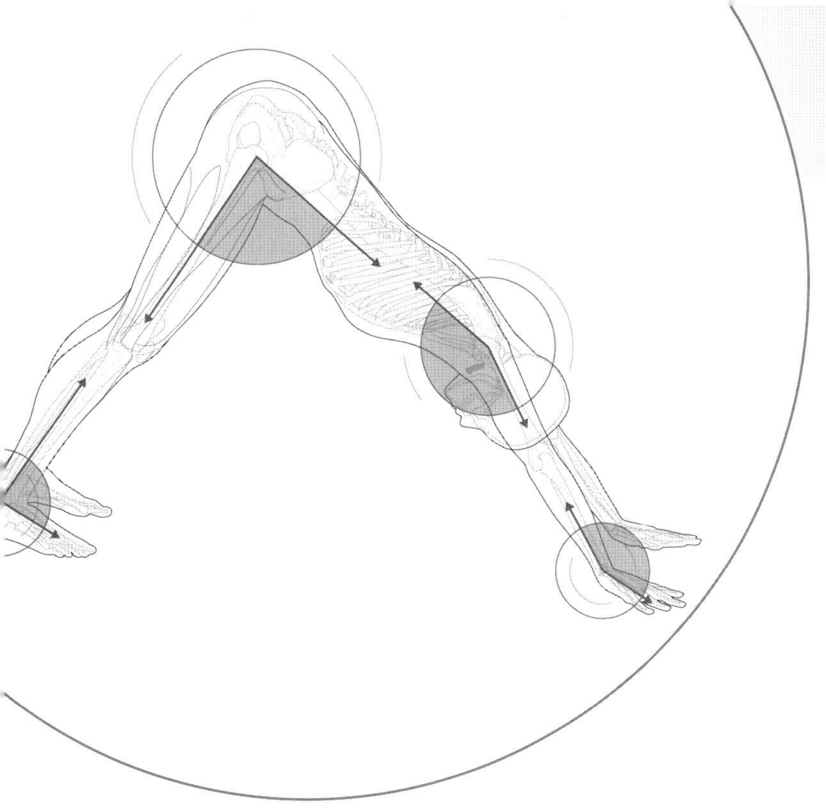

Contents

Acknowledgments

The final copy of this book is not what I thought it would be when I started. As I answered questions, more would arise, and brief moments of understanding led me down a longer path of more questions. Curiosity slowed me down, but the people in my life kept me going.

For the ability to be ever inquisitive, I thank my late parents who showed me the value of education and the dedication it requires. My father was an engineer who instilled in me a love of math, physics, and design. My mother was a university professor and author who showed me what life as a researcher, writer, and teacher is like. I am keenly aware of how their combined influence is abundantly apparent in my work.

My professors over the years (and years) I was in school further nourished my love of education. First and foremost is Dr. Jill Crussemeyer, who gave me the freedom to explore beyond the rote curriculum in my graduate program. She saw what was ahead of me when I didn't and offered me the road map. Dr. Brigitte Waldorf invited me to do graduate work when I was still an undergraduate. She also saw where I was going, before I did, and showed me the way. A humanities professor gave me philosophical insight into what calculus was, and a math professor explained calculus as a philosophy. At every academic turn, I was always encouraged to explore both the contemplative arts and hard sciences.

Thank you to all my yoga teachers over the years, who are far too many to list here. Leeann Carey showed me the value of intuition and taught me what is, in my opinion, the purest form of yoga there is; no stylistic bias, just yoga. Kathleen Grace Santor ran her yoga school with the most integrity I've seen thus far, she set the bar for me on day one. Every teacher I have ever had, including those whose class I may have only taken once, have all contributed to my ideas today. To every friend or colleague willing to talk shop with me and swap ideas, even when we disagree, and every teacher who has attended my courses and challenged me with questions, you remind me that I'm not alone in the quest for knowledge.

Tony Berlant, my friend, coach, and editor. Without him, this book would never have been written; even though he will deny it. When I was so lost in my ideas I couldn't see a single step ahead, we would meet over coffee and he would ask me where I wanted to go.

His probing questions would get me excited again, and before long I'd be yelling my ideas at him. Apologies to everyone at Starbucks who was forced to hear about the state of yoga today.

And most importantly, I give love and thanks to my family. My partner Jeff Homolya gave me the space to complete this monster of a project. He took less of me, so I could get it done, at a time when he needed more of me. I love you and always will. To my sister Marla, my rock, my best friend, my other half, thank you for taking me in and letting me be me; having you as my sister is the greatest privilege of my life. Lastly, to GOB, our beloved cat who slept endlessly on my stacks of research; he eventually died, perhaps of boredom, the week before I submitted the manuscript. When I was fretting over deadlines and word counts, his presence reminded me that the book would be complete when it was complete.

Jules Mitchell

Preface

I discovered the practice of yoga in college in the early 1990s. The first pose in the first class I ever took was Legs-Up-the-Wall. I'm pretty sure we were only in the pose a few minutes, but at the time it seemed like twenty minutes. I didn't realize that the invitation to lie on the floor in a room full of other people would quickly become an invitation to be with myself, to turn inward. The initial enthusiasm I felt for doing my first yoga pose quickly turned to fear. Since fear is not an emotion this 20-year-old was skilled at facing head on, I disguised it with insecurity. I could do insecurity, so I did. I giggled the entire time in an awkward and embarrassing display of immaturity. During the whole class, I saw myself differently, however, as if I had never before considered who I was. Fear and insecurity soon turned into fascination.

Coming out on the other side of that first yoga experience, I instantly understood what yoga was to me. It was and is a practice devoted to the inquiry of self and to one's relationship with existence. That's a vast, vague description, which is why yoga appears in many forms, with many paths, many lineages, and many teachers. I spent decades in pursuit of a subsequent yoga experience that could awaken my spirit – one that could disrupt who I was as abruptly as that first experience. Being a western white woman in an urban area, opportunities were of a certain type of privilege that included teacher trainings, retreats, university coursework in yoga philosophy and Sanskrit, traveling to attend workshops with popular teachers, and even trips to India. I fell in love with all of it.

I eventually became a yoga teacher and being a yoga teacher in the USA usually means teaching *āsana*. All my studies, however, seemed to confuse my understanding of *āsana*, not elevate it. The amount of contradiction across styles and teachers was profoundly unexpected. Some were trivial contradictions, like whether Downward Facing Dog is a rest pose or pose to work in; others were more substantial, like whether stretching connective tissue is safe or unsafe, essential or contraindicated. It seemed the more people I asked, the more answers I would receive, but none helped me to understand. In the face of all the uncertainty, I was losing my spirit.

Then I met my teacher, Leeann Carey, and she had a no-nonsense intuitive approach to *āsana* I found refreshing. She used to always say to me, "Don't worry about it" when she saw that my need to know all the answers was interfering with my ability to teach. Yoga does not need to be so cerebral. She was correct, and she taught me volumes.

I made my way to graduate school, not particularly in pursuit of one specific question. I knew I would always attend graduate school because I come from a family of academics. I taught yoga, so I figured I should pursue something in the realm of kinesiology, and because I had a strong background in math and engineering, the department head suggested I study biomechanics. I didn't actually know what biomechanics was, initially. In my first human tissue mechanics class, my jaw literally hung open in astonishment. I could not believe scientists have been studying connective tissue behavior for decades. Equations and graphs, all supported by research! I knew instantly this was the disruption for which I had been looking. My spirit was once again awake.

What I learned in graduate school was that my questions were premature. I couldn't quite articulate what I wanted to know because I lacked a foundation in biomechanics and scientific literacy. I learned to critically apply both to yoga while improving my process of inquiry. Today, I continue my pursuit of refining questions. I realize I can't ever know what is the absolute truth, but staying current with the research will allow me to see what might be true.

Based on my experience and my credentials, this book is unapologetically about *āsana* and the musculoskeletal system. Critics will argue that yoga is more than *āsana*, and I wholeheartedly agree. Critics will argue that *āsana* affects more the musculoskeletal system, and I wholeheartedly agree. The teachings of yoga are vast, far beyond what can be encompassed in a specialty book such as this one. If we remain open and receptive, however, we might be surprised to find the pursuit of scientific discovery is rich with the inquiry of self, and of one's relationship with existence.

Biomechanics is a physical science, and a natural complement to yoga *āsana*. Both are empirical, both deal with the forces of nature, and both are vast branches of study. There are many ways one could apply biomechanics to *āsana*, just as there are many ways one could apply philosophy to ways of being. How I apply biomechanics to *āsana* is what is covered in this book, and it thoroughly reflects where my personal and professional interests have led me. There is a little bit of math and geometry, some safety concerns, basic anatomy, some alignment scrutiny, and quite a bit of science.

A major subtext of the book, after yoga and biomechanics, is research literacy and critical thinking. This is not to crush the magic of yoga, rather to emphasize it. The scientific process is complex and uncertain, but it also holds space for awe and wonderment. One could say the same holds true for *āsana*. Everything I cover in this book is *what may be*, not *what is*. Theories are never proven, they are only supported. As an educator, I believe it is my job to present to you theories that you can apply to your own experience and, eventually, improve upon them. What I do not cover in this book, therefore, is a script for teaching or practicing *āsana*. I encourage curiosity, paying attention, the pursuit of knowledge, and a willingness to accept there are things we may never truly know. Ideally, when you turn the last page of this book, you will discover that you now have even more, distinguishing questions than you have answers.

Jules Mitchell MS, CMT, ERYT500
March 2018

Foreword by Greg Lehman

Wow. Just wow. What a wonderful book. I write "book" but I could just as easily write "books". This is a text that goes far beyond the subject of its title, Yoga Biomechanics. The appendix alone (essentially a pictorial guide to exercise, yoga, stretching, and strength training) is a book in and of itself. Then there are the sections which I expected to be dry and more academically oriented on tissue biomechanics and biomechanical principles. In those chapters we get a great treatise on those important biomechanical concepts but they are always explained in a way that makes them relevant to your own personal yoga practice, to your students, and even to those people you work with in pain. Further, as the concepts are taught they are put under a broader critical thinking lens, where the reader is taught to digest, critique, and synthesize the research. It is not just a biomechanical knowledge dump but rather an explanation of what we know, how we know what we know, and why it is relevant to you.

All of the sections of this book repeat these very important themes. The sections consistently describe the scientific underpinning of stretching, human function, and human anatomy – and always make this information relevant to a yoga practice.

One final point I would like to make is that one area that is handled especially well is that of the natural debates and uncertainties we have about human function. Those difficulties are not glossed over. Different sides of the debate are presented and it is easy to see how this text could be updated every decade to include new information without the existing material seeming irrelevant. This book sets an excellent framework that should be used as a reference and regularly reviewed text for all students of human function and movement.

Greg Lehman BKin, MSc, DC, MScPT
January 2019
Clinical Educator, Physiotherapist & Chiropractor
Strength and Conditioning Specialist
www.greglehman.ca
Course Creator: Reconciling Biomechanics with Pain Science
Course Creator: Running Resiliency: Best practice sport injury management for the runner

Foreword by Carrie Owerko

I first met Jules Mitchell in Australia, which was odd as we both reside in the United States. I had taken a few of her online courses and was thrilled to discover that we were both teaching in Australia around the same time, so I made sure to have time to spend a few days with her. I had a feeling this change of plans would be well worth my while, and it certainly was! I have been reading her writings, listening to her podcasts, and taking all of her online offerings ever since.

Yoga Biomechanics is like having all these experiences distilled, condensed, organized and annotated in one volume. Of course, a book does not replace the intimacy, spontaneity, and dimension of an in-person learning situation. However, Jules is as excellent a writer as she is a teacher. In fact, she is one of the most effective communicators and educators I have come across.

One of the things I most appreciated when I met Jules was how open-minded and non-dogmatic she was. Her teaching was as in-depth and thought-provoking as it was compassionate. She manages to teach this science-minded and evidenced-based approach with humility and respect – for the learner and for all that we don't yet know. She holds space for knowledge and for the mysterious nature of wholeness. Her teaching acknowledges the power of doing what is meaningful, one's beliefs, and that things might work for reasons known and unknown.

There can be as much dogma, fear mongering, and self-righteousness in yoga as there is in any discipline, but in her person as well as her teaching Jules is none of these things. This is evident in her book as well. She embodies what is best about yoga and the learning process: that it can help us live our lives in a way that makes our existence (and our relationship with our body and with each other) a little better.

In my opinion, *Yoga Biomechanics* is unique in the world of yoga books. Jules takes us on a journey where we become better educated in basic scientific literacy. She clarifies many scientific terms that are easily and often misused in the context of a yoga or movement class. For instance, we learn the difference between applied anatomy and biomechanics as these are often misunderstood. Jules focus is on biomechanics and its application to the practice of yoga. Her tutorials on tissue mechanics provide valuable insights and perspectives for those who are yoga teachers, educators, and movement enthusiasts. You will learn how to think critically and question many cherished notions of how things should be. This is important because in the yoga world there are many things that tradition does not usually question, but simply accepts.

This book encourages the reader to be curious and ask questions. It satisfies the seasoned body nerd as well as the interested lay person. It goes from the macro to the micro, all in service of the practical. Jules is interested not only in the accuracy of the science she presents, but in how that science will help you, the practitioner or teacher, to evaluate, teach, move, and live better.

If you are interested in what an evidence-based yoga practice might offer, this book will inspire you. If you think that yoga works for reasons that we still do not fully understand, this book will also be of interest to you. Jules will help you learn to ask questions rather than search for fixed and forever answers – and go on to ask even better questions!

Another thing that makes *Yoga Biomechanics* a breath of fresh air is the open-mindedness of its author. Jules reminds us that she is always capable of changing her mind if and when new evidence requires that she do so, and she encourages us to do the same. This 'zone of open-mindedness' is yoga at its best.

Finally, one of the things I love the most about this book is that Jules is a movement optimist. I too am a movement optimist. Decades of practice, study, and teaching in the Iyengar tradition have brought me to a place of tremendous optimism regarding the potential of our movement practices. I am optimistic about the robustness and resiliency of our bodies and our minds. I am optimistic about the power of movement (and yoga) to improve the quality of our lives in numerous ways. We are better off moving than not moving at all. And we are better off educating ourselves to think critically rather than blindly accepting what we have been told by a teacher or authority figure.

Yoga is, of course, more than just a set of movements, postures, and traditional practices. It includes profound breath, meditative, or mindfulness practices. At its heart – at its core – yoga is about awareness. It is an awareness practice. It is also about consistency – and about variability. You don't have to have perfect 'alignment' and you don't have to find the 'right way' to do a certain pose or movement. You do need to be willing to be present, to engage and inhabit your body in both familiar and novel ways. You also need a willingness to learn, and to accept that there is much that we do not know. This book examines all of this – the known and unknown, the familiar and the less familiar.

In *Yoga Biomechanics* Jules gives us theory, practice suggestions and variations, potent lines of inquiry, and her optimism. You will have wonderful questions to ponder, and a book that will continue to be a valuable resource and a source of inspiration for years to come. We need more educators like Jules, both in the yoga world and in the world in general. Learning to think for oneself, and having the tools to do so, is invaluable. This book provides essential tools. Thank you, Jules!

Carrie Owerko, BFA, CMA, CYIT, C-IAYT, FRCms
January 2019
Carrie Owerko is a Laban Movement Analyst, Certified Senior Teacher of Iyengar Yoga, and a Functional Range Conditioning Mobility Specialist
For more information see Carrieowerko.com

BIOMECHANICS

1

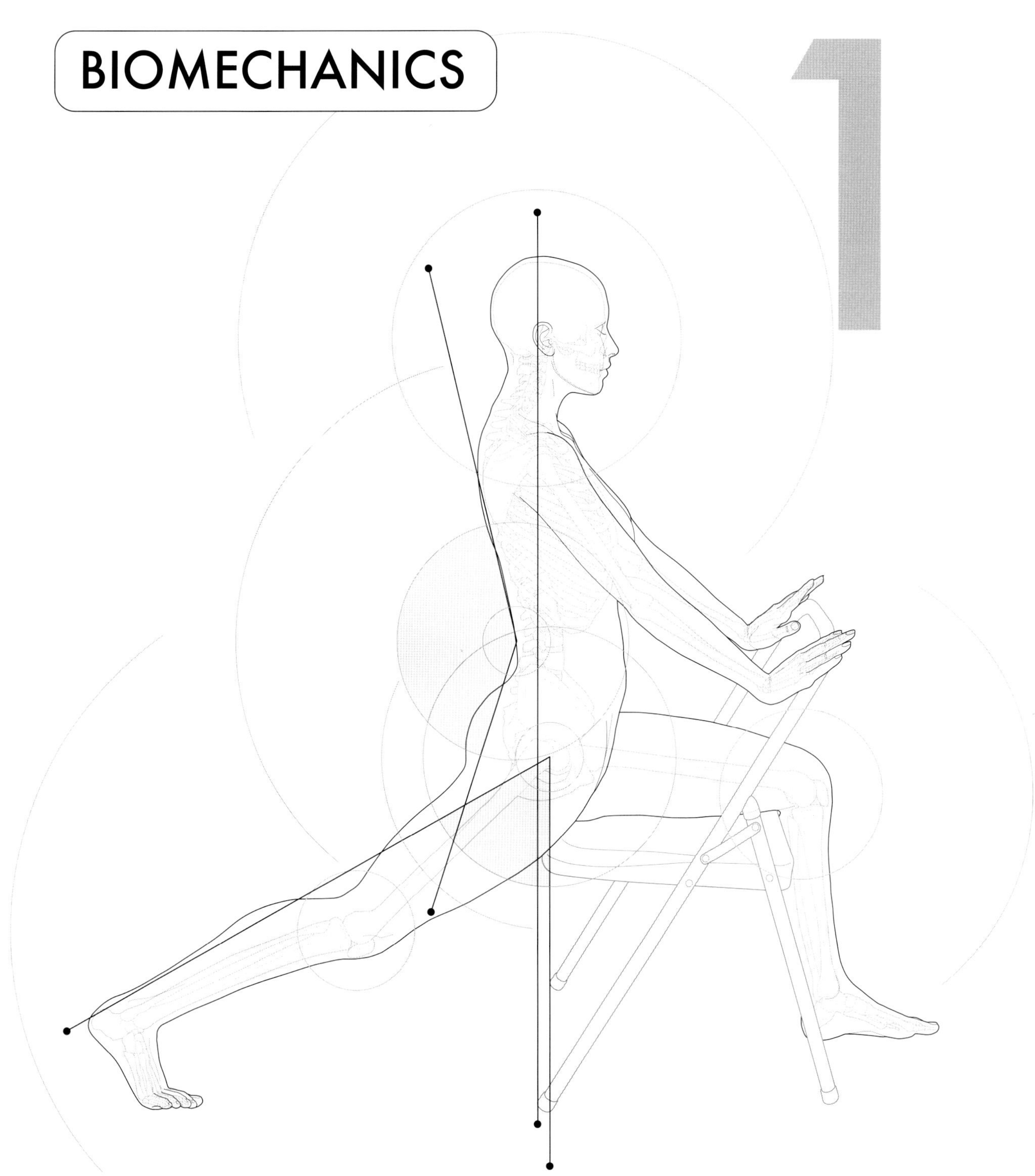

Biomechanics is defined as the study of how force affects biological systems. It is classified as a division of kinesiology, which is the study of human movement and includes many branches. A student of kinesiology may study anything from the art of dance to coaching football; the metabolic effects of cardiovascular activity to the psychology of sport; human performance to injury rehabilitation; or the development and sustainability of human movement from infancy to old age and in special populations.

Biomechanics, although it is a division of this broader field of kinesiology, still covers a wide scope of applications. A biomechanist may design ergonomic office furniture, equipment, or footwear and sports equipment. A biomechanist may work for sports teams in either the training or the rehabilitation division, or both. A biomechanist could work in a laboratory and engineer artificial tissues to replicate the behavior of human tissues for surgical procedures. Therefore, biomechanics itself has many of its own subdivisions and includes specific areas of study that not all other divisions of kinesiology require (Table 1.1). In spite of the variety of disciplines biomechanics encompasses, one specific topic is the focus of this book: mechanical forces and how they apply to the human body.

Force

Force is the operative word in the definition of biomechanics; not anatomy, not alignment, not movement cueing. The term biomechanics can be misleading, as only an engineer or physicist would assume the mechanics portion of the term implies force. Yoga teachers often associate mechanics with joint position (e.g. "knee over the ankle") or limb position (e.g. "arms alongside the ears") because that is what yoga teachers are typically taught. Most pose instructions are, in fact, applied anatomy: "heel-to-arch alignment" is an example of applied anatomy, or what is referred to as alignment in yoga. Biomechanics considers the effects of force in the context of anatomical position, placement, posture, and movement.

Table 1.1
Areas of Study in Biomechanics

Field	Role in biomechanics
Biology	The study of living organisms
Anatomy	The study of the structure and parts of an organism
Physiology	The study of function in living systems
Histology	The study of cells and living tissues
Chemistry	The study of structure, properties, and changes of matter
Physics	The study of matter and motion through space
Kinematics	The properties of motion independent of force and mass
Kinetics	The study of forces during motion
Hydraulics	The study of fluid mechanics
Engineering	The application of science in design and innovation

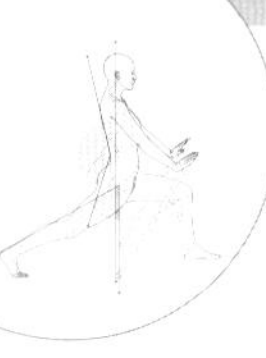

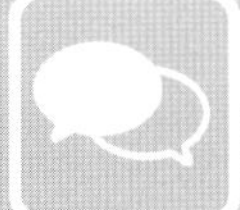

Thought Provoker

Biomechanics of Yoga

If I were to ask you "what are the biomechanics of Downward Facing Dog Pose?", what would your answer be? Perhaps jot some notes down, as I'll ask you again later in the book and you might enjoy comparing your answers.

Occasionally a conventional yoga cue inadvertently hints at the effect of force (e.g. "in Tree Pose, place the foot above or below the knee"). This instruction, however, is incomplete, reflecting applied anatomy and some inaccurate force assumptions. Yoga teachers often learn that the knee is a hinge joint and based on such anatomical classification, a seemingly logical assumption is formed. That is, a hinge operates in a single plane, and so they conclude that even a small amount of lateral pressure on the knee is dangerous. In actuality, the knee joint is a bicondylar joint (e.g. imagine two ball and socket joints side by side) capable of a small degree of rotation (Fig. 1.1). More importantly, the knee is continually exposed to lateral forces in everyday movements, including walking. Based on its location, structure, and degrees of freedom (i.e. capable directions of motion), the knee functions to accommodate and mediate lateral and rotational forces, rather than entirely avoid them. Therefore, a biomechanical cue should take these factors into account.

Biomechanics is the study of the effect of mechanical forces on the structure, function, and movement of the human body; it affects anatomy, physiology, and their applications.

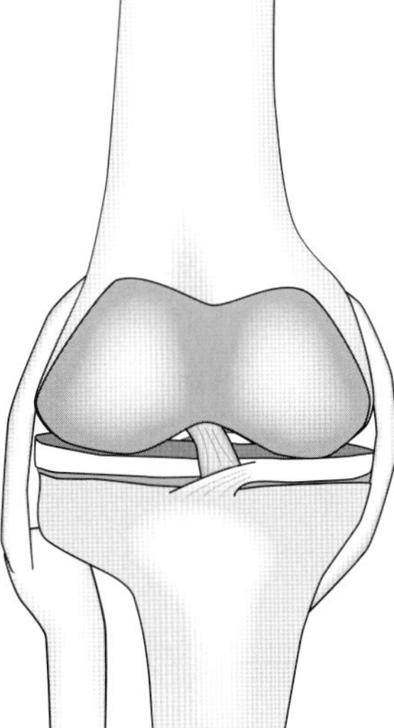

Fig. 1.1
The knee is a bicondylar joint capable of small amounts of rotation in addition to flexion and extension.

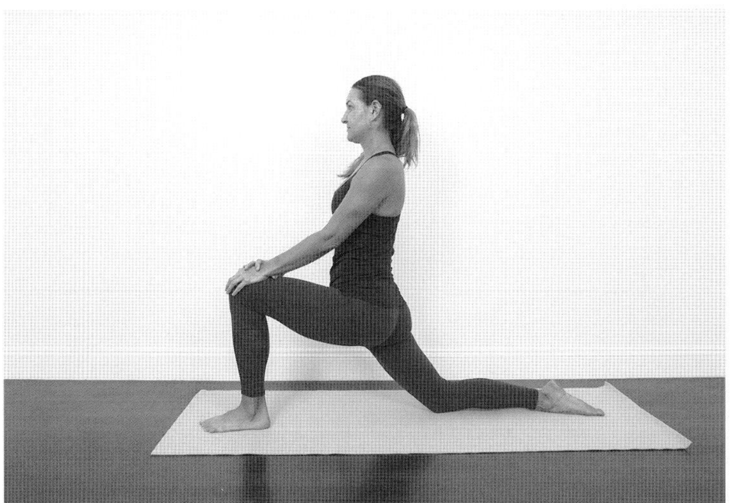

Fig. 1.2
Knee over the ankle in a Lunge position.

Reexamining some of the aforementioned yoga examples in the context of biomechanics, the cue for a static Lunge , "knee over the ankle," should consider all the directional forces at the knee and ankle joint specific to that position (Fig. 1.2), as well as the unique biology of the individual. Biomechanical analysis considers the resilience of one's soft tissues (e.g. ligaments or tendons), how well they hold up under the forces at this knee angle, and whether this alignment is beneficial or precarious for this individual's tissues. Forces on supportive tissues (e.g. bones and cartilage) must also be considered as their position might influence whether these tissues get stronger or weaker. Notice I make no implication of an absolute correctness or incorrectness, there is no line in the sand separating right from wrong. Biomechanics simply considers the benefits and risks of the forces involved in the position.

Cueing "heel-to-arch alignment," in Warrior II Pose (Fig. 1.3), for example, one must consider the forces on the ankle, knee, and hip associated with this foot placement. The external forces acting on the joints based on the geometry of the pose will be met with corresponding internal forces (bones, ligaments, muscles) in order to maintain balance and equilibrium. Since the angles of the femur bones in relationship to gravity, and relative to the knee and hip, are different than when standing in neutral, the muscles are recruited differently, and the bones and joints respond differently. The degree to which different muscles activate will vary by individual, and within an individual, based on an infinite number of external and internal conditions. Biomechanical considerations are not about doing a pose the right way, they are about what is happening in the pose, in that particular way, at that moment.

"Avoiding the knee" in Tree Pose (Fig. 1.4) reflects a misunderstanding and misrepresentation of how force affects the body. It somehow implies that force is dangerous, and it should be avoided. First, force can't be avoided – we live on a planet with a gravitational pull. Second, we obviously can get stronger when we are exposed to force.

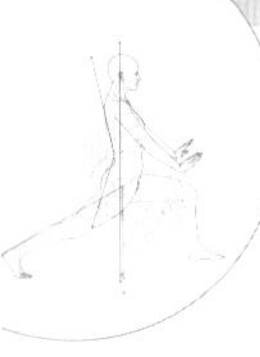

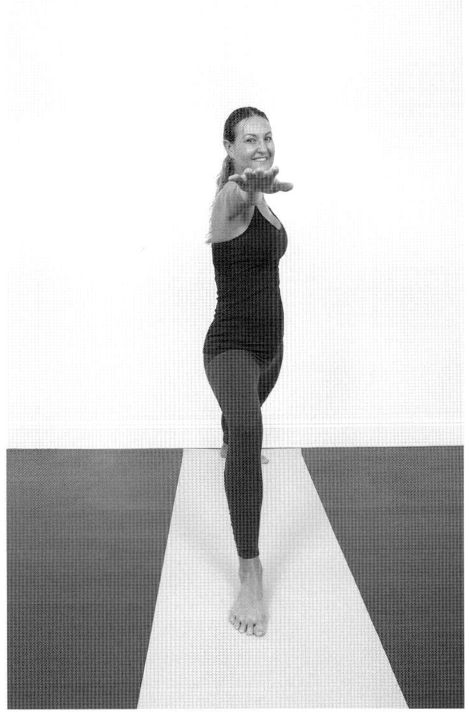

Fig. 1.3
Heel-to-arch alignment in Warrior II.

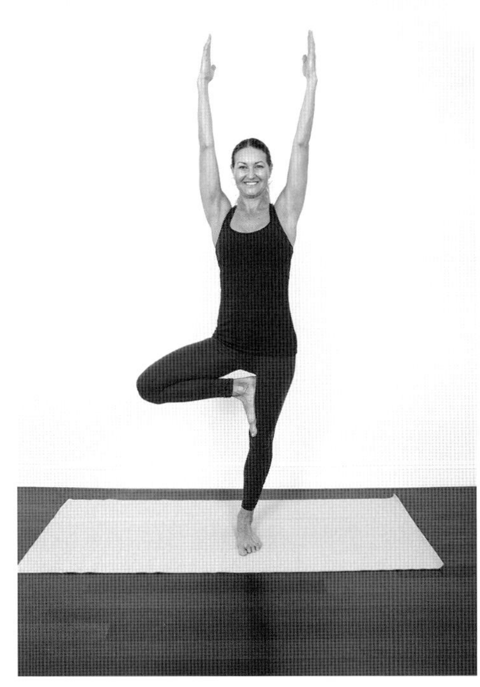

Fig. 1.4
Opposite foot applies frontal plane forces on the medial aspect of the knee in tree pose.

We require it actually. Are there reasons to avoid the knee? Sure. A biomechanical reason for avoiding the knee might include the diminished resilience of one's ligaments and cartilage in the knee, rendering it unable to withstand the force applied by the opposite foot. But that may also be a biomechanical reason for placing the foot directly on the knee – to increase the ability of the knee to withstand force. If placing the foot on the knee were fundamentally incorrect, dangerous, or even slightly precarious, you would not find those exact instructions in the Stork Test (i.e. an orthopedic test designed to identify pathologies of the lumbar or sacral regions of the spine) (Fig. 1.5).

Now is a good time to point out the trap of logical fallacies. I just presented one above by appealing to an authority as evidence. I validated my case for placing the foot on the knee as not being problematic by arguing that because medical professionals do it, it must be okay. The common yoga cue, "place the foot above or below the knee to protect it," also appeals to authority, albeit a yogic one. Instead, it may appeal to tradition as evidence, another example of a logical fallacy. Just because this is how we always do it doesn't make it valid. In order to cue the most scientifically sound instructions for Tree Pose, we need evidence.

Although the biomechanical research on yoga is sparse, one paper provides some insight into the frontal plane forces on the knee in Tree Pose (Yu et al., 2012).

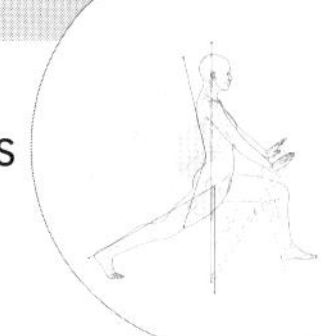

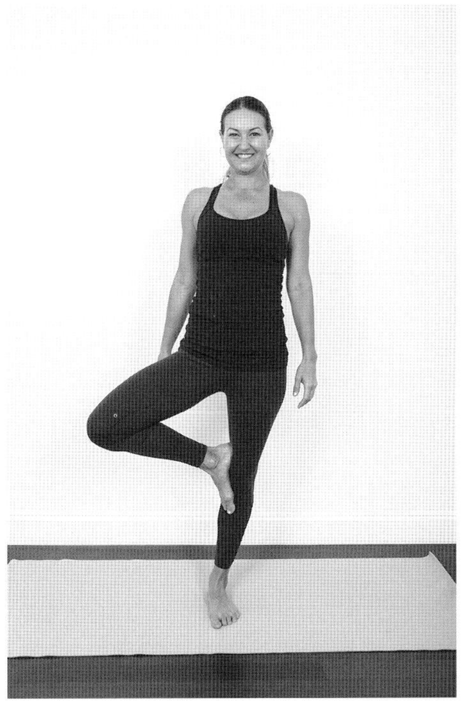

Fig. 1.5
The Stork Test: "The subject stands on one leg with the sole of the nonweightbearing foot resting on the medial aspect of the knee of the weightbearing limb" (Konin et al., 2006).

The subjects included six men and 14 women averaging 70.7 years in age. It compared: 1) the opposite foot positioned on the floor with wall support, versus, 2) the opposite foot positioned below the knee with wall support, versus, 3) the latter without wall support. The research team found that the first version resulted in 54–71% lower knee abductor joint moment of force over the knee than the second or third. They also reported that the second and third positions (i.e. the foot not touching the floor) produced 8–20% greater knee abductor joint moment of force than during the stance phase of walking at a self-selected pace. What conclusions are you inclined to make about Tree Pose in light of this evidence?

If you're looking for binary yes/no answers, there are none. I only wish to present to you force as a variable and any relevant research so that you may make informed choices when practicing. I can tell you that your conclusion about this paper will be colored by your bias. If you believe that forces on joints cause osteoarthritis (OA), you may never practice Tree Pose again without the opposite foot anchored to the floor. If you believe force on joints stimulates and nourishes them, you may choose to practice Tree Pose with the opposite foot directly over the knee, as in the Stork Test. The answer probably lies somewhere in-between. Moreover, the researchers did not test for the presence or development of OA, they tested only for the quantification of forces in three different static positions. Thus the effects of Tree Pose on OA cannot be determined. Without more research we will never know. Even with more research we may never know.

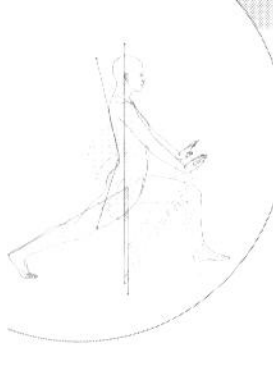

Scientific Literacy

Evidence-Based Teaching

An evidence-based teaching is a practice that combines competency in the related field of research, yoga education and teaching experience, and the unique needs of the individual student/client. Decision-making should consider all three components.

Evidence-based teaching, also called evidence-informed practice, is typically the method by which healthcare professionals make treatment choices. As yoga edges its way into the realm of therapy through organizations certifying yoga therapists, evidence-based teaching is having its moment in the spotlight (Moonaz, Jeter and Schmalzl, 2017).

Even for yoga teachers who do not identify as yoga therapists, evidence-based teaching is becoming more relevant. The rise of the internet in this millennium has led to the bombardment of information and misinformation. Research literacy is the single most important skill in deciphering fact from fiction, data from anecdote, and evidence from hearsay.

In addition to providing an education in biomechanics, this book intends to empower its readers with decision-making skills that follow those of an evidence-based practitioner. The reader is invited to consider the arguments presented here and employ skepticism when claims are unsubstantiated, as well as to be willing to change position when the evidence is compelling. It may not be fun or easy to do, but it is certainly satisfying!

What can be concluded, which was reported in the researchers' conclusion, is that instructor (and researcher) intuition is not always supported by data. The paper highlights a false assumption by revealing that using the wall for support is no gentler on the standing limb than tree in the middle of the room. By considering force, doing your research, and applying the knowledge you have gained to your practical experience, I believe you will then make well-informed choices for yourself and/or your students.

The component of force in the term "mechanics" should now be more apparent. As previously stated, engineers would easily understand the force variable because the field of mechanical engineering requires an understanding of the effect of force on the structures, devices, and widgets they design. Mechanical engineers study physics to learn how motion affects the integrity of these designs. Engineers comprehend more than the names of the components and how they assemble, but also how the components behave in certain configurations when exposed to gravity, an applied force, and movement.

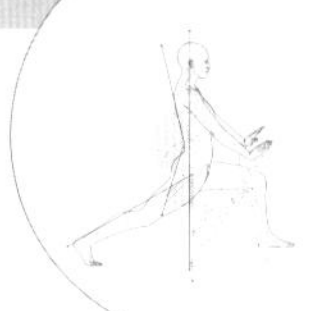

Scientific Literacy

Science and Research

Science is a process, an approach to discovery about observable phenomena in our world. Science does not tell us what is certain; rather we form models, theories, and, finally, laws when experimentation provides sufficient evidence. There really is no such thing as scientific proof, only scientific knowledge, as the models, theories, and laws represent the most accepted explanation available and are always tentative and mutable. Additionally, there are rules as to what is deemed sufficient evidence.

Scientific evidence demands a systemic process of identifying a phenomenon or problem, forming a question, and collecting data. It is an empirical process where data sets are observed, but also one that commands logic when conclusions are formed based on the data analysis. Finally, research must be replicable such that other researchers, when repeating the same test in identical conditions, can reproduce the results.

Most importantly, the scientific process requires open-mindedness. We must be willing to change our minds when new evidence challenges previous assertions. In fact, a well-designed study sets out to find evidence to oppose the hypothesized results. It is far too easy, especially in the age of social media, to surround ourselves with information that only confirms our bias. Unfortunately, science is also a business, and scientific journals are publications with expenses. Research that does not result in significant findings may get less visibility at best, and not be published at worst, subjecting even science to economic and political influence. But knowing this shouldn't deter you from appreciating the complexities of science and research, and embracing them as the most effective tool we have for understanding the world.

Politics aside, many yoga schools in the US are compelled to register their teacher training programs with an organization whose guidelines currently suggest the "bio-" component of education provides only 20 hours of anatomy and physiology (although at the time of this writing, the educational standards are under review). These schools tend to leave the mechanics component out of the already limited kinesiology content. As a result, most yoga teachers have a limited understanding of what biomechanics actually means, and as the term biomechanics gains more recognition, so does its misuse and misapplication. Yoga, arguably an oral tradition, is particularly susceptible to logical fallacies, intuition, and faulty reasoning. Shared misinformation develops deep roots, and the willingness to unlearn what you have learned is paramount to changing the course of modern western postural yoga.

Just as scientists must consider data that challenge their confirmation bias, you are invited to consider how the evidence presented in this book challenges (as well as confirms) your beliefs and previous yoga education. Often when I arrive to teach a weekend yoga course I quickly discover that many assume biomechanics to be a synonym for alignment, and where there is alignment, there is misalignment. But, can we automatically assume misalignment is unsafe or faulty? Alternatively, in biomechanics, we have adaptation and maladaptation. Both adaptation and maladaptation can, and do, occur through either alignment, misalignment, or both. These concepts will be deconstructed here, possibly creating some cognitive dissonance. You will be encouraged to question or challenge the teachings and oral tradition of modern yoga, not out of disrespect, but in an effort to uphold the evolution of the practice. Presenting evidence to the contrary is the foundation of good science. Therefore, this book, in addition to driving the biomechanics conversation forward, intends to advance scientific literacy and critical thinking skills so that you may be given permission to question, without judgment, what you have learned before. Consider this an opportunity to forward the process of unlearning and to disrupt the previously uninterruptable with the goal of becoming a more confident teacher/student of yoga.

At this point, we have established that force is central to the study of biomechanics. We have further established how biomechanics fits into yoga by way of several examples using

Scientific Literacy

Reading a Research Paper

Research articles published in scientific journals follow a general format that resembles the process researchers used to identify and solve a problem, known as the scientific method. While it may be easiest to read the online abstract (and more cost effective as the rest of the paper is often behind a paywall), the abstract is not intended to provide sufficient information about the research results and limitations. Unfortunately, many of us make assumptions based on the bare bones data provided in the abstract and forget to question the rest. Understanding the importance of each step makes it easier to think critically about the research process.

Introduction

The first step in conducting research is identifying the problem and establishing the research question. High-quality research bases this question on a developed theory that drives the purpose of the paper. In the introduction the researchers explain a problem they have observed, discuss the current theories on the topic, and provide evidence of past studies that support (and refute!) their explanation. In some cases, there may be a lack of prior evidence, therefore identifying a new problem, and surrounding research is cited to help develop an argument for why this problem

Continued on next page

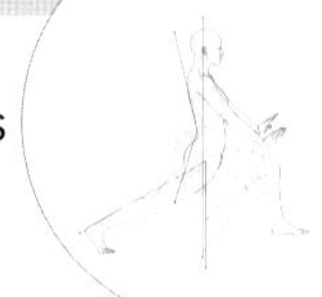

Continued from previous page

should be studied. The introduction is a condensed review of the available literature on the topic, thus familiarizing the reader with the theory at hand. At or near the end of this section, the hypothesis is stated. The hypothesis represents the specific outcome the researchers expect to find based on previous evidence.

Methods

In the methods section the researchers explain their study design. Here you will find out who the subjects were, how they were recruited, what conditions excluded them from participation, what the parameters for inclusion entailed, how many dropped out during the course of the study, etc. The researchers explain in full detail each step of data collection, any pre- and post-measurements, the specifics of the intervention vs the control group, even the make and model of the laboratory equipment that was used.

Results

In research, results are raw data and statistics. You will often find tables and charts depicting relationships between variables in conjunction with text reporting values along with their standard deviations. Here the type of statistical analysis is explained, and significance is determined. All interpretations of these data are reserved for the final sections of the article.

Discussion/Conclusion/Limitations

The final section(s) of the research paper assess the meaning of the data and how they may or may not have an effect in a real-world setting. Citations of other relevant papers support any conclusions made, limitations in the study design point to further research needs, and implications of the particular outcomes are proposed. The theory on which the paper is designed is either supported or challenged. It is important to note theories are never proved, rather research provides evidence to support it. Gravity is a theory, albeit a very well supported one.

common instructions in popular poses. Although the biomechanics research on yoga, specifically, is limited and often inconclusive, a vast library on the effects of force in sport and injury exists, providing support for the ideas proposed in this book. Before we can progress the conversation, we must first spend some time learning more about force, the terminology surrounding it, where it comes from, and how it presents in our physical world.

Communicating in Force

Every industry has its jargon. In yoga, many teachers insert the language of Sanskrit into the middle of an English sentence, speak in metaphors that defy the laws of physics, and use anatomical analogies that would baffle anyone in the medical industry. Somehow

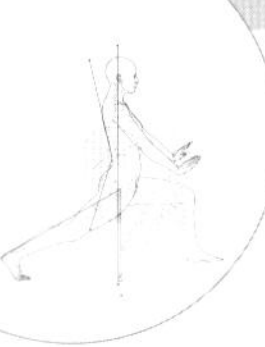

though, we understand each other. Jargon, despite the negative connotation, reflects the acceptance and normalization of specialized terminology within an industry. We agree that using a word like *prāṇāyāma* is more suitable than breathing (a weak English translation) because it has complexity, many subparts, and multiple layers of meaning which we have thoughtfully considered and philosophically examined. Our jargon is poetic, but may seem vague to an outsider, just as poetry can be difficult for a novice to interpret. Likewise, when a novice tries to write poetry, or insert random Sanskrit words into conversation, the complexity is lost.

Many yoga teachers also often use terms from exercise science and insert them as yoga jargon. We are still implying multiple layers of meaning through metaphor, but in the absence of the investigation these words require, once again, we come across as the novice poet. Words like stretching, stressing, and strengthening lack a communally agreed upon translation, are used interchangeably with energetic metaphors (e.g. a pec stretch becomes a heart opener) and are consequently reinforced through repetition, in spite of insufficient contemplation. We dilute, rather than enrichen, the definitions of these specialized terms.

Imagine if we spent as much time exploring the words in the realm of physics (force) as we did in that of social ethics (*yama*) and personal ethics (*niyama*). A well-developed vocabulary could lead to richer conversations about how stretching works, the measurable benefits of *āsana*, and which variables affect which outcomes. We would understand that while we always lack some degree of certainty, the more specific our questions are, the more accurate our answers will be. Currently, it seems that our conversation about asana and stretching starts and ends with: 1) asana strengthens and tones the body; and 2) yoga makes you flexible. That would be like the study of yamas and the niyamas consisting of: 1) do good things; and 2) be a good person. Neither is inaccurate; they are just incomplete.

Just as Sanskrit is central to the study of yoga, Latin is central to communicating in anatomy. We use Sanskrit liberally when teaching yoga. Not just to name poses, but also to describe qualities of matter (*guna*), our energies/constitutions (*doṣa*), and the layers/sheaths of our existence (*koṣa*). In anatomy, the etymology of most terms is Latin and a basic proficiency in Latin accelerates the learning of the names of most bones, joints, and muscles. The language we use in biomechanics is force, and terms such as *mass* and *acceleration* make up the vocabulary.

The language of force is communicated in units of measurement using the International System of Units (SI). Scientists and the rest of the world (with the exception of the US) all use the metric system (i.e. meters, grams, liters, degrees Celsius). Therefore, it takes some practice for many Americans to conceptualize SI values in practical applications. Many would not know that 35°C is a hot summer day, 100 kilometers per hour is slower than most people drive on a freeway, or that a 30 kg suitcase is considered overweight by current TSA regulations. Fortunately, SI familiarity is not a prerequisite for the theoretical study of force, but for clarity and consistency we will discuss force in the units of measure consistent with the scientific community.

In each of the three fields of study above (i.e. yoga, anatomy, and biomechanics), language is enhanced through art, graphics, and other non-verbal aids. In yoga, we build altars with avatars, symbols, and textiles. Many anatomy text books are filled with drawings and images, sometimes even outnumbering text. To best study biomechanics, we occasionally will depend on graphs or mathematical equations to better

Scientific Literacy

Variables

In math and science, a variable is a sometimes known, sometimes unknown quantity or quality. In research, variables are further defined as dependent (i.e. affected by some other variable), and independent (i.e. considered unaffected by another variable). The independent variables are generally set and implemented in the study design process, and the dependent variables are usually measured and analyzed as part the results phase of the study. Variables can be subjective, open to interpretation, or objective, measurable and quantifiable.

In yoga research, for example, some variables could include:

Type of yoga (Hatha, Ashtanga, etc.)

Frequency of practice (3 per week, 1 per day, etc.)

Duration of the study (6 weeks, 12 weeks, etc.)

Subjective outcome measures (qualitative) include:

Quality of life (scored by a survey)

Pain (scored on the 1–10 Visual Analog Scale)

Objective outcome measures variables (quantitative) include:

Range of motion (measured with goniometer)

Bone density scan (measured with technological equipment)

depict relationships between variables. Depending on your propensity for numbers, formulas, and geometric relationships, you will either curse or thank me. I'll do my best to highlight the artistic beauty of the Cartesian coordinate system for those less mathematically inclined.

Newtonian Physics

Any introductory biomechanics course at a university will typically begin with a lesson in Newtonian physics. Isaac Newton invented three physical laws (Table 1.2) to describe how he observed forces acting on a body (not necessarily a human body, but an object of some sort) and the motion that occurs, or doesn't occur, as a result of those forces.

The full understanding of these three laws is not something every yoga teacher needs to strive to achieve, but they tell a story about the physical world in which we live. The first law tells us that initiation, changing, and stopping motion requires force. The second law gives us a mathematical capability of calculating force, mass, or acceleration provided two of these values are known. The third law, explains the force relationship

Table 1.2
Newton's Laws of Motion

First law	An object at rest stays at rest, and an object in motion remains in motion, at a constant velocity, and in a constant direction, unless acted on by an external force
Second law	A force (F) on an object is equal to its mass (m) times its acceleration (a). That is F=ma
Third law	When one object exerts a force on a second object, that second object exerts an equal and opposite force on the first

between bodies acting on one another. It is important to remember that forces are everywhere, even when we can't see them with the naked eye (e.g. friction, either created by air acting on a moving object or between two surfaces like your palm and a sticky mat).

To illustrate how these laws fit into the study of yoga, let's compare Warrior II Pose practiced in a yoga studio to that in the shallow end of a swimming pool (think water aerobics). Water is denser than air, therefore, all things being equal (i.e. time to get into the pose), moving into Warrior II Pose while standing in a pool would require more muscle force than being on deck because water resistance is greater than air resistance. Conversely, since water provides buoyancy, the arms, for example, could conceivably float into abduction with less effort, albeit more slowly. Additionally, immersed in water, the body will seemingly weigh less due to buoyancy and the impact on the bottom of the pool will be less. The conclusion here is that practicing yoga in a pool may provide lesser ground impact, but greater overall resistance than yoga on your mat. Might you now see alignment-focused cues without any consideration of all the internal and external forces being applied is somewhat remiss?

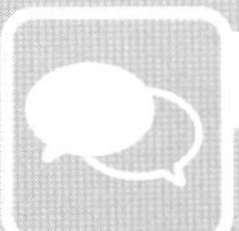

Thought Provoker

Acceleration

Velocity is the technical word for speed. It represents a constant rate calculated by displacement over time (v= d/t). If you are traveling on the freeway at a speed of 125 kilometers per hour, 125 km/h is your velocity. Acceleration is the rate of *change* of your speed. If you go from 125 km/h to 135 km/h (change of 10 km/h) in 5 seconds (1/720 h), your *acceleration* is 7200 km/h^2.

Question: If you were to decelerate from 85 km/h to 75 km/h in 5 seconds, what would your acceleration be?

Answer: -7200 km/h^2

Newton's laws of physics are quantifiable and all of the above can be measured, calculated, and verified. As a math lover, I fell in love with biomechanics when I started my graduate program. I dreamed of long romantic evenings by the fire, setting up equations and calculating forces. My academic endeavors fulfilled such scenarios, but when it comes to teaching yoga classes, the mastery of algebra and trigonometry does not translate to better teaching. When it comes to educating yoga teachers about biomechanics in a weekend course, for example, it does translate to me being a somewhat better teacher, but only by a fraction more (pun intended), because I can validate my conclusions when the discussion warrants it. What matters is our ability to translate the theory behind the calculations in a compassionate, non-threatening way, so that all of us who teach classes can make educated choices about the poses based on application of biomechanical theory, not application of mathematics. As the saying goes, give a person a fish, and she eats for a day, but teach that person to fish and she eats for a lifetime. So it is with teaching yoga. I can teach you how to teach a pose, and you can teach the pose to others, but if I teach you how forces operate in human movement, you can adapt any pose to any student (or maybe even a fish) to satisfy a specific outcome. In other words, the theory behind Newtonian physics is important, even if you don't actually perform the calculations (and even when contemporary theories challenge the accuracy of such calculations as they pertain to the human body).

Gravity

Force, as stated in Newton's second law, is calculated by multiplying a **mass** by its **acceleration** (F=ma). Mass is the measure of matter in an object and is measured in kilograms (kg). Acceleration is the measure of a change in velocity (colloquially, speed), and is measured in meters per second squared (m/s^2). It's no coincidence that the units of force are measured in a unit with the name Newtons (N). A Newton is the product of kg and m/s^2 ($N=kg*m/s^2$) and 1N is equal to the force needed for 1 kg to accelerate at 1 m/s^2. If this were a physics textbook, you would now be working through dozens of mathematical problems, setting up calculations, and solving for unknown variables. If that excites you, pick up any used introductory biomechanics, or physics, textbook and go nuts. Regardless, what is important here is that you understand that force is determined by the variables, m and a, and is most often expressed in N.

We are constantly interacting with a force of attraction to Earth that we call **gravity**. While, technically, gravity is not a force, we often refer to it as such. Gravity explains the attraction between two bodies (objects), planets, or particles (how it works requires a discussion on Einstein's Theory of Relativity, but this would derail us from our purpose). Bodies on the Earth's surface are attracted to its center at a constant acceleration of 9.8 m/s^2. This value is determined by the Earth's mass and the distance to the center; therefore, altitude affects gravitational acceleration. How this is so is certainly useful for aerospace engineering, but we can safely assume gravity is pretty much the same during a yoga practice at sea level and a yoga practice at most higher altitudes.

If gravity is expressed by an acceleration of 9.8 m/s^2, we can use this value to determine the force acting on a body. When you stand in Mountain Pose, your mass multiplied by the acceleration of 9.8 m/s^2 is the force acting on the Earth. According to Newton's third law, the Earth is acting on you with an equal and opposite force. Because gravity on Earth is a constant value of 9.8 m/s^2, a body with a greater mass will produce a greater force than a body with less mass. You may recognize this as weight, which is technically a measure of force. If you independently weigh two objects of differing mass, the scale would show the object of greater mass to weigh more than that of lesser mass. The scale is actually measuring force because it is taking gravity into account. If you independently weigh the same two objects of differing mass on the same scale but in a zero-gravity environment, they would both weigh nothing, despite their mass. Weight depends on gravity; mass does not. Your household scale automatically converts weight to mass (under the assumption of Earth's gravitational acceleration) such that the reading expresses your mass (kg), unless you live in the US where scales measure in pounds (lb).

In the biomechanics laboratory, force is measured by stepping on a force plate – a small square platform shaped very much like a bathroom scale but connected to a computer. When you stand on the force plate, the computer reports your weight (force) in N and you must perform the calculation yourself ($m=F/a$) if you want to determine your mass (kg). The value essentially reflects what you weigh on a scale but is expressed in units of force instead of units of mass. If you were to jump onto a force plate, the force reading would be higher at the moment of contact. You do not suddenly "weigh" more because you have spontaneously increased your mass. You suddenly "weigh" more because you have increased your distance from the surface of attraction, thus increasing your rate of acceleration and in turn increasing your force. But, after the initial moment of contact, once you are again statically positioned on the force plate, the reading would show your normal weight as acceleration returns to 9.8 m/s^2.

So, a body on Earth that appears still, is in fact, experiencing gravitational acceleration. While you may not look or feel like you are descending into the Earth's core when you are standing on a force plate, you are being "pulled" toward it. Simultaneously, according to Newton's 3rd law (i.e. for every action there is an equal and opposite reaction) the force plate is actually "pushing" back up at you with an equal force keeping you on its surface. If you were to measure this reaction force in water, it would be less, and if gravitational acceleration were to disappear entirely, the reaction force would be zero. In spite

Thought Provoker

Handstand

Question: If you were in a handstand and placed a scale upside down on your feet, what would the number on the scale reflect? What if the scale were right side up?

Answer: Upside down, the scale would read the "weight" of the scale expressed by the mass of the scale times the acceleration of gravity. If it were right side up, it would read zero.

of your unchanged mass, the force plate would not react to you, and you would appear "weightless." Interestingly, the absence of gravity, and thus force, can have detrimental effects. For example, astronauts lose tendon strength and bone density in as little as just 90 days when in zero-gravity environments. We'll discuss this in greater depth soon.

Because of the omnipresence of gravity we are always interacting with it. Infants learning the most basic movements – rolling over, crawling, standing, and walking – are primarily learning to interact with gravity. More importantly, force is fundamental to the development of the body's musculoskeletal tissues. Children run, climb, hop, and jump because they are in training to become resilient adults with bones and joints of great capacity. As you can see, force is essential to the human experience on Earth, and you, literally, are a force to be reckoned with.

Applied Loads

Force, we have established, is a measurement of the interaction between two bodies; between them exists a force and an equal and opposite reaction force. In biomechanics, we are also interested in the effect of a force exerted on a body. When that is the case, it is termed **load** or, more specifically, an applied load. As explained, activities such as walking, running, jumping, and even yoga vary the measure of force and reaction force between the person and the surface of attraction. The reaction force acting on the individual is

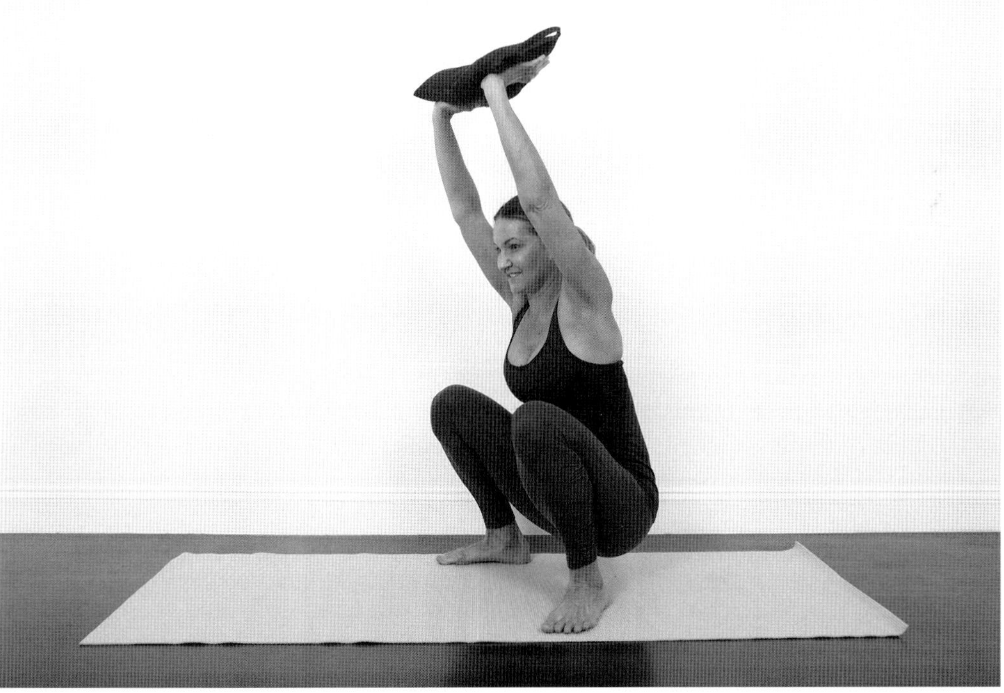

Fig. 1.6
A sandbag can be used in Garland Pose (Deep Squat) to apply an external load through the shoulders, spine, and hips.

considered an applied load. Diving deeper, if you put a separate force plate under each foot in Warrior II Pose, the readings would differ. Determined by the asymmetrical geometry of the pose, your limb lengths, and your mass, the reading of the force plate under the front foot would differ from that of the back foot. Therefore, the applied loads to the lower extremity in Warrior II Pose are not equally distributed between the front and back leg. Again, mastering the mathematical equations is not necessary here. The key is that applied loads are always changing as you change positions, direction, and acceleration.

We experience a great number of externally applied loads (i.e. loads applied by one or more additional objects or bodies other than your own). These loads come from a wide variety of sources. Examples include holding a weighted barbell in the gym, carrying a graduate student's backpack, a high-speed collision in sport, a therapeutic manual manipulation (e.g. massage), an assisted stretch, a yoga adjustment, or a yoga prop (Fig. 1.6). When used deliberately, an adjustment or prop can provide a purposeful external force, diversifying the exposure to loads in any given pose. Not all loads, however, are externally applied.

The human body also produces and transmits forces internally. Muscle force is an internal force resulting when an electrical impulse from one's nervous system converts to a chemical signal at the neuromuscular junction, whereupon proteins within the muscle cell interact to produce a muscle contraction. During a muscle contraction, the resulting tension (i.e. mechanical force) is transmitted through the tendon, across a joint (or many), and to a bone. Other examples of internal loads include ligaments pulling on bones, changes in intrathoracic pressure resulting from the contractions of the diaphragm, and hydrostatic pressure on synovial fluid inside the joints.

Movement, or the prevention of movement (e.g. holding a static yoga pose), is the integration and interaction of multiple and varying internally and externally applied loads. This is essentially an application of Newton's 1st law, where motion, as well as the interruption of motion, requires an application of force. Borrowing an example from a classical motor control theory, let's explore the process of picking up a wine glass. While the wine glass example is historically about sensory feedback, reaction times, and recall of maintaining proper grip when you sense a wine glass slipping out of your hand, we will, for fun, apply the wine glass example to biomechanics where many loads are acting on many objects. Simply holding your wine glass in a fixed position is an example of your internally created forces counteracting an external load. When you want to sip your wine, the force initiated by your muscles acts directly on your tendons and bones, as well as on the glass. Your outstretched arm itself imposes a load on the shoulder joint in addition to the load of the wine glass. As you bend your elbow to bring the glass to your mouth, the lever length of your arm changes, reducing the demand on the shoulder muscles. After you sip your wine, the mass of the wine glass has decreased, changing the load in your grasp and the muscle force needed to elevate it. It's a silly example, I know, but sometimes simple events lead to great leaps in understanding (as the fictitious legend of an apple falling from a tree led to Newton's discovery of gravity). Life, however, consists of more than just sipping wine, and thus we are compelled to explore applied loads in greater depth.

In a biomechanics laboratory, the force plate can be used to quantify applied loads acting on the human body. The aforementioned reaction force is referred to as the

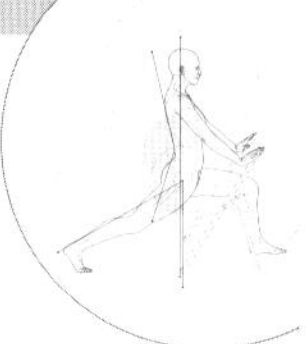

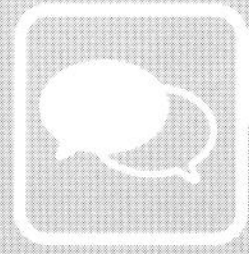

Thought Provoker

Weight-Bearing Exercises

Most yoga teachers have heard the phrase "weight-bearing exercises improve bone density," and are even more likely to have heard that yoga is good for bone health and may even reverse osteoporosis. Is this assertion dose-dependent? Might it depend on the subject? Can you think of specific styles of yoga, certain transitions, or added props/equipment that might result in higher GRFs than others?

ground reaction force (GRF). In a laboratory, researchers can ask subjects to engage in physical activity on top of a force plate and collect data about the associated GRFs with those movements. Your walking GRFs are generally 1.0–1.5 times your standing GRF (i.e. body weight), depending on your acceleration. Due to the greater acceleration at the moment of impact, running provides GRFs of approximately 2.5–3.5 times your standing GRF. What if we did yoga on a force plate? Research tells us the GRFs of a Hatha flow-style practice are comparable to walking but do not typically reach those of running or jumping (Wilcox et al., 2012). How does this align with your own understanding, or your own intuition?

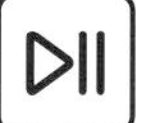

Pause and turn to page 36 for a summary of related research.

The relevance in GRFs lies in the long-term changes to musculoskeletal tissues in response to these various loads. In zero-gravity environments where surface attractions are absent, astronauts exercise on specially designed equipment to offset the external load deficiency. Bones thrive, as assessed by elevated bone mass density (BMD), in the presence of ever increasing forces. Sport science tells us that the lower-limb bones in runners are denser than in sedentary individuals, and the racket arm of a tennis player is denser than the non-racket arm. Just as load carries the propensity to build resilience (e.g. jumping off a 3-foot box), load also carries the propensity for injury (e.g. jumping out of a three-story building). The distinction between them is not always clear, and never absolute. The long-term adaptive changes to an applied load are relative to the individual and are dose-dependent. Applied loads are measurable and quantifiable; further, the ways in which these loads can be applied can be more narrowly defined.

Load Parameters

Loads must be further described by their parameters because they can be applied with great variety. Just walk into the weight room at your local gym, and you'll find dumbbells of different weights, machines with pulleys at varying angles of resistance, members performing a wide range of repetitions, and runners on treadmills at different speeds.

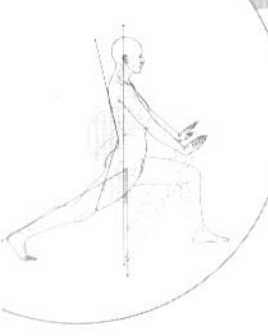

By selecting different parameters, the individual can customize a workout to select a certain physical response to the load. Personal trainers do this all the time. We do this in yoga as well. The body responds differently to a Vinyasa flow-style class than to a gentle seated practice. Mechanical load is shaped by quantity, position, time, and rate parameters.

Continuing with bone as our example (mainly because it is easy to conceptualize for most people new to biomechanics), consider the long bones of the arms and legs. We could vary the applied load simply by adjusting the parameters. By adding a sandbag to the soles of the feet in Legs-Up-the-Wall Pose, you increase the magnitude of load on the legs. Placing the hands directly beneath the shoulder in Plank Pose versus placing the hands wider than shoulder distance would impose different internal and external loads on the arms because of geometry. Load can further be described by duration, as in the length of time holding Downward Facing Dog Pose; by frequency, as in how many Downward Facing Dog Poses per day, per month, per year; or any combination of the two. Finally, the rate at which any external load makes impact with a bone matters, as in jumping versus stepping back to Plank Pose or Four-Limbed Staff Pose from Downward Facing Dog Pose, or brisk walking versus slow walking. To illustrate this, we can consider the task of driving a nail into a wooden board. If we rest the hammer on the nail, the nail may never penetrate the wood. We make progress if the hammer contacts the nail at a slight acceleration, and even more progress with greater acceleration. The mass of the hammer can also be taken into account, which explains why toy hammers don't make effective construction tools. Thankfully, bones do not behave exactly like wood or else high-speed activities like sprinting and hurdling would produce debilitating effects to the femur bone, but the example serves to explain that slowly or quickly applied loads have different results. Later, we examine the behavior of human tissues, but, the key points to recognize here are that load parameters (Table 1.3) are changeable and responses are variable.

You might find yourself reflecting on how adjusting these variables shapes a yoga class. A sequence of postures individually held for 45 seconds reflects different loading parameters from the same sequence of postures flowed through in 5 repetitions without any prolonged time spent in each pose. Even though the selection of postures is identical, the

Table 1.3
Load Parameters

Magnitude	How much?
Location	Where?
Direction	At what angle?
Duration	How long?
Frequency	How often?
Velocity	How fast?
Acceleration	What rate of change in velocity?

time under load is not, and the response is very likely not, as well. A more detailed conversation of how the body responds to different load parameters lies ahead. At this point, I am only bringing to the foreground the concept that simply identifying a pose by name tells us very little about the loading parameters. I hope that when you now hear a statement suggesting that a certain yoga posture is good for a condition such as osteoporosis, you immediately wonder which loading parameters might satisfy that statement.

Response to Load

A **stressor** is by definition any stimulus that triggers a response. You can stress your body in variety of ways, including, but not limited to, chemically, thermally, psychologically, and mechanically. Colloquially, stress has a negative connotation, but not all stressing stimuli are negative. *Distress* refers to bad stress, but *eustress* refers to good stress. While a 200 kg (440 lb) deadlift may be distressing for a novice it is likely eustressing for an Olympic weightlifter. How well stress is tolerated is, therefore, relative to the dose and the individual, rather than absolute.

When a material is loaded, its stress is determined by how it deforms. When first hearing the word, **deformation**, it is easy to think it has a negative connotation. In materials science engineers use the term deform to merely denote a change in form or shape when exposed to load. Some deformations are *elastic*, meaning they return to the unloaded shape when load is removed. Other deformations are *plastic*, meaning the deformation is permanent. Stress is the measure of a material's concurrent resistance to deformation when exposed to an external force.

The capacity to surrender to and resist deformation describes a material's behavior. Behavior is just one aspect of a material's properties – composition (i.e. components of which the material is made) and structure (i.e. the arrangement of parts) also contribute. Just as materials science is the field of study where engineers investigate the behavior of a material they may use to construct a bridge, tissue mechanics is the field of study where biomechanists study the behavior of human tissues. The exciting details of this field are covered in a future chapter. For now, understanding that tissue behavior is the relationship between load and deformation is sufficient.

Resistance to deformation is often confused with strength and it is subsequently assumed that materials that deform are weak and materials that do not are strong. This assumption would lead you describe glass as strong because it does not bend and copper wire as weak because it does. Glass is brittle, however, and therefore does not tolerate stress well, whereas copper is ductile and tolerates stress quite well. Human tissues, neither as brittle as glass nor as ductile as copper, are evaluated for their capacity to tolerate stress. Human musculoskeletal connective tissues are able to maintain structural integrity because they have the ability to undergo large deformations while simultaneously absorbing force at a capacity similar to that of stainless steel. Colloquially, one may say they have tremendous strength, but we now know that implies they have tremendous capacity to tolerate stress.

Externally applied loads and the resulting deformations are mostly described as tensile, compressive, torsional, bending, or shearing (Fig. 1.7). *Tensile* loading pulls an object in opposing directions, "stretching" or lengthening the material. *Compressive* loading squeezes an object together, sometimes causing bulging as the matter seeks

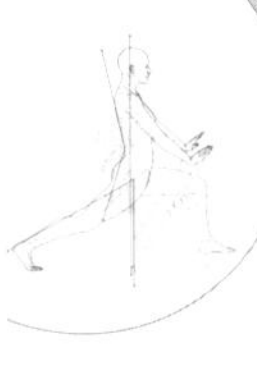

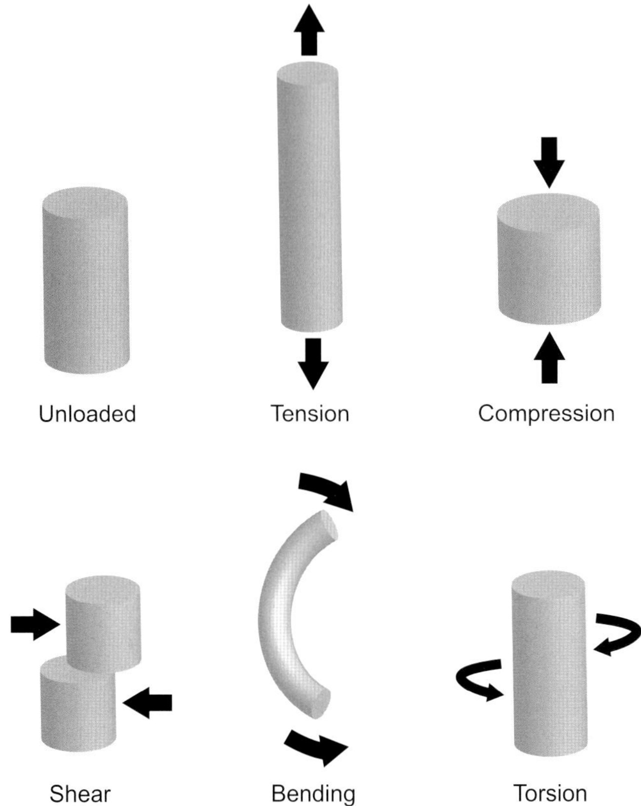

Fig. 1.7
Various types of loading and deformations.

to take up space in any available direction. The remaining three are a combination of tensile and compressive forces. *Torsion* results in twisting or rotation, *bending* curves an object, and *shearing* slides surfaces parallel to one another. For the purposes of this book, although I may occasionally reference torsional, bending, or shearing, with the exception of compressive stress on bone and cartilage, we will primarily investigate tensile stress.

To highlight resistance to deformation during tension, let's consider a stretched material. Imagine you and your friends were hiking and came upon a suspension bridge made of nylon ropes and wooden planks. From a materials science perspective we would want to know how many of your friends the rope has the capacity to hold before the rope tears and sends you falling at 9.8 m/s^2 acceleration (i.e. gravity). Keep in mind that the rope may give a little while loaded and return to its unloaded length (i.e. elastic deformation) when you have all successfully crossed to the other side. If too many of you cross at once, however, you risk the rope exceeding its load-bearing capacity. How many bodies the rope can withstand depends on how well it tolerates stress. Depending on the mechanical properties of the nylon rope, the maximum capacity may vary.
It may deform a lot (i.e. sag close to the ground) or deform very little (i.e. maintain its

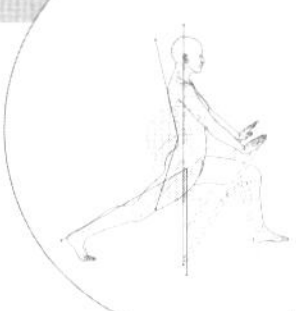

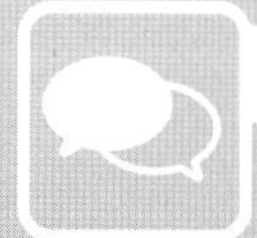

Thought Provoker

Compression and Tension

Compression and tension are terms often used casually in a yoga setting, causing confusion when learning the mechanical definitions as they relate to tissue mechanics. Compression is often described as end range of motion due to bone structure. For example, when the femur head makes contact with the acetabulum in hip flexion, external rotation, and abduction, there is no more range of motion available. Tension is described as end range of motion due to soft tissue restriction, where range of motion is still available because the bone morphology is not the limit. The tissue would only need to be stretched farther to achieve the available range of motion.

These explanations are technically correct from a range of motion perspective, but they give us no indication of the tissue's capacity to bear load and resist deformation. It is implied that compression may as well be avoided because there is no foreseeable benefit and tension is an obstacle that should be overcome. When the conversation takes a mechanical turn, these misleading implications carry over.

Our present conversation about yoga and biomechanics evaluates the behavior of the tissue and its ability to adapt. The common application of compression and tension in yoga is a perfect example of how the casual use of biomechanical language develops into yoga-jargon. When we lack a communally agreed upon definition, we only impede clarity and comprehension, diluting the power of our words. Can you think of any mechanically oriented words that we use in yoga that may not accurately reflect the properties which they are intended to describe?

unloaded shape), but if the structural integrity of the material remains intact (i.e. the material does not tear), the rope would be considered "strong" in both situations.

To highlight resistance to deformation during compression we will return to bones, which are continually compressed between the force created by your body mass and gravity, and the opposing GRF. If your bones could not absorb compressive load and resist deformation, you would shorten with each step. Bones do have a limit, however. When loading parameters exceed the bone's capacity, they are overloaded, and may be at risk for compression fractures. Often this leads to fear of high-impact activities where bones are exposed to higher magnitude and rates of compressive loading; however, improving the capacity of your bones to absorb compression, and resist deformation, requires a gradual increase in the magnitude of load! It's a biomechanical conundrum.

Adaptation

Where materials only tolerate stress, biological tissues can tolerate, and also adapt to, stress. A load-bearing wall in your apartment will not develop a greater capacity to bear load due to the time or rate of exposure, but human bone will. The concept of adaptability was first described in the 1800s when the German anatomist Julius Wolff identified that osseous tissue (bone) adapts to exposed loads. Today biomechanists accept Wolff's Law as a validated theory that applies to all non-pathological bones. The lesser known corollary to Wolff's Law, called Davis' Law, refers to the adaptable nature of the soft connective tissues surrounding bones. Despite the relatively infrequent reference to Davis' Law, the connective tissue research supporting the theory is abundant. Unfortunately, the public perception of how we adapt to "stretching" does not yet reflect these physiological principles.

Most people believe their limited range of motion could be rectified by "stretching out." First, it relies on an assumption that the tissue is short. Second, it relies on a subsequent assumption that stretching makes tissue longer. The laws of adaptability suggest that stressing biological tissues can improve their tolerance to stress, not permanently deform them. I often joke that if stretching your hamstrings made them longer, my hamstrings would be dragging on the floor behind me due to 20 years of yoga and hamstring stretching. I confess this is an unreasonable and inflated comparison, but changing perceptions sometimes requires a bit of humor and self-deprecation.

If you consider a stretch to be a tissue loaded in tension and you apply Davis' Law, you'd find the conclusion dubious, at best. The law of adaptability tells us stretching a soft connective tissue should increase its capacity to resist tensile loading, not make it longer, nor decrease its resistance to tension. Just like Wolff's Law, where osseous tissue loaded in compression does not make it shorter, nor less resistant to compression. Quite the opposite, in fact.

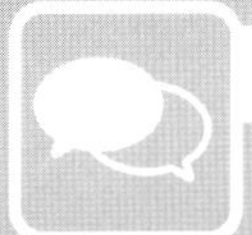

Thought Provoker

Scope of Practice

A scope of practice outlines a set of services a healthcare professional may provide under their regulatory professional license. While yoga teachers do not answer to any regulatory body, we can all agree within our unwritten professional code of conduct that our scope of practice is limited to areas in which we have adequate training and experience.

Therefore, yoga teachers will neither diagnose nor treat any pathology (unless they are licensed to do so under an appropriate regulatory body). Yoga teachers do, however, teach movement and movement affects tissues. Providing deliberate modifications, variations, and alternatives to poses is well within their scope. Additionally, it is acceptable for yoga teachers to work with a student to promote positive changes in certain components of fitness (e.g. strength, balance, flexibility). Problem solving on an individual basis is a useful skill in satisfying these student outcomes.

Can you identify a situation, hypothetical or real, where you should refer a student/client out because her needs are beyond your scope of practice? What additional training or licensing, if any, would you need to work with this student/client in the future?

At this point, you should be referring back to the previous section and asking yourself which loading parameters might incite these adaptations. In bone, the most obvious quality is size, or magnitude, of load. GRFs are most often studied by magnitude. Using the hammer and nail analogy, the magnitude of force is a product of acceleration and hammer mass (F=ma) and is more important than the duration of the hammer's contact with the nail. Hitting the nail hard is far more effective than resting the hammer on the nail and waiting for time to drive the nail into the wall. Since human tissues don't behave like wood, the analogy isn't perfect; analogies never are.

Frequency may be another load parameter that comes to mind when considering adaptation. Perhaps you have heard or even repeated the phrase, "weight-bearing exercises increase bone density." If you understand the nature of adaptation, you will know that a single input is not sufficient to strengthen bone, just as single training bout at the gym is not enough to build bulging biceps. Inputs need to be frequently applied and of a high enough magnitude to make this statement true.

In sport science, the notion that the body adapts to the movements most frequently performed (or loads most frequently applied) is referred to as the SAID principle (Specific Adaptations to Imposed Demands). A tennis player will develop denser bone in the racket arm than the non-racket arm just as a high jumper will develop Achilles tendon properties that promote better performance in high jumping. The improved cardiovascular capacity gained from running may prepare a cyclist for a long ride but running is still not a suitable replacement for cycle training. Running will improve lower-limb bone density, however. In contrast, the body maladapts to the absence of imposed demands, as we identified earlier in astronauts. The SAID principle can also be applied to skill acquisition.

Adaptation is one of the reasons why it is so difficult to determine which yoga poses are "safe." A mostly sedentary office worker may find a ninety-minute yoga class filled with hand and wrist weight-bearing poses aggravating while a seasoned yoga student might not. Not loading the hands and wrists, however, is not the best solution either, as the best way to improve the capacity for bearing weight on the hands is to ... wait for it ... bear weight on the hands. It seems so obvious, yet our language and our instruction often contradict the principles of adaptation. Our protective instincts lead us to advise students to avoid load when we are uncertain. We consider a yoga class for healthy wrists one where we avoid bearing weight on the hands, but if we want to promote healthy adaptation we would want to gradually expose the wrists to load.

I acknowledge how difficult it is to choose just how much exposure to offer an under-loaded structure, particularly in a group class setting where no two students share a loading history. I also understand that avoiding load is often the safest appearing and least controversial option. To be clear, I'm not advising we throw caution to the wind and start exposing untrained students to load without discernment. I am, however, clarifying that just because we may advise against load to protect students from potential aggravation (and ourselves from liability), this choice does not reflect the principles of adaption. If our students are coming to yoga with the goal of improving their capacity to practice yoga asana, then the principles of exercise science must apply. Becoming informed about how the body adapts to load is the first step in having another choice, one other than avoidance.

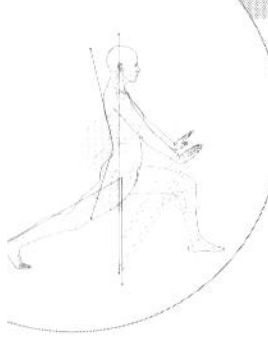

Scientific Literacy

Burden of Proof and Anecdotal Evidence

The burden of proof refers to the person with whom the responsibility of providing evidence to support or refute a claim resides. In general, the person making a claim should provide the evidence, as the null hypothesis is the default position.

Let me explain.

Years ago I was on a social media thread discussing the passive forward fold version of One-Legged King Pigeon Pose (i.e. Single Pigeon). We were debating its merits at a time in which I expressed a more negative judgment of passive stretching than I do now (the change of position is the effect of challenging my bias). I was suggesting more active alternatives when one of the commenters said she was not willing to change the way she taught the pose because it cured a student's back pain and was, therefore, effective as a passive pose. So:

The research question is: Does a passive Single Pigeon eliminate back pain?

Based on the theory: Single Pigeon stretches the hips and low back, and stretching alleviates pain.

The hypothesis is: Passive Single Pigeon does eliminate back pain.

The null hypothesis is: Passive Single Pigeon does not eliminate back pain.

The burden of proof lies on the person making the claim that passive Single Pigeon cures back pain. Until she presents sufficient evidence, the null hypothesis is the default position – we cannot claim that this pose cures back pain because we think it does.

This brings us to the topic of anecdotal evidence.

Anecdotal evidence is evidence in the form of personal experience, or third party testimony. Anecdotal evidence may feel very real, but because it is not conducted in a controlled research setting, it cannot be accepted as data. In the Pigeon Pose example here, we have no way of knowing if the person who was relieved of back pain engaged in any other activities that could have resulted in the same outcome. For example, the person could have changed jobs, started sleeping more, joined a gym, or changed her diet. Or maybe, she would have improved even if she had done nothing. With no controls in place, we have no way of knowing. Anecdotal evidence is therefore generally not accepted as reliable evidence.

This fact is at the heart of the popular phrase: "The plural of anecdote is not data."

Continued on next page

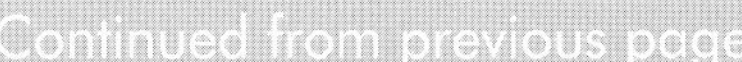
Continued from previous page

Finally, in the spirit of full disclosure, I, too, was making an unsupported claim about Single Pigeon. I don't recall exactly what my claim was, but I can guess that I was making some sort of fear-mongering statement about the perils of passive stretching and the damaging effect it has on the hip and knee joints in this position. The burden of proof to provide such evidence was on me, as I was making the claim.

At that time, I had a dismal view of passive stretching, fueled by anecdotal evidence, which, in turn clouded my ability to interpret the literature without bias. In the absence of compelling evidence to support my claim about Single Pigeon, had someone challenged me, I may have been forced to change my position. As it turns out, over the years, I learned more about my personal bias, was willing to be challenged, and, eventually, did change my position.

If all contributors to social media threads were well-versed in where the burden of proof lies, that anecdotal evidence is not research evidence, and could recognize their personal bias, we could save a lot of time in our debates. Seeking knowledge through scientific discovery means little tolerance for defending personal beliefs and not taking personal offense when your claim is challenged. When these basic principles are not in place, social media disputes can seem futile.

Yoga and Performance

Yoga for athletic performance is a marketable product and even professional sports teams report including yoga in their training repertoires. We want yoga to make a profound impact, and so we are quick to credit yoga for improved performance, in spite of the contradiction set forth by the SAID principle. In the absence of a high-quality, blinded, randomized controlled trials (RCT), such assumptions are belief-based and not scientifically validated. Claiming yoga improves performance because you've witnessed a team improve after yoga is the equivalent of claiming your team won the game because you wore their jersey on game day – it could be true, but the vigor of the scientific process has not enabled us to narrow our understanding enough to make the correlation with confidence.

If a high quality research study on the effects of yoga and sports performance were to exist, I might suggest an RCT that would divide the subjects of the study into a minimum of two groups. One would receive the yoga intervention, the other(s) another type of intervention, or none at all. All other variables would be controlled for as best as possible (i.e. sleep, diet, sport specific training, total training hours, etc.). The subjects would be randomized into the groups (to ensure assignments are by chance only) and the investigators and coaches would be blind to knowing which subject is in which group to avoid influencing the study design. A clear performance outcome measure would be defined ahead of time, and preferably objective (i.e. range of motion, jump height, speed) rather than subjective (i.e. athlete's/coach's opinions on performance). Moreover, the study design would need to include some method

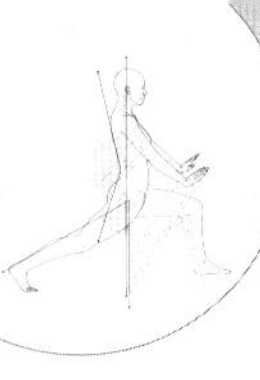

Scientific Literacy

Randomized Controlled Trials

Randomized controlled trials (RCTs) are experimental studies where a sample of subjects is randomly selected and assigned to two or more groups. At least one of these groups is a control group (a neutral group from which to compare) while the other group(s) are assigned an intervention. Blinding is when the subjects are unaware of which intervention they are receiving in order to mitigate for any potential bias that may influence the results. Double-blinding is when the investigators are unaware of which subjects are assigned which intervention reducing the potential of observer bias.

Yoga research is difficult to blind because it is virtually impossible to disguise a yoga intervention. Imagine we collected a sample of subjects with low back pain through a local medical practice. After screening each subject for exclusionary factors (e.g. certain medications, recent surgeries, specific conditions) we randomly assigned each subject an intervention. One group received a yoga intervention, another group received a fitness intervention, and the control group did nothing at all. It would be difficult to convince the yoga group they weren't practicing yoga. If the experiment were measuring the effectiveness of a new low back pain drug, all three groups could take a similar-looking pill even if the first group was taking the experimental drug, the second group was taking an already established drug, and the third group was taking a placebo (i.e. no active ingredient). But in our hypothetical yoga study, subjects would know if they were practicing yoga, doing a general fitness routine, or doing nothing at all. Therefore their preconceived ideas about yoga and low back pain may influence their reported effects.

RCTs are considered high-quality research and blinding improves the study's validity (how likely the results of a study reflect the intended outcome measure). Reliability measures how likely the results of a study are to be reproducible. In the imagined yoga study above, depending on the population from which the sample was drawn, cultural bias may produce different results. If the study was conducted in a community where yoga is promoted as a superior alternative treatment, then replicated in a community where yoga is widely considered a sham treatment, and the results reflected this bias, then we would deem the study unreliable. Further, these results would suggest that the outcome measured the beliefs of the subjects more than the actual effect of the intervention and would therefore question the study's validity.

of determining how any improvements in objective measures translate to sport performance (e.g. improved range of motion does not automatically imply skillful use of this new range). Unfortunately, at the time of this writing, no such study exists.

I feel compelled to note here that yoga has many other suggested benefits beyond objective sports measures listed above. Mental acuity due to the meditative aspects may, in fact, be a major contributor to improved sports performance. Here we are simply applying the SAID principle and how the practice of physical asana affects physical performance.

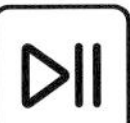

Pause and turn to page 36 for a summary of related research.

Optimal Loading

Returning to load adaptation, we have established that human tissue is biologically active, and changes occur in response to load. The musculoskeletal system is always building, repairing, or degenerating in response to the dose of mechanical input. This raises the question: Is there an optimal load? Which raises yet another question: For what outcome? With the mutable nature of human tissue, the best we can do is learn about all the potential ways in which loading leads to favorable physiological adaptations and make informed decisions from there.

The last statement above goes against common musculoskeletal contraindications to exercise. For example, seniors with low bone density are often advised to avoid high-intensity loads to best prevent compression fractures. Yet Wolff's Law states loading bone triggers physiological adaptations which increase the bone's capacity to withstand more load. Recent research at a bone clinic in Brisbane has shown safe and effective improvements in bone density in women over 60 with osteoporosis in response to heavy lifting, which challenges conventional thought about the adaptability of bone over a certain age (Watson et al., 2015). Another example states that stacking bones is the safest position and imposes the least amount of stress on the joints. Yet Davis' Law states that stressing connective tissue improves its capacity to tolerate greater loads. These positions are clearly in contradiction to each other.

It turns out both positions are right and both positions are somewhat wrong. Evidence exists to support the pervasive idea that high training loads cause injury. Evidence also exists to support the opposite idea that high training loads protect against injury (Gabbett, 2016). If one of the goals of a yoga teacher is to teach in a safe and sustainable manner, then the pursuit of optimal loading is warranted. And, as we've learned, loads are applied with different parameters and are, therefore, not all equal. Thus, the best way to answer the questions the above information raises – Is there an optimal load? and For what outcome? – is to study the demands of a given activity (i.e. yoga), the properties of the affected tissues, and their adaptive responses.

Progressive Overload

In terms of magnitude, the principle of progressive overload is the golden rule of loading, with the keyword being progressive (Fig. 1.8). The biomechanical phenomenon states that loading must progressively increase above normal loading patterns to stimulate growth. Conversely, underloading will have the opposite effect, and tissue will adaptively diminish. The magnitude of the optimal load is not absolute, it is relative to the typical loading patterns of the individual. This explains why bicep curls with a 5 kg barbell sufficiently develops strength in a novice but is insufficient for

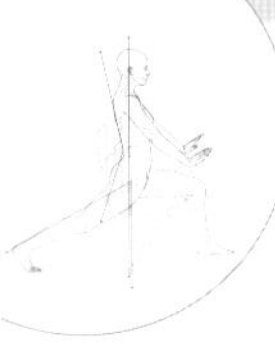

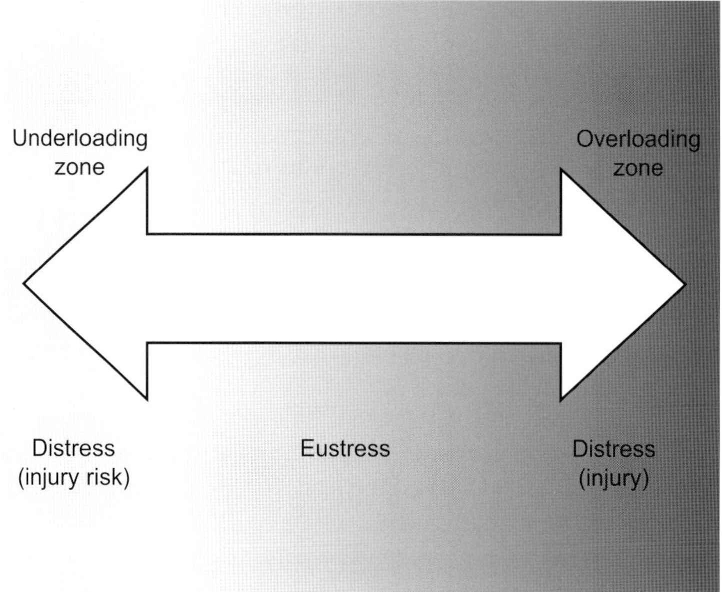

Fig. 1.8
The principle of progressive overload.

someone who regularly curls 50 kg, all other load parameters being equal. The load must progressively stress the targeted tissue to favorably adapt it.

In weight lifting, the most common progressive adjustments to load are the number of repetitions (reps) and/or the percentage of maximum capacity. These variables are often referred to as volume and intensity, respectively. Volume, however, is better defined as a product of the number of sets, the number of reps in a set, and weight being lifted. If you were to curl 1 set of 10 kg for 8 reps and then 2 sets of 12 kg for 6 reps, your total volume would be $(10 \times 8) + 2(12 \times 6) = 224$ kg.

Intensity may refer to load or a percentage of aerobic/endurance capacity, therefore, it's best to be specific. Simply saying "high-intensity exercise" tells us very little. In terms of load intensity during weight lifting, percentage of maximum capacity is discussed in terms of 1 repetition maximum (1RM). The most weight you can lift one time is your 1RM and load intensity (i.e. magnitude) is determined by using a percentage of this amount. The higher the percentage of 1RM, the higher the intensity, and the lower number of reps can be accomplished, usually.

In order to progressively overload, one would gradually increase the volume by increasing the reps, the sets, the percent 1RM, or all. Spikes in training, or rapid fluctuations in load, are associated with an increased risk for injury (Soligard et al., 2016). For this reason, 1RM is most often not measured by testing how much one is able to lift once, but rather is calculated by the number of reps that can be achieved with good form at a certain weight (you can easily find an online calculator to do this for you). The strength and conditioning research contains an abundance of data analyzing the effects of loading repertoires. Here is not the place to review, or debate, the methodologies – any textbook can get you started if you have further interest.

The point here is to understand the importance of slow but consistent progression, as well as the importance of acknowledging deconditioning. An everyday runner who still feels fit, but has taken 3 months off for whatever reason, should probably not reintroduce running at the volume at which she was running previously. Another important consideration is that relative load may refer to more than just a measurable volume. Psychological stressors are another variable which must be included.

Quantifying psychosocial stress (subjective) in combination with mechanical stress (objective) poses a challenge. A frequently used method among coaches is to assess the rate of perceived exertion (RPE) for each individual athlete. To calculate RPE, the time in training is multiplied by an exertion score on a scale of 1–10. Since the exertion scale is subjective, it is better suited to account for stressors of daily life that may contribute to fatigue. RPE isn't perfect, however. A 45-minute hot yoga flow class

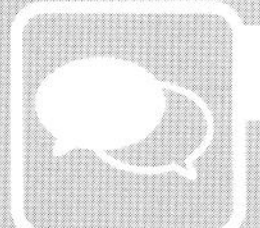

Thought Provoker

Load Exposure

Modern yoga follows many different paths and is expressed by a wide variety of sequencing and class styling. In some of the larger urban areas where I have practiced, Downward Facing Dog Pose is very popular. It often begins class, separates flow sequences, and is offered as a resting posture. Many students who frequent these classes have adequate exposure to load, including weight training, upper body centric sports, and advanced arm balancing practices, for the time spent in the pose to be a non-issue.

A private client, new to yoga, asks for your professional assistance. She has been to the local group yoga class and she says it makes her wrists feel sensitive during class and sometimes soreness lingers into the next day. She feels fine otherwise, has no history of wrist pain, and has a clean bill of health from her physician. When she spoke to the teacher, the teacher told her to rest in child's pose instead of doing all the Downward Facing Dog Poses. The client expressed that she felt intimidated that she couldn't participate in class and was hoping some private lessons were a better environment for her to start and then improve to attend classes. Her immediate goal is to attend one group class per week while working with you, eventually attending class regularly and participating fully.

As we know, the best way to increase the capacity to bear load is through load exposure. Thus was the teacher's recommendation potentially detrimental to the student's progression? What poses would you work on with her? Any variations? Any homework? For her group class, in addition to unloading the wrists by resting in child's pose, what alternatives might you offer her to work on while allowing her to feel like she is participating with the group?

with an RPE of 8 versus a 90-minute inversion workshop with an RPE of 4 both yield a total RPE of 360, whereas the differences in loading profiles are likely to pose different injury risks. Regardless, the theory can be generally applied if comparing similar types of loading profiles to avoid spikes in training. The mantra "listen to your body" takes on entirely new, practical, measurable meaning when assessed in the context of RPE and should be honored.

The principle of progressive overload clearly states the importance of load, but not too much load (and not too little load!). The examples provided were mostly in the context of muscle adaptation, because that is where volume and intensity are most often played with. When we start looking at other structures (e.g. bones, ligaments, tendons), we see that other load parameters are especially important to consider.

Variable Loading

Back to the concept of what optimal loading might be; in addition to specific and progressive, loads should be variable. Specificity is important for targeted training. In the previous example with the runner who took 3 months off, assume the runner was instead cycling for those 3 months. The runner may not have become aerobically deconditioned and feels fit enough to pick up running at the volume where she left off. The bones and ligaments in her foot, or her Achilles tendon, may have become deconditioned, possibly putting her at risk for a stress fracture or tendinopathy. Loading the foot through progressive exposure to specifically running, in combination with additional exposure to variable load helps promote positive adaptation. A trainer or coach might suggest exercises such as foot and ankle mobility drills, calf raises, and squats. A yoga teacher might add standing poses and single-leg balancing postures. In this example, specificity requires that the foot and ankle be loaded, as opposed to the wrist and hand, but variable loading allows for a wider net of a stressors to be cast. Less important than the exact exercises or poses is the biomechanical principle, variable loading, and supporting the selection.

Bones and connective tissue are especially responsive to variable loading and novel stimuli. In early stages of training, or recovery from acute injury, slowly and systematically applied loads are best. In later stages of training, changes in the rate of loading, and variable direction are imperative in the progressive overload model. The benefits of variable loading are two-fold; it reduces the potential for repetitive stress while simultaneously preparing the tissue for unpredictable load exposure (Glasgow, Phillips and Bleakley, 2015). This recommendation goes against the conventional safety rules we hear in yoga, where the right way is the only safe way. Perhaps there is a favorable way to anatomically position the body to satisfy the alignment of a certain pose. Perhaps the alignment requirements of the pose are novel, thereby introducing variable loading. To conflate the shape of the poses with avoiding injury is too simplistic for the complex molecular, cellular, and structural factors considered in optimal loading.

Future discussions on optimal loading are aimed at advocating for a deeper understanding of yoga asana. Through detailed study of the mechanical demands of yoga poses alongside the adaptive nature of tissue properties we may elevate the conversation from a binary model where right or wrong prevails, to a multi-dimensional model that considers intent, evidence, experience, and skepticism. Optimal loading, as a construct, is evolving, mutable, and negotiable, but one that is only accessible when we expand beyond the narrow perception of correctness or incorrectness.

Yoga and Biomechanics

Our working definition of biomechanics, the study of how force affects biological systems, is quite broad and now warrants deeper discussion. A large portion of biomechanical research is in the fields of kinetics and kinematics. Both terms describe human movement, but in different ways. Kinetics is a branch of biomechanics that considers how forces act on masses to cause motion and includes both internally and externally applied loads. A kinetic analysis could be linear or angular (e.g. a rotational movement around a joint). Kinetics examines forces in terms of mass and acceleration, including variables such as gravity, friction, and anthropometrics. Force is not measurable with the naked eye, however, and so laboratory equipment such as video analysis software, electromyography (EMG), and force plates are usually needed. Kinematics is a branch of biomechanics that examines the appearance of motion but disregards the forces that cause movement. Kinematic calculations are mostly geometrical equations that examine the form or pattern of motion with respect to variables such as time, velocity, and displacement. Both apply the laws of physics and concepts in engineering to describe sport and daily activity and are dynamic branches of study.

We know a living body is never truly static, but on their surface, yoga postures appear static and lacking motion. The postures are achieved and then held, mostly evaluated by teachers in the static stage. In yoga, it is not uncommon to hear the name of the pose, execute it, and then continue to be offered extensive kinematic instructions (tilt, rotate, extend) while holding the pose. These cues tend to be aesthetically derived, not taking into account variables such as length of moment arms (note: it's not a called moment leg when studying the lower limbs, it's always just called the moment arm), angular forces around an axis of rotation, or frictional forces supplied by a sticky mat.

When I started studying biomechanics, I spent several semesters solving equations for these types of variables in different yoga poses. One of my class projects involved a photo of me from the side (i.e. in the sagittal plane) in Downward Facing Dog Pose, uploaded into software to measure angles, followed by four pages of calculations to determine reaction forces, torques, and how they would change if I were to make small adjustments to the pose. I was looking for that binary answer, that one best way to do Downward Facing Dog Pose, not aesthetically speaking, but biomechanically speaking. It didn't work out so well.

In my pursuit, I discovered many shortcomings. First, it was not uncommon for me to list a dozen assumptions and limitations in order to validate the equations as accurate. A free body diagram (upon which such equations are written) is a two-dimensional sketch representing theoretical conditions that cannot possibly capture the complexity of the forces involved in human movement (Fig. 1.9). More importantly, assigning any meaning to the results was the biggest challenge. In sports, players are moving at extremely high speeds, jumping great distances, and propelling objects of substantial mass (including their own bodies), all while being evaluated by quantifiable performance

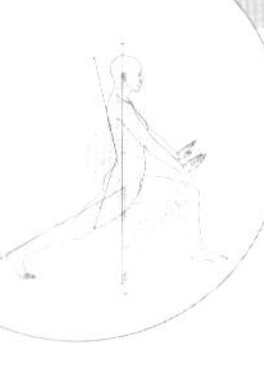

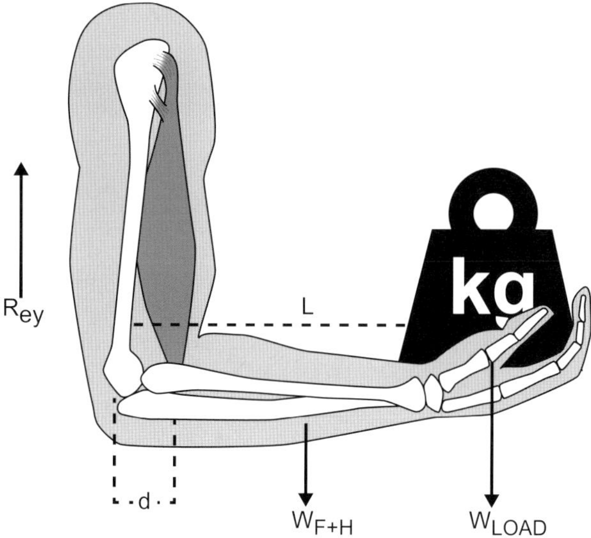

Fig. 1.9

An example of a free body diagram. Reaction force (R_{ey}) required by the bicep muscle to offset the load of the dumbbell can be calculated as $R_{ey}=(W_{load})+(W_{F+H})$ where W_{load} represents the external force or load applied by the dumbbell, and W_{F+H} represents the internal force applied by the forearm and hand. Other important variables include distance between the center of joint rotation and biceps insertion (d), and the length of the forearm and hand (L). Torque (rotational force) at the elbow in the units Newton*meter (Nm) can also be calculated if the segment centers of gravity are known: $T_e=(T_{load})+(T_{F+H})$.

measures. A coach might utilize this information to specifically target training for an athlete to improve performance. In yoga, we typically don't try to maximize speed, power, or strength, nor is there is any winning of the game with the best score. Most of us are looking for a little body-weight strength, some improvements in mobility (kinematics), and a little stretching, all while trying to stay safe. These calculations, albeit interesting, in terms of teaching provide little to no value. Knowing how to calculate how much force the hamstrings needed to produce in order for a student to hold Downward Facing Dog Pose didn't help me teach it to someone.

As it turns out, much of the laboratory-conducted research has similar shortcomings. Knowing the degree to which the abdominal muscles activate during Upward Facing Dog Pose (Beazley et al., 2017), or that lower limb muscles are more active in a single-leg standing pose than in a double-leg standing pose (Kelley, Slattery and Apollo, 2017), or that the patterns of muscle activation during a series of postures are inconsistent across practitioner experience levels (Ni et al., 2014) does not immediately transfer to the teaching of poses, particularly in a group class setting. At best, these data may provide some insight into pose selection for a specific individual with a specific goal in mind. Most published papers claim the importance of the study lies in improving pose selection for rehabilitation purposes, but how the collected data translate into an effective rehabilitation program is generally not studied. Moreover, the theoretical assumptions and methodological limitations noted in these papers warrant critical analysis before accepting their conclusions, which tend to be rooted in the "avoiding load to avoid injury" model. Biomechanics can still inform general yoga practice; however, only from a different angle.

This brings me to another emphasis in the interdisciplinary field of biomechanics: the study of tissue mechanics. Here we apply principles of materials science and mechanical engineering to biological tissues. Just as engineers must understand the properties of structural materials like steel, concrete, and wood, biomechanists must understand the properties of biological structures. With the exception of a brief discussion of muscle physiology in the chapter on stretching, the tissues of interest here are the collagenous connective tissues such as bone, cartilage, joint capsules, ligaments, tendons, and, in some cases, fascia. Of the variety of ways biomechanics can be applied to the teaching of yoga, I find the mechanical properties of these tissues to be the most practical.

At the time of this writing, the overall spirit of yoga asana has entered new territory. In my earlier years of study, prior to the advent of social media, yoga was the panacea for just about any musculoskeletal ache or pain. It was always "therapeutic," and it would do you no harm. As more people joined the practice of yoga, fueled by internet communication, we started hearing about more injuries, specifically connective tissue injuries, that might have been caused by yoga. Concurrently, although in a different industry, sports scientists started publishing research refuting the anecdotal benefits of stretching. Soon enough, yoga experienced its fall from grace, and stretching and extreme yoga posture became vilified.

This brings me back to biomechanics and, specifically, tissue mechanics. If we are truly committed to a safe and sustainable yoga practice, we can benefit the most from understanding how load affects structure. The aesthetic cues rooted in postural assessment, limb placement, and alignment are insufficient for this goal, as are many of the kinetic and kinematic data. What might translate into safer teaching is the study of *how* active and passive loads affect tissue properties. With this education, the poses are released from the binary realm of safe/injurious or correct/incorrect and placed into the realm of "it depends." How exactly "it depends" is complicated and simultaneously fascinating and is precisely what this book sets out to explain.

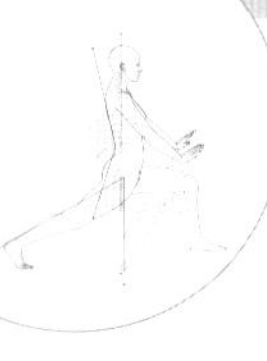

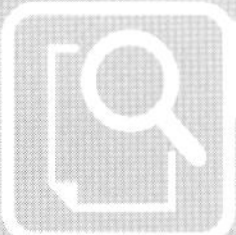

Research Summary

Ground Reaction Forces in Yoga

Ground Reaction Forces Generated by Twenty-eight Hatha Yoga Postures (Wilcox et al., 2012)

Background

Consumer media implies that yoga is good for bone health, but at the time of this publication there was insufficient research to support this claim. The article references one book on yoga and bone health in particular, although there are certainly others. In order to begin to substantiate the benefits of yoga on bone health, it would be helpful to know the magnitude of ground reaction forces (GRFs) associated with yoga postures and transitions.

Purpose

This study aims to establish the level of impact yoga provides by measuring GRFs in common yoga poses. The authors reference several articles suggesting that high-impact sports (e.g. running and jumping) and lower-impact resistance training (e.g. weight lifting) both have positive effects on bone-mass density (BMD) and hypothesize yoga as an activity that would fall into the lower-impact category (resulting in less than two times individual body weight of the subjects). They further hypothesize GRFs would be consistent across all subjects, as data were reported in percentages of body weight and not in absolute values.

Methods

12 women and 8 men participated in the intervention. A sticky mat placed over a force plate, after ensuring the mat didn't interfere with the technology, was the method of measurement. Sun Salutations, all the Warrior Poses, several common standing poses, single-leg balancing poses, and beginner arm balances (28 unique poses, 32 total poses) were verbally cued and performed in a set sequence. Three of those times they stepped onto the mat to perform the postures and the other three times they began on the mat so that GRFs on both upper and lower extremity could be measured for all the poses.

Results

GRFs were less than two times body weight for the duration of the sequence for all the participants. The highest GRF was from jumping forward to Standing Forward Bend in the Sun Salutation.

Continued on next page

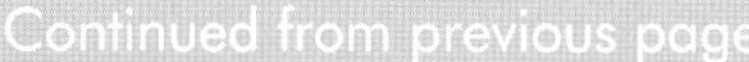

Continued from previous page

Discussion

Since the study only measured GRF and not actual BMD, it is difficult to conclude that yoga is sufficient for improving BMD. Additionally, the GRFs only measure the magnitude of force, which is only one loading parameter to consider in the development of BMD. Given the obviousness of the low-impact nature of yoga, these results are somewhat underwhelming, yet it is important not to make assumptions based on seemingly obvious information. This study, while not overwhelmingly useful, achieved its purpose to quantify the magnitude of GRFs in 28 Hatha yoga postures. Based on the research question, we can conclude a Hatha flow-type yoga practice results in similar GRFs as slow to fast walking but does not match running or jumping.

Research Summary

Yoga for Speed Skaters

Influences of a Yoga Intervention on the Postural Skills of the Italian Short Track Speed Skating Team (Brunelle et al., 2015)

Background

Speed skater efficiency depends partly on a specific posture (i.e. trunk forward and pelvis low while using hip extension and balance for push off and recovery). As the athletes increase the volume of skating sessions during off-season training, coaches observed that adaptation to these postures interfered with the quality of other training sessions both on and off the ice (e.g. running, core strengthening). The coaches wanted to counteract postural adaptations with a different type of postural training: yoga.

Purpose

The athletes were given a yoga intervention to determine if they could improve skating technique, diversify training methods without interfering with the current training schedule, and reduce injury. (Personal note: the aim does not seem to align with the background, which already reveals a flaw in the study design.) The coaches hypothesized that yoga would improve the athletes' movement repertoires, which would translate to their sport performance.

Methods

After selecting a sequence (which varied each session) of 85 approved and sport-specific yoga postures, coaches added 8 weeks of yoga to eight men and

Continued on next page

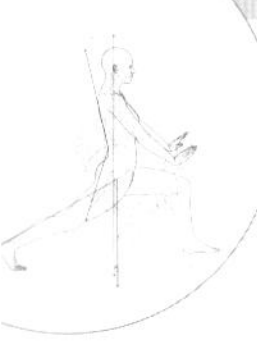

Continued from previous page

seven women on the Italian national team training for the 2014 Olympics. The 15 athletes received 36 yoga sessions (averaging 41 minutes each) in addition to their current training schedule. They measured spinal extension, shoulder mobility during trunk rotation, and a runner's Lunge position both before and after the intervention. Additionally, records were kept for total training hours (accounting for actual seconds of activity and movement for the non-cyclical training activities) and whether or not injury was the cause for any missed sessions.

Results

Joint angles increased, mostly statistically significant. Yoga sessions took about 30% of total training time and the coaches did not observe any deficits in performance of other training types. No training sessions were missed due to injury.

Discussion

Based on the results the coaches were satisfied that adding yoga to off-season training satisfied their aims. The coaches observed greater embodiment and an increased skating efficiency; however, this observation is purely subjective and was not quantified in any way. The authors concluded that these data are promising and may be an encouragement for future athletes to add yoga to their training. Personally, I agree that while the aims were satisfied, the logic for the study design is not consistent with the background information provided. Moreover, the results are not sufficient to state that yoga unequivocally improves the performance of speed skaters at the Olympic level. Overall, the study has many flaws and fails to provide any compelling reason for yoga to be implemented into their training program. This paper does suggest that future yoga research for athletes is unlikely to be harmful or have a negative impact on performance, which is probably where its greatest value lies.

STRETCHING

2

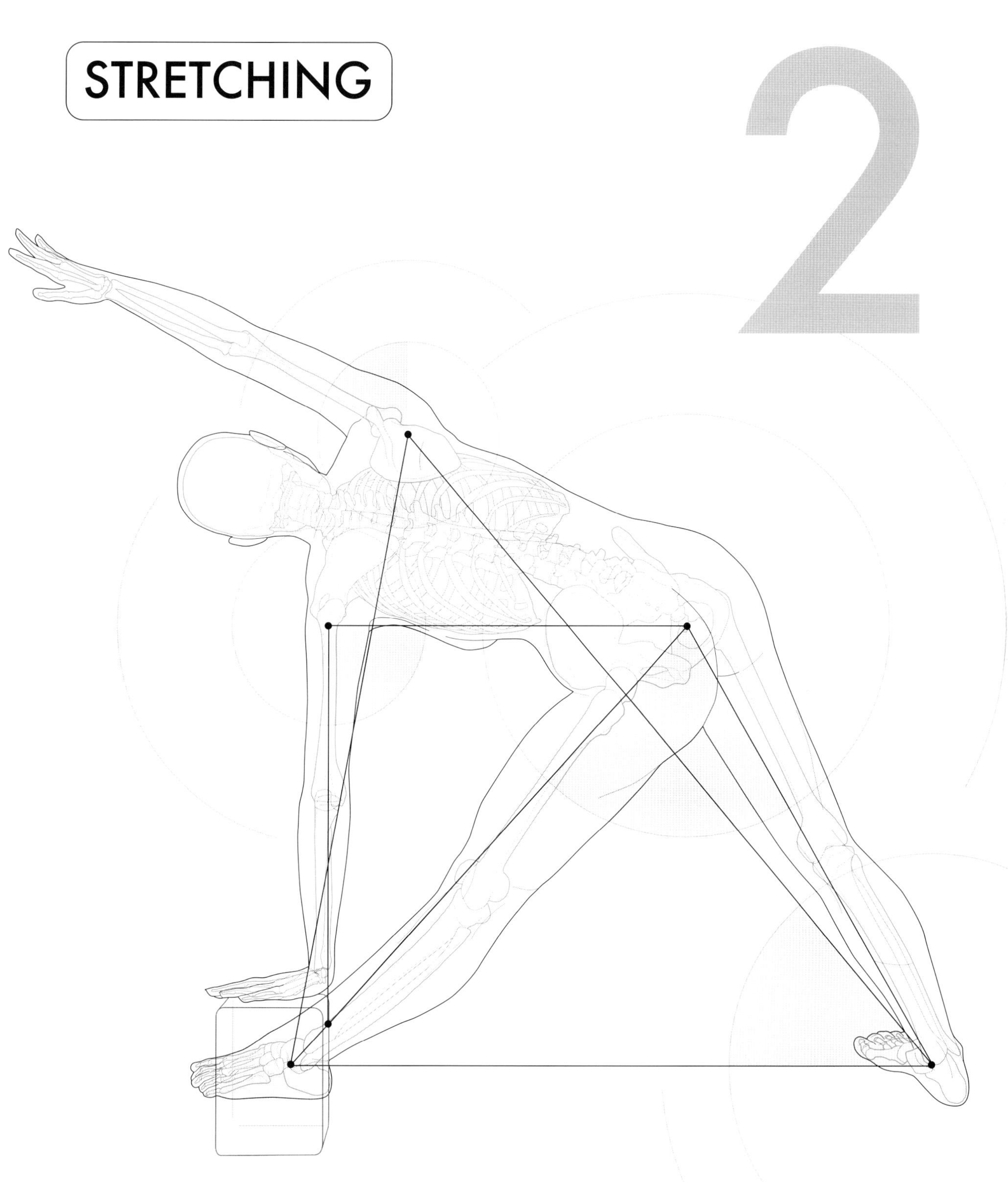

Select any yoga posture to analyze in the context of load and you will easily identify, in addition to the compressive loading on bones and cartilage, the tensile loading on the soft musculoskeletal tissues. In other words, most of the positions we place our bodies in to accommodate the shapes of yoga asana require some stretch and flexibility. Perhaps it is this reason that leads the public to associate yoga with stretching, much to the dismay of many teachers. There appears to be a divide within the yoga community – some ardently refute that yoga is stretching, while others seem to enthusiastically connect the two. My intention is not to defend either position, but to offer an alternative view of stretching so that we may move beyond the disparity and come together to have a fresh conversation on what it means to put tissues under tension.

In order to achieve this, we will need to define some terms – a lot of terms. I find that many conversations I have out in the world about stretching are inconclusive because we are all speaking the same words but with different definitions. Just recently a colleague, who is also a yoga educator, asked me a seemingly simple question about the best way to stretch tendons. My first answer did not satisfy her because she was invested in what she had already learned about the topic through her previous yoga studies. Not until we started breaking down all the components of the question for clarity and defined all the terms until we were certain we understood each other, did we make progress. At this point, we rephrased the question altogether to ask about the best way to load tendons and the discussion became quite enriching.

Incidentally, the scenario I just described is not unlike reading a research paper. Different authors use different terminology and methods, and make varying assumptions and interpretations. So, I do not wish to imply that only the yoga community falls into these communication traps. I gather it is an element of being human and a limitation of language.

In order to further the discussion on yoga, biomechanics, and load, we will spend the present chapter learning about stretching and how it may or may not be a part of yoga. This temporary diversion into the topic of stretching naturally occurs here because

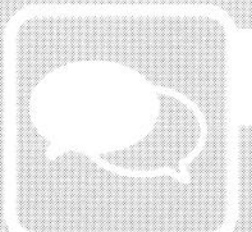

Thought Provoker

What is Stretching?

Have you ever stopped to ponder what stretching means exactly? Could you explain what stretching does, how it works, and why we do it? Could you go further and define precisely what words like mobile, flexible, tight, loose, lengthen, release, resistance, etc., mean? Take a few moments to ponder what structures are involved, what mechanism is contributing to your explanation (i.e. how it works), and how confident you would be explaining it to a room full of exercise scientists.

I encourage you to do this because it was this self-imposed exercise that led to me to many of the conclusion I will present to you. I first had to become uncomfortably aware of the fact that I was using words without a clear understanding of what they meant.

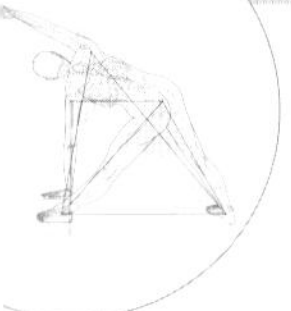

a stretched material is one subjected to tensile load. Through a careful exploration into stretching, not just whether it improves flexibility, but some of the possible mechanisms at work, we can deconstruct many stretching sound bites commonly recited in class. This will set a linguistic foundation so that, in future chapters, we may consider the benefits of stretching beyond flexibility.

Conventional Stretching

Stretching is widely accepted as an essential practice for maintaining physical activity. The general population overwhelmingly believes that stretching is good. Some commonly associated benefits may include improved athletic performance, injury prevention and, of course, flexibility. If you can reach your toes, although you probably have not acquired any sort of special skill resulting from it, you may have been the subject of "flexibility envy" on more than one occasion.

Culturally, stretching is promoted ubiquitously. My grade school physical education teacher led us through stretches before sending us off to run laps, a practice which continued through my high school soccer years. Commercial gyms provide stretching areas, some community racing events provide organized stretching often alongside the massage services, and stretching related products are sold everywhere.

For a more formal assessment of the benefits of stretching we turn to a governing body for health and fitness, the American College of Sports Medicine (ACSM). Founded in 1954, the ACSM is "the largest sports medicine and exercise science organization in the world. With more than 50,000 members and certified professionals worldwide, ACSM is dedicated to advancing and integrating scientific research to provide educational and practical applications of exercise science and sports medicine" (American College of Sports Medicine, 2017). Every several years the ACSM publishes a series of position statements. These in-depth reviews of current research in exercise and sport science serve as the gold standard for exercise recommendations in different populations. For the general population, they have selected five components of fitness (Table 2.1) (Garber et al., 2011).

Flexibility is one of the components of fitness, as is neuromuscular training. Interestingly, yoga falls under the mind-body category, not the flexibility category (although they do reference yoga in the flexibility guidelines). Yet, the number one reason the consumer chooses yoga is to become flexible (followed by stress relief,

Table 2.1
Components of Fitness

Component	Example
Cardiovascular	Running
Strength	Weight lifting
Body mass index (BMI)	Measure of body fat percentage
Flexibility	Stretching
Neuromotor fitness	Qi gong, yoga

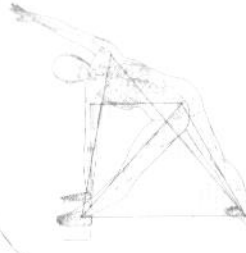

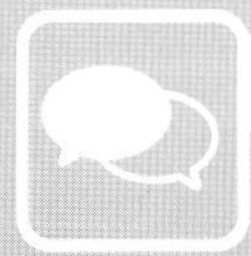

Thought Provoker

Yoga and Flexibility

For the 35 million people in the US practicing yoga in 2016, it is the desire to attain flexibility that is bringing them to their mats. Additionally, flexibility is what keeps them coming back, as it has been reported as the number one motivation to continue practicing. If yoga and conventional stretching are not related, as many argue, then perhaps yoga has a serious publicity problem.

What are your thoughts on yoga, stretching, and flexibility? What role do the mainstream media, social media, and the leaders in your own yoga community play in perceptions about yoga?

If a yoga student wants to improve her flexibility, what responsibility does the yoga teacher have to either meet the demand or change her perception?

general fitness, improvements in general health, and physical fitness), as reported in the 2016 Yoga in America study conducted by Yoga Journal magazine (Ipsos Public Affairs, 2016). Note the difference between the sport science and consumer impressions of yoga.

The ACSM classifies the activity of stretching as flexibility training. They clearly define five different approaches to achieving greater range of motion (ROM). Surprisingly, the ACSM guidelines for how to stretch and the reported benefits are somewhat underwhelming. In the 25-page position stand offering exercise guidelines, less than one page is dedicated to stretching. A full body stretching routine can be completed in under 10 minutes and 2–3 days per week should suffice (Garber et al., 2011). In the absence of a detailed and compelling argument for more than 20–30 minutes a week, tradition appears to be the driving force for the promotion of stretching.

Here, we will review in detail each type of stretching to highlight that not all stretching is the same. Just as compressive loads can vary in magnitude, rate, and time parameters, so can tensile loads. The purpose, at this time, is not to value one type of stretching over others, but to clearly outline the similarities and differences. Later, when we examine how different loading modes and parameters affect muscle and connective tissue, you will be able to determine which type of stretching satisfies a specific outcome. A mantra to which I adhere is that there is no right way to teach a yoga pose or sequence a class, as long as you can provide sound reasoning for your methods.

The first type of stretching, **ballistic stretching**, is characterized by bouncing repeatedly into a stretch. I am always reminded of the type of stretching we did in physical education class in elementary school before running a few laps; we would sit on the grass, stretch one leg out, bend the opposite leg in, and bounce repeatedly while reaching for our toes. The process looks very Jane Fonda and very 1980s. This technique fell out of fashion for some time; rumors told us bouncing was unsafe and would

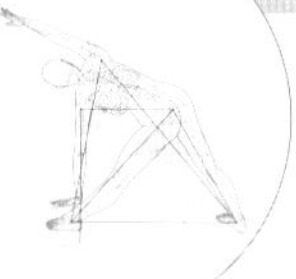

lead to injury. Lack of evidence has weakened this position and while it is now more acceptable to bounce and stretch, it is still not something we see very often. I expect someone will soon discover this untapped market, develop a system of ballistic stretching reinforced by several optimistic claims of superiority, trademark the brand, train others to teach it, charge them an annual licensing fee to be associated with the brand, and further monetize it by manufacturing widgets necessary to achieve the greatest benefits. Sound about right?

Dynamic stretching, also called slow movement stretching, is characterized by repetitive slow movements that progressively increase in range. You may relate this to joint rotations such as full shoulder circles or ankle rolls, for example. Qualities of dynamic stretching appear in the Vinyasa style of yoga where classes are often sequenced to progressively increase one's range through repetition. For example, Plank Pose becomes Downward Facing Dog Pose becomes Handstand, eventually. Or Side Angle Pose becomes Bound Side Angle Pose, which then becomes Bird of Paradise. While these configurations are far more complex than the basic and isolated joint rotations characteristic of dynamic stretching, the underlying concept is still there. Incidentally, the currently preferred (because ideas change as research progresses) method of pre-sport or pre-activity stretching among coaches and athletes is dynamic stretching (for reasons we will discuss ahead).

Static stretching encompasses a larger range of stretching styles than the previous two and is considered either *active* or *passive*. Both types of static stretching consist of holding a stretched position for a specified amount of time. The most common durations you will find in the literature are 15 second increments up to 60 seconds, but you will certainly see others, and sometimes, although rarely, upwards of 5 minutes. If you consider the average slow-breathing yoga practitioner takes approximately 12 breaths per minute, each breath would last about 5 seconds, therefore holding a yoga posture for five breaths approximates a 25 second static stretch. The category of static stretch depends on the nature of the pose.

Static stretching is most often done passively. Passive stretching requires an external force to hold the stretch. Legs-Up-the-Wall Pose, although not a pose with a central purpose of stretching the hamstrings, is technically a static passive stretch because the wall provides the support for the position (Fig. 2.1). Reclining Hand-to-Big-Toe Pose with the index and middle finger hooking the big toes or supported with a belt is a passive stretch because the arm is holding the leg in hip flexion to stretch the hamstring. Because of the ubiquity of passive stretching in the flexibility research, many papers use the terms static stretching synonymously with static passive stretching. It is prudent, therefore, to read the methods section of any paper on static stretching to reveal exactly what type of stretching the intervention entailed.

In contrast, active stretching, according to ACSM, recruits the opposing muscle group to hold the position. By this description, the active muscle is the prime mover (agonist) and the target muscle being stretched is the opposing one (antagonist). The active version of Supported Legs-Up-the-Wall Pose is Supine Double Leg Raise Pose (Fig. 2.2) and of Reclining Hand-to-Big-Toe Pose is a hands-free, prop-free, unsupported expression of the same pose. In both, the absence of any external support recruits the agonist hip

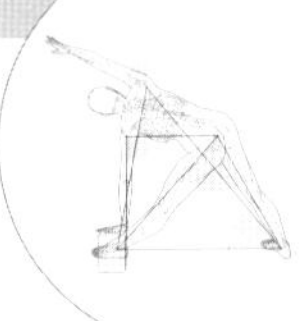

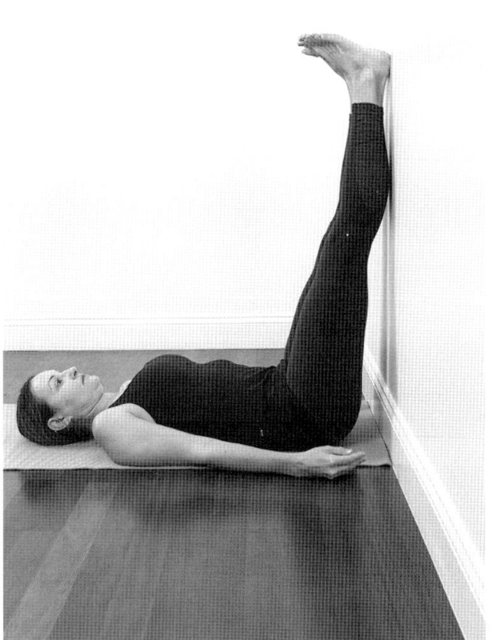

Fig. 2.1
Legs-Up-the-Wall Pose or a passive stretch supported by a wall.

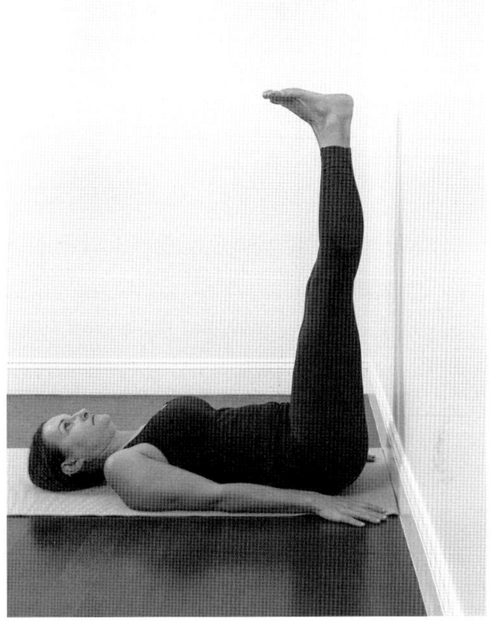

Fig. 2.2
Upward Extended Feet Pose (supine double leg raise) or an active stretch held with agonist contraction.

flexor group to hold the position, stretching the targeted antagonist hamstring group. The active stretching category is the only section in the ACSM flexibility guidelines which refers to yoga. Arguably, any standing pose in yoga held statically is an active stretch across one or more joints, as is any arm balance, inversion, or seated posture as long it recruits agonist muscle contractions.

In some seated postures, however, the distinction between active and passive stretches may be somewhat ambiguous. For example, in Seated Forward Bend Pose, one individual may effortlessly rest her trunk on her thighs and the pose would be passive (Fig. 2.3). In another person, the trunk may deviate backwards, perhaps due to the lack of a hip hinge, and the pose would be active as she works against gravity to maintain a forward leaning position (Fig. 2.4). Brace the back against a wall, however, and it would become passive again (Fig. 2.5). Therefore, the same pose may be active for one student and passive for another, determined by the source of force (i.e. internal, external). An active stretch requires internal force production on the part of the student to hold the position whereas a passive stretch is supported by any external force, including gravity.

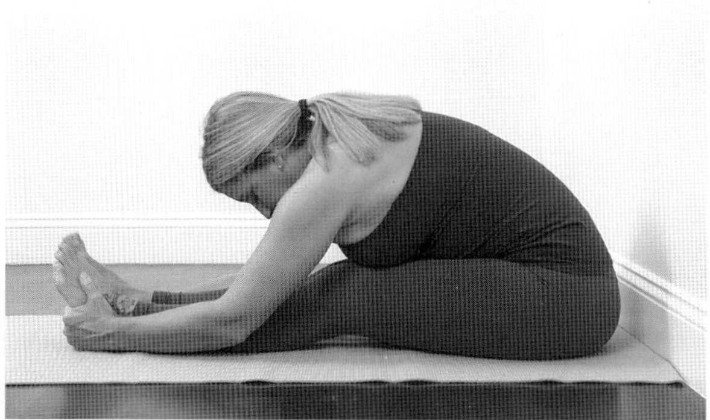

Fig. 2.3
Seated Forward Bend Pose, passive, supported by gravity.

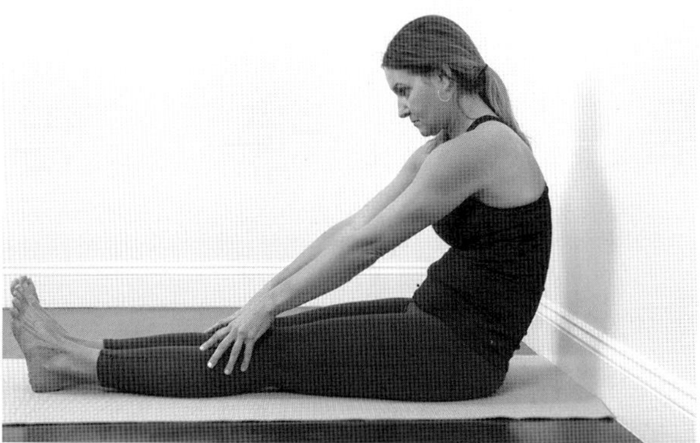

Fig. 2.4
Seated Forward Bend Pose, active, working against gravity.

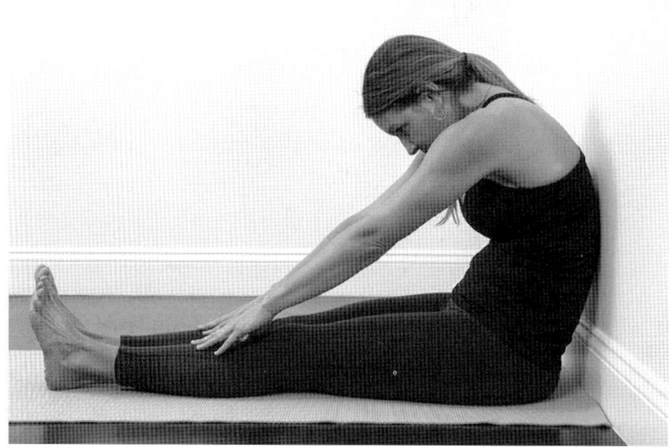

Fig. 2.5
Seated Forward Bend Pose, passive, supported by a wall with some gravitational assistance.

The fifth and final approach to stretching recognized by ACSM is **proprioceptive neuromuscular facilitation** (PNF), or as manual therapists often call it, **muscle energy technique** (MET). The stretching applications of this technique vary, mostly combining some aspect of isometric contractions with passive stretches through a given ROM. The most recognized method is probably the *contract-relax method*, where a partner takes a subject to the end range stretch of a target muscle, the subject then isometrically contracts the target muscle against the partner's resistance for a period of time (usually around 6–10 seconds), after which the subject relaxes, and the partner passively stretches the target muscle further. What is unique about contract-relax is the emphasis on the contraction of the target, or stretched, muscle instead of the opposing muscle.

Although utilized more by athletic trainers and manual therapists than yoga teachers, PNF techniques are widely accepted as an effective method of ROM training. Moreover, the immediate, albeit temporary gains in ROM make PNF an easily demonstrable technique susceptible to exaggerated claims about its benefits. Rife with assertions about the role of muscle reflex activation in flexibility, plenty of misinformation circulates around PNF. For this reason, moving forward, we will focus on the isometric component and refer to PNF and MET stretching as isometric stretches, where the target muscle is isometrically contracted for some period of time at end range. Isometric stretching is, therefore, distinct from active stretching and also from **resistance stretching**.

Resistance stretching, although not identified by the ACSM, is a method of stretching utilizing eccentric contractions. Most often performed with a partner, an inanimate external weight can also be used to apply resistance. The subject will warm-up the muscle with a few resisted concentric contractions, isometrically pause briefly at the shortened range, and then in a slow and controlled manner, lengthen the muscle with the resistance still applied. Unlike isometric stretching, this method is less about a contraction at end range, and more about a loaded controlled eccentric contraction through the entire range. Extreme ranges are usually avoided because the stretch ends when the subject loses the ability to effectively control the joint position, regardless of the subject's available passive range. Resistance stretching is not well represented in the literature, presumably because it is not commonly identified as a stretching method. Eccentric training has been extremely well studied, especially in recent years, and therefore, the eccentric training research will inform us about the effects of this particular method of tensile loading.

With so many options available, it becomes apparent why definitions are needed in a conversation about stretching. Clarification of variables is required when speaking of specific outcomes. For example, resistance stretching might essentially be eccentric loading, but it's a relatively low load eccentric contraction when compared with the types of eccentric loading used as an intervention in a study. Static stretching can be active or passive, and not all stretching types suggest the stretched muscle must be relaxed as is often assumed. Now that we have identified the different ways in which we can stretch (Table 2.2), we turn to a discussion on all the reasons why we are supposed to stretch and whether or not those reasons are satisfied by the method.

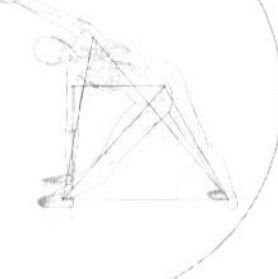

Table 2.2
Types of Stretching

Flexibility Exercise	Description	Example
Ballistic	Bouncing stretches utilizing momentum to increase range	Jane Fonda workouts
Dynamic	Slow movements gradually increasing in range	Joint circles
Static passive	Holding position using support	Legs-Up-the-Wall Pose
Static active	Holding position using opposing muscle	Supine Double Leg Raise
Proprioceptive neuromuscular facilitation (PNF)	Stretch involving some combination of isometric contractions and passive stretching	Contract-relax (isometrically contracting target muscle at end range followed by a deeper passive stretch)
Resistance stretching	Slow, controlled eccentric lengthening against resistance	A partner-assisted stretch where the person being stretched tries to concentrically contract against the partner's efforts to lengthen the muscle

Why We Stretch

Surprisingly, the bulk of the research on the effects of stretching is relatively new. In the last 10–20 years, when papers on the subject were first published, the data on static stretching began to reveal that influences on performance, injury prevention, and ROM may not be as positive as we originally assumed. This discovery caused a reversal of opinion in many fitness circles and, in some cases, stretching was even vilified. Fortunately, continued research has shown that those conclusions may have also been premature. There is still much we do not understand and, for now, the conclusions lie somewhere in the middle – stretching is sometimes good, but not that good, and when good, only under certain conditions.

What the body of literature lacks in tenure, reliability, validity, and reproducibility it makes up for in volume. Literally hundreds of papers set out to determine once and for all why we should or should not stretch. It can be quite dizzying as they examine multiple types of stretching of varying dosages against different controls on diverse populations. Fortunately, a recent collaboration between the top stretching researchers produced a systematic review summarizing the results of the high-quality RCTs published to date (Behm, Blazevich et al., 2016). This book sets out to explore how tissues behave under tension beyond the constraints

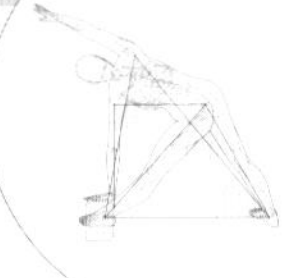

Scientific Literacy

Reviews

Literature reviews evaluate a set of published research on a given topic. Reviewers are first tasked with collecting all the available published research using a specified set of key words. The findings are then assessed for quality by a set of exclusionary and inclusionary standards. The remaining curated collection of papers is then analyzed such that conclusions are based on multiple findings and replicated data. Literature reviews can be as basic as an undergrad term paper providing an overview of a certain topic, more sophisticated like a systematic review summarizing the findings quantitatively to answer a specific question, or a meta-analysis applying statistical methods to objectively summarize the findings. Some academic journals print only reviews as these are often recognized as the highest quality research available (Fig. 2.6).

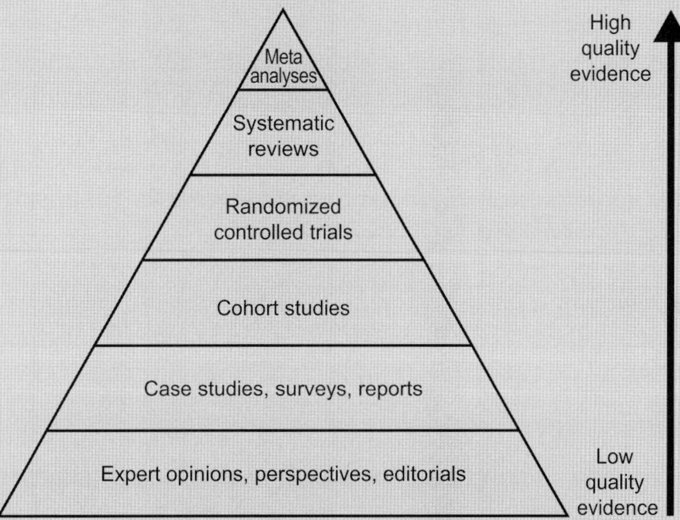

Fig. 2.6
Hierarchy of evidence.

of conventional stretching. We will rely on this current and high-quality review to provide us with a condensed, yet focused, summary of stretching outcomes so that we may move on to explore other biomechanical principles and how they fit into yoga asana.

Regarding sports performance, the researchers assembled the data into multiple configurations to establish various relationships. To begin, all types of stretching were evaluated for acute influences on overall performance (whichever specific performance outcome was being measure in any given paper). Acute effects of stretching refers to the results immediately (usually within 1 hour) after a stretching bout. Stretches under 60 seconds resulted in an average *decrease* in performance by 1.1% and stretches over 60 seconds *decreased* performance by 4.6%. Whereas both results had a negative impact, the evidence may only have clinical significance in highly competitive situations like training for the Olympics. The results may not be compelling enough to advise a recreational athlete who enjoys his stretching routine prior to his sport, and who feels better because of it, to forgo it.

When the same data were rearranged to divide performance into the categories strength and power, the numbers told a different story. The acute effects of stretching resulted in a 4.8% deficit in strength, but only a 1.3% deficit in power-speed. The caveat here is that the duration of the stretches in the strength data was longer and we have no way of determining if time in the stretch was a factor in the greater deficit. The variable, strength, is measured by how much weight someone can move, power is measured by the speed at which one can move said weight. Power has a time component to it, strength does not. In the following chapter, when we discuss the mechanical behavior of connective tissue, we may gain insight into why strength and power may respond differently to stretching.

Arranged by type of stretch, static stretching diminished overall performance by 3.7% and PNF by 4.4%, but dynamic stretching improved performance by 1.3%. Anyone familiar with the literature expects dynamic stretching to improve performance as it has been the recommended pre-activity stretching method for roughly the last decade. ACSM suggests engaging in static stretching or PNF either post-activity or entirely separate from the activity or sport.

Static stretching affected tasks requiring short range performance negatively by 10.2% but positively by 2.2% in tasks requiring long range performance. It seems that specificity, as should be expected, applies again – end range training improves end range performance.

Concerning injury, the acute effects of static stretching or PNF seem to slightly reduce injury frequency in muscle injuries relating to sprinting type activities but not endurance sports. For overuse injuries and other "all-cause" injuries, stretching did not appear to have any effect. In any case, there appeared to be no adverse effects from pre-activity static stretching, rendering the intervention harmless but only somewhat beneficial, and sometimes even slightly detrimental, depending on the performance goals.

The authors examined dozens of other configurations in addition to the few I selected above. Among the many outcome variables they examined, those I have highlighted tell us enough of the story for our purposes here. I mention this for full transparency, so it does not seem I am cherry-picking data to support my own opinions. I encourage you to read the paper in its entirety if the subject matter intrigues you (Behm, et al., 2016).

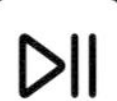

Pause and turn to page 70 for a summary of related research.

As per our discussion on why we stretch, it appears the evidence does not hold up to the popular consumer belief about performance and injury prevention. One issue with measuring performance and injury prevention as primary outcomes, however, is that there are any number of internal factors and external environmental conditions that could influence outcomes. This complicates study design for the long-term effects of stretching on performance. If the subjects continue to train, any long-term benefits could be a result of the actual training. If subjects discontinue training, we would expect to see deficits and injuries, but I'm not aware of any studies looking at the effects of stretching on injury occurrences in sedentary populations as that would seem irrelevant. I'm also unaware of any studies designed to test whether stretching causes injuries because that is not the theory sports scientists are striving to validate. The emerging yoga narrative about the stretching injuries that yoga may cause will be discussed in future chapters. We must first exhaust our investigation of conventional stretching and how the body responds and adapts to it.

Passive Resistance Torque

Torque, as you may recall, is the word for a rotational force. In ROM research, when a subject's limb is passively moved into a stretch, a torque occurs within the joint space, measurable by a torque meter. Passive resistance torque is the measurement of resistance against a joint rotation (Fig. 2.7). The deformation behavior of the soft tissue crossing the joint as it is stretched contributes to this resistance.

Imagine practicing yoga in stretchy yoga pants versus jeans. The jeans contribute greater resistance than the stretchy pants, thereby limiting ROM. Now imagine those jeans developed less resistance after several stretches. We could call that a decrease in passive resistance torque (PRT).

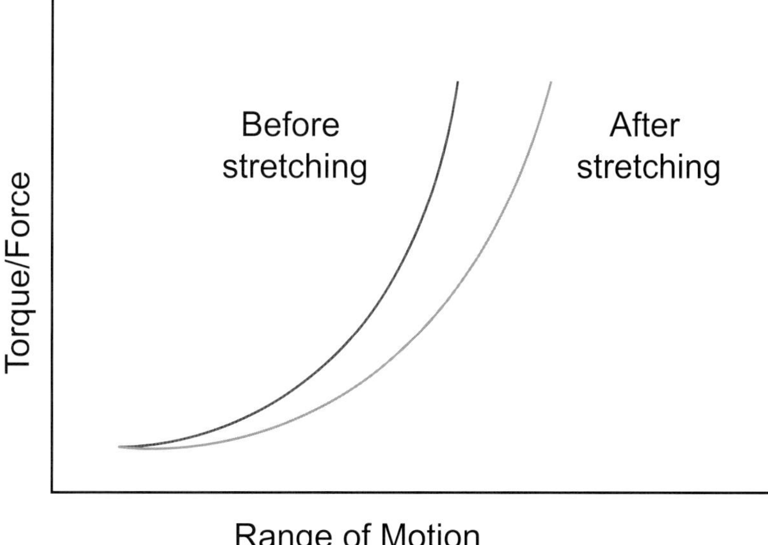

Fig. 2.7
A decrease in passive resistance torque after stretching.

The word passive implies that the movement is not initiated through an internal force, but is achieved through the application of an external force. In a biomechanics lab, this is usually a rig with a pulley. A goniometer measures joint angle and a dynamometer measures the torque. A subject with less PRT responds with less resistance than a subject with greater PRT.

Research shows acute stretching reduces PRT, thereby increasing ROM. In the early years of flexibility research, Magnusson published what is today considered a classic paper. His work established some of the testing protocols of the time, before technological advancements in ultrasound became the measurement tools of choice. One of his discoveries was that the acute changes in PRT were fleeting, lasting only about an hour. The subjects had decreased PRT with 5 × 90 second stretches, spaced 30 seconds apart. PRT returned to baseline in a follow-up test, 1 hour later (Magnusson, Simonsen, Aagaqard and Kjaer, 1996). His work has been replicated, and also refuted, by many over the years, including himself.

Chronic stretching has also been shown to reduce PRT. A 4-week protocol of 2 × 60 second stretches twice per day resulted in a decline of PRT at the end of the intervention. Final PRT measurements were taken 24 hours after the last stretching dose, indicating that reductions in PRT last more than an hour when stretching is consistently performed. No follow-up test was conducted in the weeks or months after the daily stretching protocol, providing no indication of the lasting duration of change (Nakamura et al., 2012).

Finally, long-held stretches also have an acute effect on PRT. Subjects held a passive stretch for 1, 2, 3, 4, and 5 minutes. After 1 minute, PRT was not yet significantly lower than baseline, but every additional minute thereafter, it was. The 4 and 5-minute stretches resulted in significantly lower PRT than the 1 minute. Moreover, the 5-minute stretch was significantly lower in PRT than the 2-minute one (Nakamura et al., 2013). We can conclude that in men averaging 20 years of age, a 5-minute static stretch should reduce passive resistance in ankle dorsiflexion more than a 2-minute stretch will. In sports science, it is a long-held belief that diminishing returns do not warrant holding a stretch longer than about 30–60 seconds (which is still the ASCM recommendation). This paper suggests that changes might continue to occur 3–5 minutes into the stretch, which is interesting because certain types of yoga are characterized by long-held stretches, although their practice is only anecdotally supported. I must note here, we cannot extrapolate these results to just any yoga posture, or even to all other joints or populations because those variables were not accounted for in this particular study.

The significance of PRT is that we see changes in mechanical properties in response to various static stretching parameters. Some changes are temporary, some are longer lasting. We will learn more about mechanical properties and their influencing factors in future chapters. For now, we will consider possible neural adaptations to stretching.

Stretch Tolerance

Stretch tolerance describes the limit to which an individual can "tolerate" the discomfort associated with a deepening stretch. A purely "sensory" theory, its basis lies in an individual adapting to and becoming less sensitized to what most consider the painful experience associated with stretching, or finding the sensation becoming less offensive, or more tolerable, after repeated exposure. The theory emerged because all human trials measuring end ROM will always stop at an individual's tolerance. Unlike animal studies where tissues can be extracted and mechanical limits tested ex vivo, ROM studies on humans are limited by the subject's request to stop the stretch in the presence of pain and discomfort. The main premise of the sensory theory is that changes in ROM are not due to alterations in tissue properties, but in sensory tolerance.

In the early years of flexibility research, Magnusson, again, published a second classic paper. This time, he looked at the effects of a 3-week stretching intervention on tissue properties as opposed to those immediately following a stretch. His testing protocols were twofold. One measured PRT at a predetermined range assessed by the sensation of tightness. The other was similar but progressed into a painful range. Yoga teachers may understand this distinction via the popular cue – to enter the pose "to the point of discomfort but not to the point of pain." After the completion of the intervention, the investigators found no alterations in tissue properties, concluding tolerance to be the mechanism of change in ROM (Magnusson, Simonsen, Aagaard, Sørensen et al., 1996). Note, Magnusson published both the previously cited paper on the transient changes in tissue properties in response to acute stretching and this paper on the absence of tissue property changes in response to chronic stretching in the same year. It was an important year for stretching science.

These papers launched a debate among the mechanical and sensory theorists, and the subsequent publication of multiple papers defending either position or both. Magnusson continued to publish, and 14 years later coauthored a perspective paper proposing that the sensory theory explains the inconsistencies across the literature resulting from the challenges posed in attempts to control for all variables (Weppler and Magnusson, 2010). In spite of these methodological challenges, today, the evidence is compelling enough for us to validate both theories concurrently, but there is still much we do not know.

For example, we do not understand the neurophysiology behind tolerance and how it is regulated in the nervous system. We do have some limited research on the topic of anesthesia and ROM. Subjects undergoing knee surgery were tested on the "healthy leg"

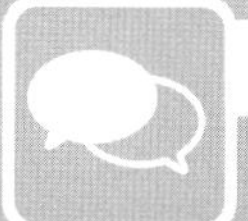

Thought Provoker

Tightness

How do you explain the feeling of tightness that compels people to stretch?

Do you think tightness is a function of mechanical tissue properties or a sensory experience?

How can you determine if a muscle is tight; would it require a laboratory setting? Does this method of measurement support your explanation of tight?

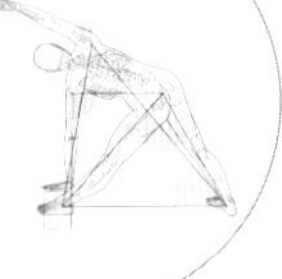

(i.e. the leg not operated on). ROM during a passive hamstring stretch was tested pre-, intra-, and post-operatively. The aim was to compare four variables: spinal anesthesia, general anesthesia, a nerve blocker, and an epidural. In all cases, the intra-operative ROM was significantly greater than the pre- and post-operative measurements, which did not change significantly. The spinal anesthesia resulted in the greatest increase in ROM, suggesting neural regulation of stretching may occur at the level of the spinal cord (Krabak et al., 2001). In another study focusing on the role of pain in ROM, subjects undergoing total knee arthroscopic surgery as a treatment for osteoarthritis were tested. The operative knee was measured for maximal knee flexion and extension prior to surgery and during surgery after a spinal anesthesia followed by a femoral and sciatic nerve blocker (which blocks nerve impulses, not feeling). Average passive ROM across 141 subjects was greater by 13.4 degrees in flexion and 3 degrees in extension under anesthesia (Bennett et al., 2009). Whether stretch tolerance or other painful symptoms are the limiting factor in ROM, we have support for a sensory theory that warrants further research.

At this point, we are treading dangerously close to the field of neuromechanics, which is not the title of this book. The neuromechanical aspects of stretching and ROM would require an in-depth study of the nervous system, stretch reflexes, electromyograph amplitudes, and even neurological disorders such as cerebral palsy, stroke, and

Scientific Literacy

Opinions and Perspectives

Some published research is the expert opinion of a single author, or more than one author, on a topic on which they are highly informed. These types of papers, also referred to as perspectives or editorials, are neither experimental nor observational and are void of subjects, materials, and methods. Although considered the lowest quality of research, they have their place in science. In my personal work, I find expert opinion papers are most useful when authored by researchers from whom I have read multiple experimental papers. If I am well read on the work of the researchers, a written perspective can help me integrate the data with their expert knowledge, which reflects all of their insight including that which is beyond what has made it to print. Of course, clinicians (who do not work in an experimental laboratory) can also provide useful expert opinions, particularly in the realm of decision-making in evidence-based teaching.

If we had to categorize this book, we would call it an opinion piece. Years of teaching, combined with competency in the related field of research, have enabled me to assemble some opinions on yoga and biomechanics. It includes a basic literature review, does not set out to test a specific theory through experimentation, and offers a well-rounded critical analysis of relevant themes. The sequences I provide at the end of this book have not been tested experimentally (although I would love to see that happen one day). They are a product of my professional and academic experience.

spinal injuries. The neurophysiology of pain is also beyond our scope here, although we will return to the topic of pain and its relationship to injury later. Since the biomechanical aspects of stretching focuses on load, tissue structure, and mechanical behaviors, we will stay within those boundaries. Any improvements in ROM as a result of loading are incidental in this context. It is my position that influences in ROM are likely a function of both sensory and mechanical mechanisms, but exactly how, when, or why each is a factor, we don't yet understand. Thus, where my interest lies is in the question of how, when and why tissues adapt their mechanical properties when loaded in tension. We will delve into the topic of muscle length to elucidate this point.

Muscle Length

As muscles are being stretched, they naturally resist deformation. Some muscles seem to resist deformation stubbornly well, while others tend to yield quite easily. We are apt to call those unyielding muscles tight. Colloquially, the definition for tight implies something pulled taut. If tight muscles are wound up like guitar strings, then an additional tension would not result in any further deformation. Alas, muscles are not wound up like guitar strings, and the term tight is derived more from imagery than mechanical behavior.

We might conclude the resistance to deformation occurs due to a structurally shortened muscle, one that has developed a diminished length of tissue between the two attachment points (i.e. origin and insertion). If this were true, then the opposing muscles would have inadvertently been fixed in a lengthened position, and one would expect them to have developed an excessive length of tissue between attachment points. I often hear this regarding the hip flexors. Clients, students, even yoga teachers have all told me they have "tight" hip flexors and "weak" glutes, considering this to be the reason why they stand in Mountain Pose with an anteriorly tilted pelvis. Less often, but still frequently, I hear the opposite. They explain to me their hamstrings are "short" and their hip flexors are "overstretched." I'd like to deconstruct these scenarios in terms of muscle length.

The first problematic issue with the binary short/long line of thinking is that it further assumes that shorter muscles must be strong/tight and longer muscles must be weak/loose. Muscles, however, don't get strong by being held in shortened position. They become stronger when exposed to progressive loads. Likewise, muscles don't become weak from stretching. They become weak when loads are insufficient. Also, strong muscles are not always tight. Olympic weightlifters have incredible ROM including full overhead shoulder flexion and ankle/knee/hip flexion needed for a full squat, yet are arguably the strongest athletes in the Olympics. Gymnasts also demonstrate extreme flexibility, but are not lacking in strength and power, defying the presumed long/weak relationship.

Looking at the inverse relationship, the false assumption is that strong muscles adaptively shorten, and weak muscles adaptively lengthen. I tend to blame bodybuilders for the former impression. The primary training goal of a bodybuilder is aesthetic, to put on muscle mass, and bulk up, not to get stronger. The training methods for building muscle to those extremes are very specific, and while they do get stronger, strength

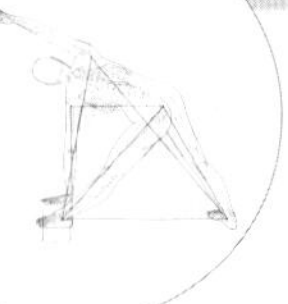

training methods are somewhat different. Therefore, the classic image of a bodybuilder who can't straighten her arms or reach overhead is often the result of anatomical barriers, not strength. The latter impression, that weaker muscles adaptively lengthen cannot possible be true or a sedentary desk job would result in the longest muscles in the office!

The second concern with this assertion is the widespread acceptance that stretching and/or exercise corrects postural deviations. It is an attractive concept to embrace, partly because of its simplicity and partly because of what we have all witnessed, but biology is rarely simple, and assessing a student in Mountain Pose, identifying muscles as either short or long, and assigning stretching or strengthening exercises to correct them is the epitome of simple. Perhaps, several decades ago, when we knew far less, the theory served us well, but today, the evidence forces us to reconsider (Hrysomallis and Goodman, 2001; Hrysomallis, 2010; Borman, Trudelle-Jackson and Smith, 2011). One of my friends and colleagues who also leads teacher trainings attended a course of mine where we elaborated on this idea. She shared with us that on day one of her trainings, everyone takes a photo of themselves in Mountain Pose. Then, months later, at the end of the training, they take a second photo for comparison, and share with the group the change they see in themselves. As would be expected, everyone is standing "taller," yet they *always* attribute it to psychological factors such as confidence, joy, and fulfillment. It is far easier to assume that the yoga stretched out a short tissue when you are looking at a static photo of a body without the context of human experience. There is no denying we have all witnessed such personal case studies where yoga has improved posture, but we must ask ourselves how much is attributable to actual muscle shortages or surpluses.

I can continue to deconstruct these postulations about muscle length, but I find it difficult to do so without falling into a logical fallacy trap. In part, this is because I don't really understand the logic behind these assumptions, which have been only explained to me through unsupported conclusions, based in weak reasoning and anecdotal evidence. These conjectures are difficult to refute with evidence when the theories have not, thus far, been validated. Recall with whom the burden of proof lies; she who is making the claim should provide the evidence. It is difficult to refute a claim that Shoulderstand is the "panacea to most common ailments" (Iyengar, 1979) when no credible evidence is provided to support the claim. Additionally, many are invested in the long/short line of thinking and have been using language in their teaching to support it. It's never easy to change beliefs, even when evidence to the contrary is compelling. In the spirit of critical thinking, as you continue to read, I ask you to consider any number of other possible mechanisms that might contribute to the experience of muscle or joint tightness, "faulty" posture, or other states of being we seem to want stretching to "correct."

To further explore the topic of muscle length, it will be useful to define a few more terms. It is often argued that stretching muscle will make it longer. We have already explained that stretching a muscle will decrease resistance torque and will improve tolerance for the stretch, but what are the components of muscle that might adaptively lengthen when loaded under tension? Let us next begin with the study of muscle structure.

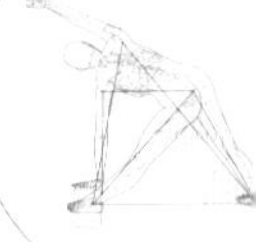

Scientific Literacy

Case Study

A case study is a type of descriptive research that examines a single participant in order to gain insight into other similar participants. The participant is often an individual, but a case study could technically examine any type of subject matter including concepts, organizations, and programs. The methodology is considerably speculative as an in-depth review of the circumstances and results of an individual case is then assumed to be reflected in the behavior cases. A case study, however, is not intended to be used to make generalizations, but rather to help to develop a broader theory.

There are multiple approaches to the design of a case study and methodology tends to be rather vague; therefore, the reader must approach this form of research with a critical eye. Let's create a hypothetical case study where a yoga student experienced a sudden sharp shoulder pain during class and a subsequent visit to the orthopedist resulted in a radiographic image of a partial tear of a rotator cuff tendon. As researchers we would want to establish the details surrounding the student's yoga practice (how long, how often, which style, which pose caused the pain, etc.). It would be responsible to include in the assessment other potential factors, such as prior history of injury and/or pain and other activities that require the student to use this shoulder. Perhaps we further reported that after a complete course of physical therapy the student reported improvement and returned to yoga. We would then begin to build a theory based on these details. But case studies are not free from bias. One researcher may see this case study as support for the theory that yoga poses a risk for rotator cuff injuries. But another may caution that we have no evidence that the rotator cuff tear was a result of the yoga practice since there was no radiographic imaging before the incident. Moreover, we know that tissue damage and pain are poorly correlated, thus there may be some other contributing factors to the incident.

It must be noted that case studies are a form of anecdotal evidence used to develop a theory. Even though a subject can be tested and studied, the results represent weak evidence, at best. Case studies can be useful in the furthering of ideas and are excellent citations for developing research questions to test in a randomized control trial. Therefore, case studies have value in the field of research and conclusions can be made in spite of their limitations, but they must be accepted for what they are.

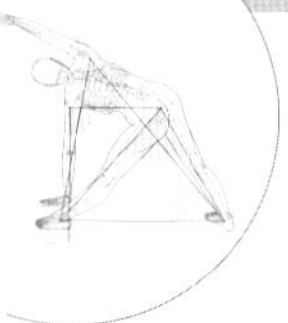

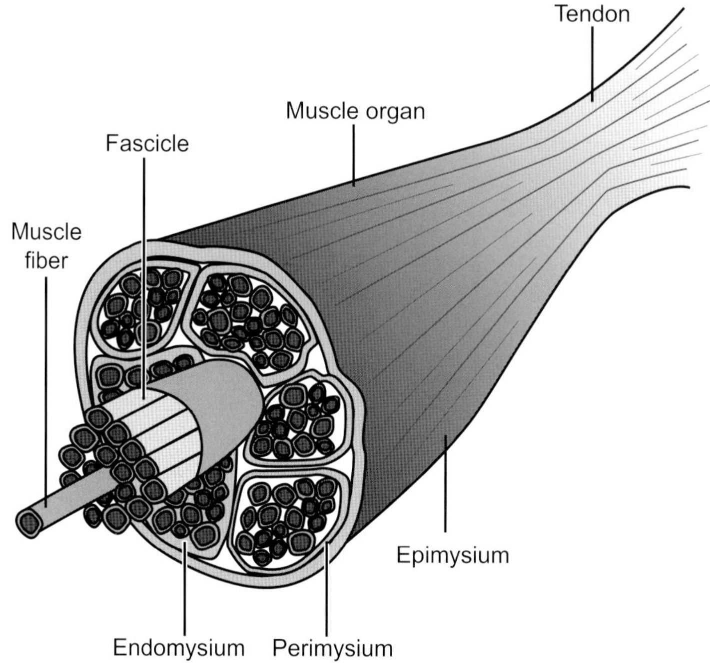

Fig. 2.8
Muscle structure depicting the deep to superficial endomysium, perimysium, and epimysium.

Skeletal muscle is made of muscle cells, also called *muscle fibers* because of their long threadlike structure, and surrounding connective tissue, called the myofascia. Three layers of connective tissue help define the shape of the muscle body. At the deepest layer, the endomysium envelops each individual fiber. Bundled together, these fibers form *fascicles*, encased by the next connective tissue layer, the perimysium. Finally, these fascicles bundled together to form the muscle organ, enclosed by the epimysium. These fascial layers contour and give shape to the muscle organ (Fig. 2.8).

A commonly used and convincing analogy is that of an orange. Underneath the outer peel, the white pithy layer which contains the spherical shape of the orange is likened to the epimysium. The thinner skin that contains each wedge resembles the perimysium which contains the fascicles. Finally, the individual pockets of juice are contained by an even thinner skin just as the fibers are enveloped by the endomysium.

The muscle fiber itself is made up of smaller myofibrils, which are made up of myofilments (Fig. 2.9). These filaments are made up of proteins organized into *sarcomeres*. Sarcomeres are known to be the smallest contractile functional unit of a muscle, although some muscle physiologists have recently proposed that it might be the half-sarcomere. Sarcomeres are arranged in series, end to end, to form the long fibrils. Sarcomeres are a few microns (one millionth of a meter) in length. For perspective, the width of a strand of human hair is about 25 times wider than a sarcomere is long!

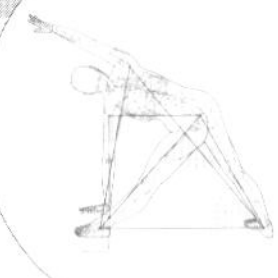

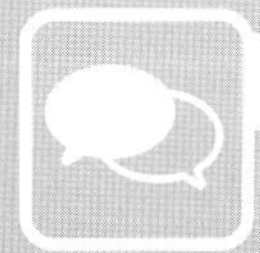

Thought Provoker

Stretching Resistance

If you were to try to stretch an orange wedge, would the resistance you have to overcome come from the juice inside or from the surrounding connective tissue, or both?

If applied to muscle, when you stretch a muscle, is the resistance coming from the bags of connective tissue, or the proteins within, or both?

The proteins within the contractile sarcomere (*actin*, *myosin*, and *titin*) interact together to generate muscle force. According to the Sliding Filament Theory, actin and myosin link together to form cross-bridges. Through consecutive linking and unlinking, cross-bridge formations pull the actin toward the centrally located myosin to create a concentric contraction. During an isometric contraction, the cross-bridges still generate a force, but the sarcomere lengths remain the same. Finally, during an eccentric

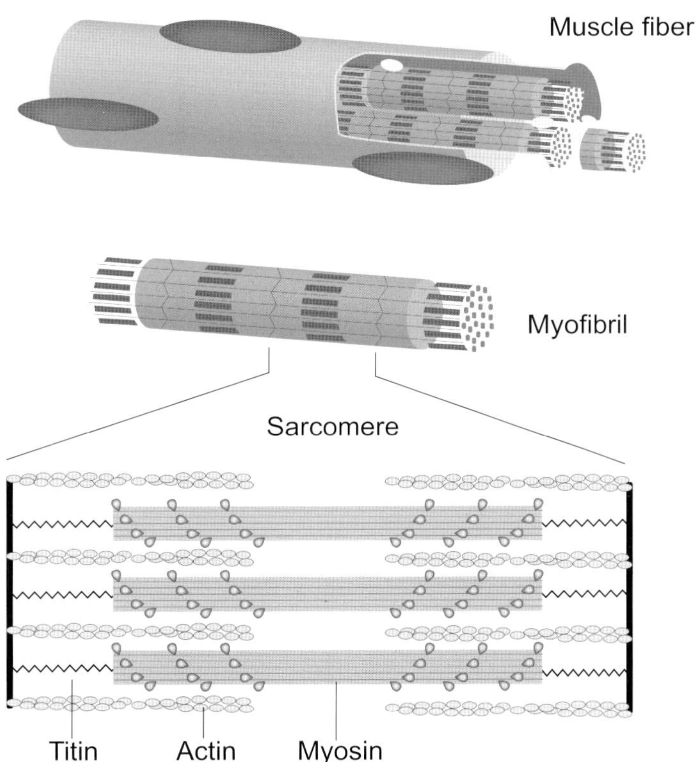

Fig. 2.9
Muscle structure depicting the macro to micro fiber, myofibril, and myofilaments (actin, myosin, titin).

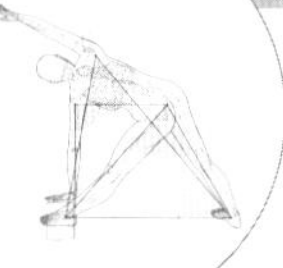

Table 2.3
Muscle Contraction Types

Contraction Type	Change in Length
Concentric	Sarcomeres shorten
Isometric	Sarcomeres do not change length
Eccentric	Sarcomeres lengthen

contraction, an opposing force greater than the force generated by muscle pulls the actin away from the center, lengthening the sarcomeres (Table 2.3). When the sarcomere is actively stretched (possibly even beyond cross-bridge formation), titin interacts with calcium and maybe even actin to contribute to force production (Herzog et al., 2016).

In recent years, the role of titin has shed light onto the previously uncertain and unexplainable mechanisms of eccentric contractions. At the risk of veering off topic, the significance for investigating eccentrics here is to grasp that muscles do generate force in the absence of cross-bridge formations. Although, since the introduction of the Sliding Filament Theory in the 1950s, concentric contractions have been explained thoroughly, lengthening contractions have not been so well understood. Perhaps it is this uncertainty which led to the speculation that lengthening a muscle is a factor of relaxing a muscle and that fewer cross-bridges would make for less resistance to the stretch. The reevaluation of titin's role (it was originally considered a passive element, holding the sarcomere together when stretched beyond the actin-myosin overlap) has advanced our understanding of muscle force production from a two filament model (actin and myosin) to a three filament model (Herzog et al., 2016).

Admittedly, these last few paragraphs provide only a gross oversimplification of muscle physiology. Additionally, the Three Filament Model, at the time of this writing, is just a proposed possible mechanism for eccentric contractions by a select group of researchers – the theory is still new, somewhat controversial, and has yet to make its way into kinesiology textbooks. As this is not a muscle physiology textbook, I believe it is okay to offer new perspectives, as long as I am transparent about their overall position in the scientific community, and I offer this perspective here in an effort to define terms, which, as I've argued, is essential to clear communication. Simplified, sarcomeres are contractile functional units that produce force via actin–myosin binding at shorter lengths and actin–titin binding at longer lengths (Herzog et al., 2016).

Now that we understand the structural components of muscle we can study how they are arranged. Muscle morphology explains how muscle fascicles are positioned in relation to the tendon (Fig. 2.10). Some run parallel to the tendon (at a 0 degree angle) and some run at a pennation angle. In parallel muscles, 100% of the longitudinally transmitted force transfers to the tendon. In pennate muscles (Fig. 2.11), if the pennation angle is given, a trigonometric equation can determine the percentage of longitudinal force transferred to the tendon. An example of this force transfer is attempting to move an object horizontally by pushing on it directly from the side versus pushing it at an angle

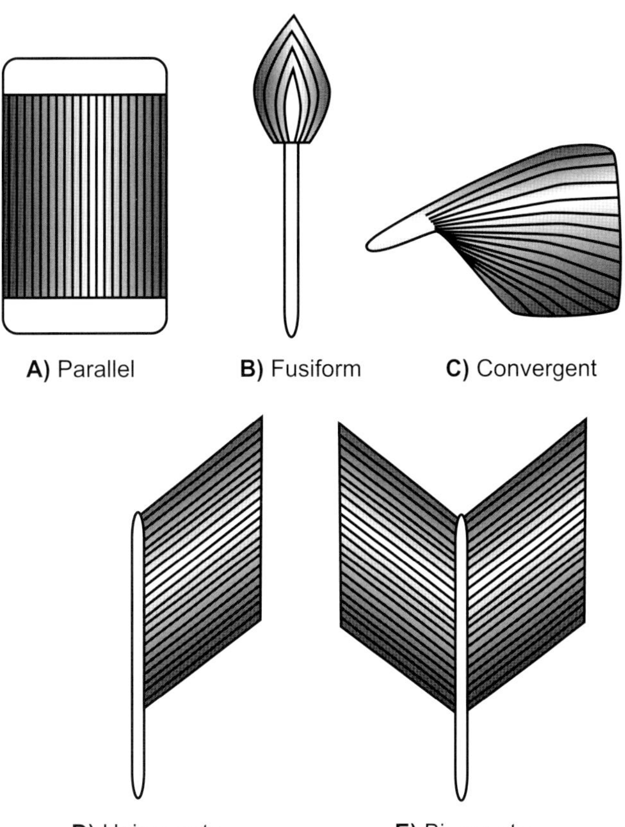

Fig. 2.10

Some examples of different types of muscle morphology: (A) parallel, e.g. sartorius; (B) fusiform, e.g. biceps brachii; (C) convergent, e.g. pectoralis major; (D) unipennate, e.g. extensor digitorum longus; (E) bipennate, e.g. rectus femoris.

from the top of the object. Both methods can displace the object horizontally, but the amount of force transfer is determined by the angle of application.

Practically speaking, pennate muscles accommodate more muscle fibers into their oblique architecture than parallel muscles, thereby increasing their capacity to produce greater overall force. The amount of force not transferred to the tendon is minimal compared to the amount of total force gained by the pennate morphology. Most muscles are morphologically pennate, the significance regarding muscle length being that most muscle fibers are obliquely oriented. An increase in muscle fiber length, therefore, is not always a purely longitudinal growth with respect to attachments points. If the pennation angle also increases, the additional length is even further away from the longitudinal axis relative to the tendon (and attachment points). Ultimately, the amount of additional muscle tissue length between the two tendon–bone attachments is geometrically determined.

In this regard, muscle length is defined by the length of the muscle fascicles. If we expanded our definition of "muscle" to include the entirety of the muscle organ,

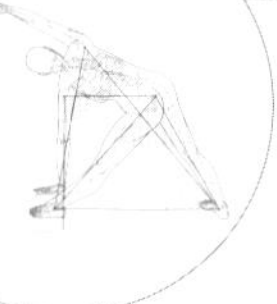

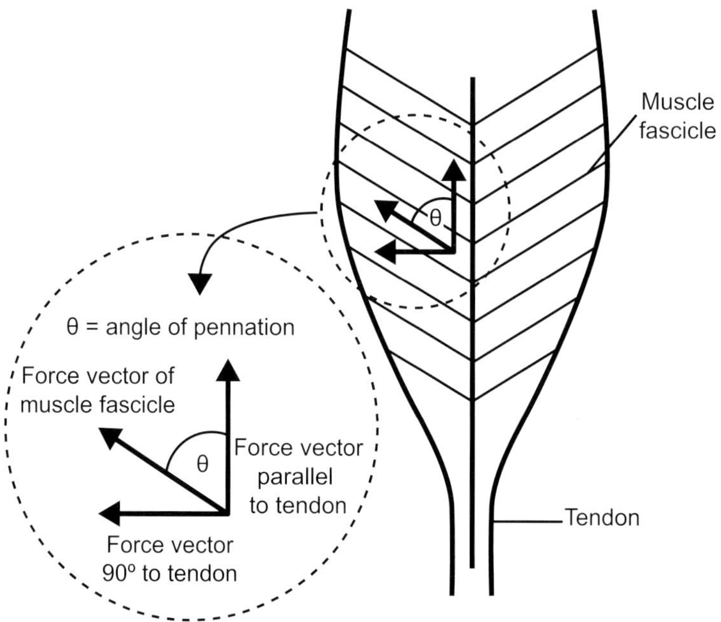

Fig. 2.11
Muscle architecture of a bipennate muscle. Longitudinal force transmitted to tendon is determined by the pennation angle. Most often, a greater Θ is paired with a shorter fascicle length, resulting in less force transmission to tendon.

which includes the connective tissue layers that merge to become a tendon where the ends of muscle fibers do not reach, we end up with a slightly different interpretation of muscle length. Using the orange analogy, the former definition only accounts for the juice inside the bulbs, whereas the latter accounts for the surrounding materials as well.

Interestingly, during development, if a limb is immobilized, it will present with a greater proportion of tendon length than mobilized limbs (Heslinga, te Kronnie and Huijing, 1995). In other words, when muscle fibers are not growing longer, connective tissue replaces it. Again, using the orange analogy, if a bulb were to lose some juice at one end, the space would be filled with extra enveloping material. The envelope itself would not become architecturally smaller, only the proportion of outer material to inner material. Is it possible then that when muscle lengthens, the fibers fill more length of the connective tissue envelope rather than expanding the entirety of the envelope?

I've been insinuating that muscle proliferates to meet rising demand. Hypertrophy, the enlargement of muscle fibers, is the muscle growth that occurs when we load muscles (i.e. lifting weights). *Sarcomerogenesis*, the addition of sarcomeres in series, occurs when we load muscles eccentrically. *Sarcomerolysis*, the removal of sarcomeres in series, occurs when we load muscles concentrically (Butterfield et al., 2005). Unsurprisingly, muscle architecture adaptations are load dependent.

Sarcomerogenesis is regulated by chronic stretch. As bones grow longer during development (provided immobilization is not a condition, as noted above), the growth spurt is met with sarcomerogenesis, meeting the movement demands of the child for optimum function (Herbert, 2005). Other examples of chronic stretch include surgical limb lengthening and casting to specific joint angles (Zöllner et al., 2012). Conversely, during deconditioning or immobilization, sarcomeres are lost, and excess connective tissue accumulates (Williams and Catanese, 1988). In spite of what you may read online, passive stretching alone may not be enough to preserve, or increase, sarcomeres.

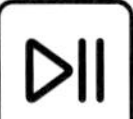

Pause and turn to page 72 for a summary of related research.

Biomechanics tells us load matters. Muscle contractions, of any type, are needed to regulate sarcomere quantity, presumably because of their energetic expense. Contractile tissue is expensive to operate – it requires an energy source to function. Muscles burn calories. In the evolution of human existence, having enough calories to survive is a modern luxury enjoyed by the privileged. The human body has evolved to conserve energy and would likely not preserve unused tissues with a high energy cost.

A passive stretch is a tensile load indeed, but when muscle contractions are paired with stretching, the load parameters are more effective in regulating sarcomere production and loss (van Dyke, Bain and Riley, 2012). A recent meta-analysis concluded that stretch training alone produced "trivial" changes in fascicle length and angle, reinforcing previous statements I've made (Freitas, Mendes and Andrade, 2017). We know stretching does influence muscle architecture, but not as much as it may seem.

Arguably, muscle architecture plays a greater role in mobility than flexibility since muscles produce the internal force to create movement. If flexibility is measured passively, mobility is measured by how someone performs through a ROM. It has been shown that increased passive ROM does not transfer to twist and reach activities or improvements on an elliptical machine (i.e. functional tasks) (Moreside and McGill, 2013). What, then, is the benefit of improved flexibility without training in these new ranges? At surface level, it is easy to accept that ROM is limited by an insufficient length of tissue (i.e. short muscles). It is also easy to explain without a detailed conversation about muscle architecture and physiology or differences between flexibility and mobility. When these factors are taken into consideration, however, it challenges the idea short muscles are the sole cause of limited flexibility.

Whereas a number of studies do show improvements in ROM simultaneous to increases in fascicle length, many do not. Muscle extensibility (think "stretchability" of the tissue) has been shown to increase 13% after a stretch training intervention with no changes in fascicle length or amount of tendon deformation (Blazevich et al., 2014). In other words, the muscle portion of the entire organ (inclusive of the enveloping connective tissue layers) resisted the stretch less, while the tendon portion did not become more pliable. Unless the definition of muscle length as an architectural adaptation is clarified, increased pliability could easily be falsely interpreted as a sarcomeric muscle lengthening.

Moreover, increased ROM has been shown to be altered by many activities other than stretching. In addition to the effects of anesthesia and tolerance on ROM discussed earlier, core endurance activities (Moreside and McGill, 2012), breathing techniques

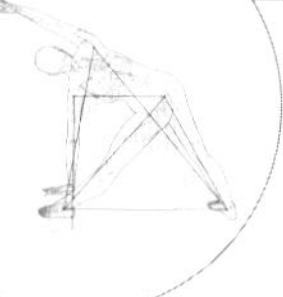

(Hamilton et al., 2015), somatic practices (Stephens et al., 2006), and foam rolling (Junker and Stöggl, 2015) have all improved ROM. Improvements have also been observed after interventions involving joint other than the target joint. Foam rolling one limb has increased ROM in the contralateral limb (Kelly and Beardsley, 2016). Static stretching of the upper limb has produced significant changes in lower limb ROM and vice versa (Behm, Cavanaugh et al., 2016). None of these activities are associated with muscle lengthening by any mechanical definitions. If adaptive tissue lengthening is not the driving factor, we are therefore left to consider other mechanisms of action.

Biomechanics, how the human body responds to and adapts to force, is the main topic here. If you recall the different types of stretching discussed, those that involve force production of the target muscles are those that include isometric and eccentric contractions. Although conventionally not discussed in terms of stretching, eccentric contractions including resisted stretches, body-weight exercises, and loaded training are all worthy of reviewing in our expanded view of stretching as a tissue under tension.

Eccentric Contractions

Eccentric contractions are lengthening contractions against a greater opposing load. Muscles cannot willingly lengthen. When a muscle contracts, an electrical signal from the nervous system, called an impulse, travels along a neuron to the muscle. At the neuromuscular junction, where the neuron meets the muscle cell membrane, the impulse prompts an electrochemical and then a mechanical sequence of events leading to cross-bridge formations. Skeletal muscle can only voluntarily concentrically contract. In order for an isometric contraction to occur, opposing forces must be equal to the force produced by the contracting muscle. In eccentric contractions, opposing forces are greater. The opposing force could come from an external load, like a free weight, or from the internal load produced by surrounding muscles.

When first learning about muscle actions, the process is often described in a binary relationship, contracting, and relaxing. For example, you may have learned that to flex the elbow, the biceps brachii concentrically contract and the triceps brachii relax. It is quite the contrary, however, because if the triceps were relaxed, the elbow would flex rapidly and clumsily without a decelerating mechanism. The triceps eccentrically contract and contribute to the ideal combination of forces necessary to achieve the given movement. It may be helpful to think of concentric contractions as accelerators and eccentric contractions as decelerators. This model of opposing actions is still a reductionist view of elbow flexion. Such a local agonist and antagonist relationship around a single joint ignores the global contractile contributions of other muscles, both proximally and distally, needed to achieve any given movement. Muscles work individually and collectively as motors, brakes, springs, and struts – they work in far more complex patterns than our experimental models have accounted for in controlled laboratory settings (Dickinson et al., 2000). Putting aside a detailed exploration of muscle mechanics, for it is somewhat off topic, we will keep our focus on the effects of eccentric training on muscle architecture.

The length–tension relationship of muscle describes the amount of force a muscle can produce at different lengths (Fig. 2.12). Muscles are generally weaker at very short and extreme long lengths and strongest in mid-range. Additionally, we are somewhat stronger eccentrically than concentrically. Graphically depicted, the length–tension curve represents the ideal length for optimum force production. In response to eccentric training, that curve shifts to the right (Brughelli and Cronin, 2007). Eccentric training improves force production capabilities at longer muscle lengths, which may be useful in activities that utilize longer end ranges (i.e. require force production at long muscle lengths) such as gymnastics, martial arts, and potentially, yoga.

Sarcomerogenesis is one of the proposed mechanisms by which the length-tension relationship shifts. It has recently been shown that fascicle length increases after a

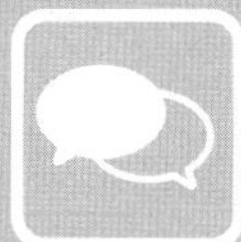

Thought Provoker

Muscle Relationships

In Standing Forward Bend Pose, an instruction we often hear is "contract your quadriceps to relax your hamstrings." In actuality, on the way into the forward bend from Mountain Pose, as in the beginning of a Sun Salutation, the hamstrings are eccentrically lengthening to control the descent. While the pose is held, the hamstrings are isometrically contracting to counterbalance the load of the trunk and prevent falling forward. What does the reciprocal relationship in the instruction inaccurately imply about how muscles work? Is there a cue you could use instead that would emphasize control of the movement rather than individual muscles?

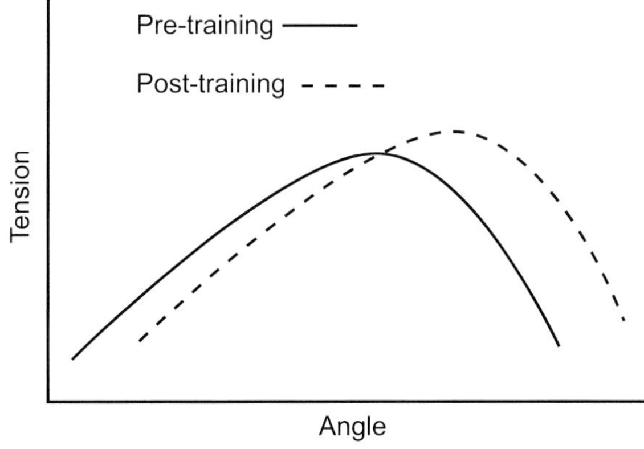

Fig. 2.12
Length–tension curve before and after eccentric training. Force production increases at longer muscle lengths (i.e. greater joint angles). Illustration modified after Brughelli and Cronin (2007).

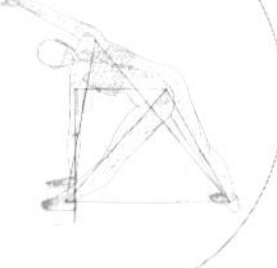

10-week eccentric intervention utilizing the high magnitude body-weight exercise (Fig. 2.13), the Nordic Hamstring Curl (Bourne et al., 2017). Body-weight eccentric exercises resembling many common yoga pose transitions, however, have been shown to not provide a great enough load magnitude to shift the curve (Orishimo and McHugh, 2015). These body-weight exercises, some of which resemble Mountain Pose to Warrior III Pose (Fig. 2.14), or gliding into and out of Hanuman's Pose (Forward Splits) (Fig. 2.15), were effective as overall strengthening exercises and, in another study, these same exercises did reduce the time to return to sport when compared with conventional exercise (Askling, Tengvar and Thorstensson, 2013). The outcomes of eccentric exercises including sarcomerogenesis appear to be load dependent as well.

That is not to suggest that eccentric exercise is the only way to improve end range force production or alter muscle architecture. Training at long muscle lengths (Guex et al., 2016) and isometric training of a muscle in a lengthened position has been shown to increase fascicle length (Noorkõiv, Nosaka and Blazevich, 2014), replicating the effects of eccentric training. In any case, the over-arching theme is that load parameters matter. It appears that contraction type (concentric, isometric, eccentric) is less important than specificity and intensity on causing changes in muscle architecture

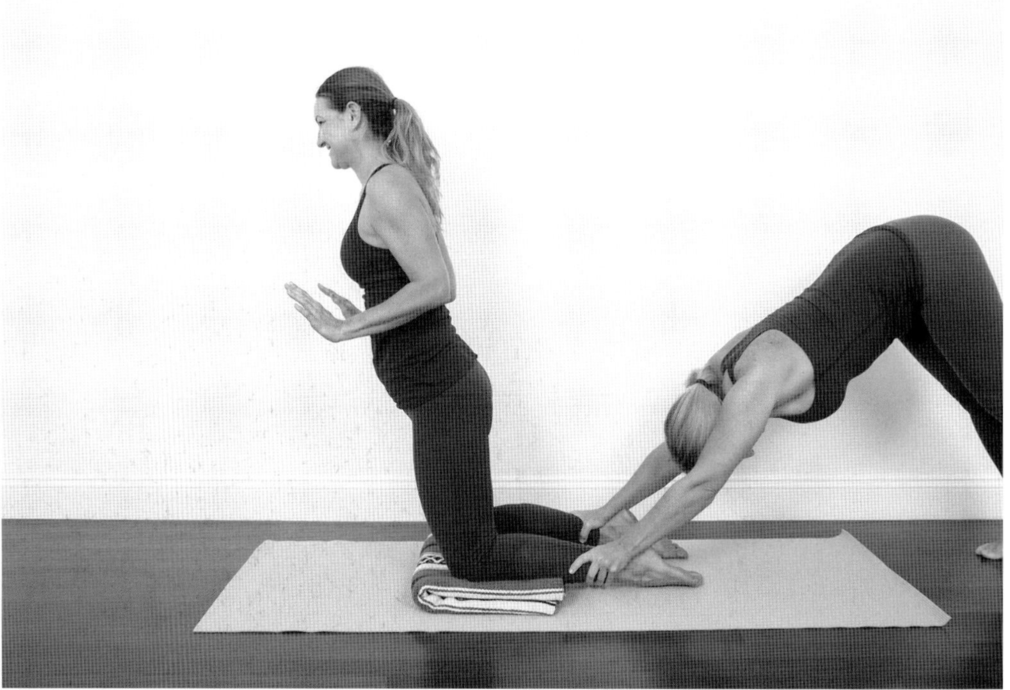

Fig. 2.13
Nordic Hamstring Curl. While the ankles are pinned to the floor, from an upright position standing on the knees, the knees begin to extend while the hips and spine remain neutral. The hamstrings eccentrically lengthen to decelerate and control the descent.

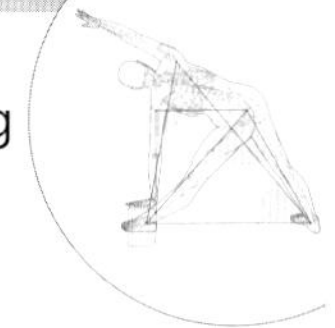

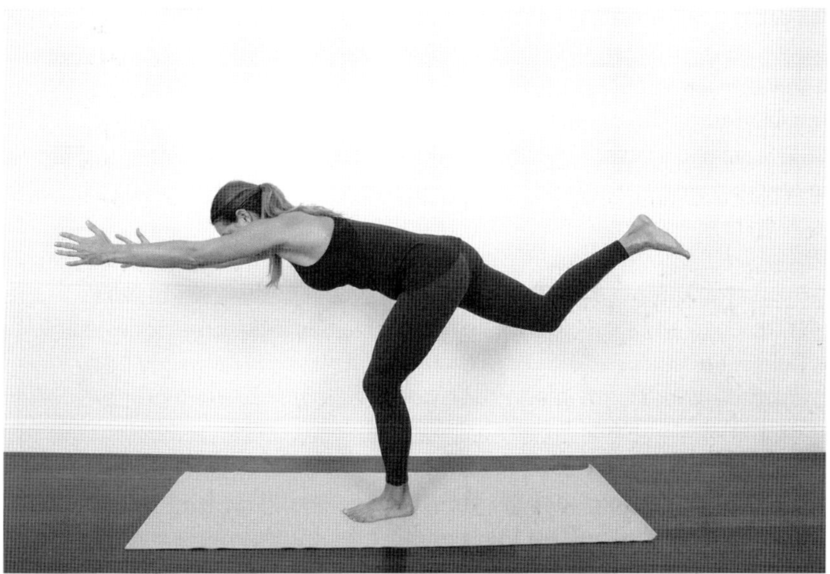

Fig. 2.14
The Diver (resembling Warrior III Pose). From an upright position, hip flexes in standing leg while slight bend in the knee is maintained, hip of lifted leg extends maximally while 90 degree bend in the knee is maintained, and arms stretch out over head.

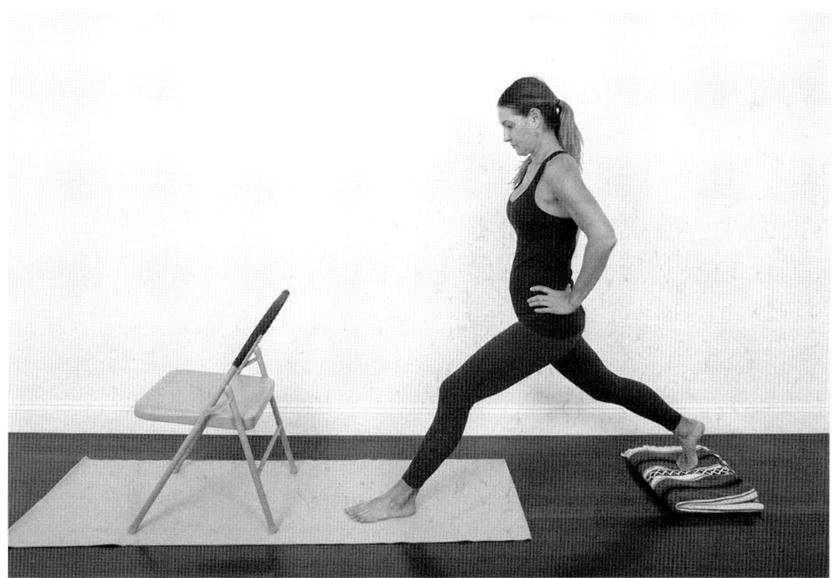

Fig. 2.15
The Glider (resembling Hanuman's Pose). From an upright position, body weight shifts to heel of standing leg while slight bend in the knee is maintained, gliding leg extends (using towel or blanket) maximally before gliding back to starting position, arms used for support (e.g. chairs or yoga blocks).

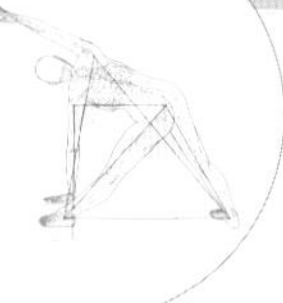

(Franchi et al., 2017) – a concept that should not be surprising at this point. Of the types of stretching previously discussed, PNF and resistance stretching utilize contractions. Based on the above evidence, whether the intensity is high enough to promote any substantial muscle remodeling is still doubtful.

Regarding yoga, we know training at long range improves long range performance, providing load parameters are sufficient. In the absence of any research examining muscle architecture and yoga asana, we are left to draw parallels using the available sport science research. If eccentric loading associated with common yoga transitions potentially improves strength but falls short of shifting the length–tension curve to the right, isometric training at end range may satisfy that specific adaptation. It certainly builds a case for holding postures while cueing to co-contract the ostensibly binary/opposing muscle groups to incite a high-magnitude isometric contraction ("hug muscles to the bone," for example).

Co-contraction can also be used to develop an internal resistance during transitions in asana. If eccentric contractions are the decelerators, these lengthening contractions can be emphasized by "putting on the brakes." Imagine you were lowering from Plank Pose all the way to the floor. The path of least resistance would be to go quickly, letting gravity take you down. But if you were to lower slowly, you would have to create some internal resistance to modulate the pull of gravity. You could further develop this internal resistance if you were to try to push your way back up into Plank Pose while simultaneously trying to pull your way to the floor. Naturally, this approach would ensure slow descent, as well. The point here, however, is not to move slowly, but to explore control through a ROM at a higher demand than that which you might be accustomed to during your yoga practice. Stretching (or lengthening) against external resistance can be used with equipment (e.g. theraband or weight), explored with a partner (e.g. resistance stretching), and in body-weight activities, like yoga, utilizing co-contraction.

My intent here is not to establish a right way of teaching asana, but rather to recognize how various approaches have different outcomes. Cueing students to relax their hamstrings under the assumption that a passive stretch is the only way to improve flexibility is incomplete. Eccentric training has been shown not only to increase flexibility, but also to increase fascicle length (O'Sullivan, McAuliffe and Deburca, 2012). Furthermore, always cueing to relax the hamstrings reinforces outdated concepts about stretching and fails to highlight beneficial principles of progressive loading, specificity, and adaptation. Equipped with this understanding, you are prepared to make educated choices in how you teach that are outcome specific and population dependent. Instead of debating with other teachers what the right way is, we can now debate about which options we think are best given a desired result.

Stretching Redefined

Some time ago, when I was developing the narrative for this book, I took an informal survey of everyone on my mailing list and asked them "what is stretching?" I intentionally made the question open-ended, hoping to get answers that weren't led by my own words. The responses varied, of course, but three distinct themes came up: ROM, tissue lengthening, and sensation. When we look at conventional stretching as it is described and studied in the research, these themes are absolutely central to the conversations of flexibility, muscle architecture, and tolerance. It seems we can all agree on some basic concepts, but where we get lost is in the details.

In my informal survey, some answers described stretching as a function of muscle relaxation with an insinuation that a stretch is the opposite of a contraction. Others described stretching as an activity designed to bring "strength," "suppleness," and "elongation" to the muscle. I'm hoping you are, at this point, asking what type of stretching would develop strength and how it is measured, while also wondering what exactly "suppleness" might mean. A clear definition for "elongation" is also needed (is it deformation, tolerance, or sarcomerogenesis?) before determining the accuracy of that perspective. Some responders separated muscle from connective tissue, implying they can be stretched separately and alluding to the notion that different approaches to yoga target different tissues. In our review of conventional stretching thus far, we have discussed very little about connective tissue outside of the fascial layers providing the structure for the muscle organ. In order to establish how stretching might affect tendons and ligaments, we would first need to define the properties of the tissue, and then the type of stretching, the load parameters, etc. In other words, the details.

I highlight these varied and sometimes contradicting perspectives for you here to explain the importance of coming together to agree on terminology. As the reader, you don't have to agree with my definitions or interpretations of the literature; however, we must at least agree on the words we use so that we can form our opinions knowing we are talking about the same thing. If you are talking about how muscle tissue behaves during a stretch and I'm talking about how the collagen in connective tissue behaves, we will always be tuned to different channels. This reminds me of the John Godfrey Saxe poem of the six blind men and the elephant. Each blind man's position near the elephant influenced how they perceived the animal. One man likened the elephant to a tree stump (feeling the leg). Another argued that the elephant is like rope (being near the tail). While yet another likened to elephant to a spear (feeling the tusk). And so on. While all the men were partially right, they were all wrong. This poem is also referenced in a research paper about spinal stability (Reeves, Narendra and Cholewicki, 2007), which we will return to in a later chapter. Regarding stretching, the poem also serves to highlight the importance of continuing to define our terms.

In order for us to discuss stretching in terms of connective tissue, it is important that we re-establish the definition of stretching as load; a tensile load. This will keep us within a framework of biomechanics while including forces that may not fit into any conventional type of stretching. For example, a concentric muscle contraction applies a tensile load to the tendon (because the force produced by a muscle pulls on the tendon, in turn pulling on the bone to create, or prevent, movement across a joint). Most would not consider a concentric contraction to be a tendon stretch, but in fact, it is. A passive stretch also applies a tensile load to a tendon, albeit a lesser load due to less muscle force. An isometric contraction at end range, which we have established is a type of conventional stretch, might apply a great tensile load to a tendon, depending on degree of muscle contraction. If we want to ascertain how a tendon responds to a stretch, we have to include all types of tensile loading, not just passive stretching. If you recall the conversation I had with my colleague about stretching tendons, these were some of the concepts we had to go over to move forward in our discussion. At the conclusion of this book, when in a conversation about stretching, it is my goal for you not to be bound by the limitations of the blind men discussing the elephant.

Incidentally, my favorite response to my stretching survey was from a medical writer who flatly declared "I have no idea how to describe stretching." It takes a vast amount of education to be willing to say, "I don't know." It also creates a perfect starting point to a discussion on the finer points of loading, stretching, and tissue adaptation. Admittedly, my "what is stretching?" probe was somewhat of a trick question.

Research Summary

Yoga and College Athletes

Impact of 10-weeks of Yoga Practice on the Flexibility and Balance of College Athletes (Polsgrove, Eggleston and Lockyer, 2016)

Background

Yoga is associated with many positive physical and health outcomes. Yoga moves the body in varied ways, differently from specificity in sport training. Yoga enhances many components of fitness simultaneously, including balance, coordination, flexibility, strength, and endurance.

Purpose

The aim is to determine "if and how yoga can impact specific components of fitness related to athletic performance." The researchers hypothesized that balance, flexibility, and joint angles would improve after the 10-week yoga intervention.

Methods

Two groups of male college age athletes were recruited. None of the participants had any yoga experience. The intervention group (yoga group) consisted of 14 soccer players averaging 19.8 years of age. The control group (non-yoga group) consisted of 12 baseball players averaging 20.3 years of age. The soccer players were led a 1-hour yoga class twice a week for 10 weeks. The baseball players did not practice yoga at all. Both teams continued to train as usual.

Prior to the start of the intervention, both teams were assessed for balance, flexibility, and joint angles. The balance test consisted of the Stork Test (resembling Tree Pose). The flexibility tests included a shoulder flexibility test (resembling the arms in Cow Face Pose) and the sit and reach test (resembling Seated Forward

Continued on next page

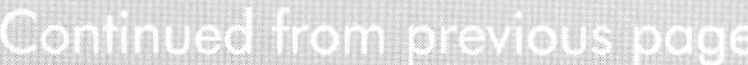

Bend Pose). The joint angle test included right forward Lunge (resembling a yoga/runner's Lunge), Downward Facing Dog Pose (they didn't even call it something else), and chair (like Chair Pose). After the intervention, both teams were tested in these same six positions.

Results

The soccer players (yoga group) significantly improved in the flexibility, balance, and joint angles tests, whereas the baseball players (non-yoga group) did not.

Discussion

I deliberately selected this paper to review because it is: a) a poor-quality study, and b) highlights some challenges in determining how improvements in flexibility carry over into performance. The comments in this discussion are my own, as I found the discussion and conclusions section of the paper illogical and unsound. The comments in the above sections were drawn from the paper, which I would like to discuss here.

Regarding the background/introduction portion of the paper, my summary is brief because it was difficult to extract any solid reasoning for study other than something akin to "yoga is supposed to be pretty good." I found concern with their logic that improvements in components of fitness automatically translated to improvements in sport. While they did raise the challenge in this assumption by outlining the importance of specificity training, they continued to suggest the variability in yoga training could have a positive impact on sport performance. Then, the aim was to show that yoga could improve components of fitness (not performance). The prior performance conversation seemed a bit misleading and incongruent with the purpose of the study.

Probably the most obvious glaring fault in the methods section is that the intervention and control group did not play the same sport. It is, literally, like comparing apples to oranges. Another issue with the study design was that the pre- and post-test positions were essentially yoga poses. The study tested the subjects in six yoga poses, gave one group 20 hours of yoga training and the other group none, and then tested the subjects in the same six yoga poses. Based on the principles of specificity and considering none of the subjects had prior experience with yoga, the results are to be expected. In order to highlight how misleading abstracts can be, I quote the original below.

Abstract (as printed in the original paper)

> "Background: With clearer evidence of its benefits, coaches, and athletes may better see that yoga has a role in optimizing performance. Aims: To determine the impact of yoga on male college athletes (N = 26).
>
> Methods: Over a 10-week period, a yoga group (YG) of athletes (n = 14) took part in biweekly yoga sessions; while a non-yoga group (NYG) of athletes

Continued on next page

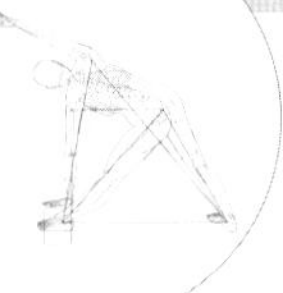

Continued from previous page

(n = 12) took part in no additional yoga activity. Performance measures were obtained immediately before and after this period. Measurements of flexibility and balance included: Sit-reach (SR), shoulder flexibility (SF), and stork stand (SS); dynamic measurements consisted of joint angles (JA) measured during the performance of three distinct yoga positions (downward dog [DD]; right foot lunge [RFL]; chair [C]).

Results: Significant gains were observed in the YG for flexibility (SR, P = 0.01; SF, P = 0.03), and balance (SS, P = 0.05). No significant differences were observed in the NYG for flexibility and balance. Significantly, greater JA were observed in the YG for: RFL (dorsiflexion, l-ankle; P = 0.04), DD (extension, r-knee, P = 0.04; r-hip; P = 0.01; flexion, r-shoulder; P = 0.01) and C (flexion, r-knee; P = 0.01). Significant JA differences were observed in the NYG for: DD (flexion, r-knee, P = 0.01: r-hip, P = 0.05; r-shoulder, P = 0.03) and C (flexion r-knee, P = 0.01; extension, r-shoulder; P = 0.05). A between group comparison revealed the significant differences for: RFL (l-ankle; P = 0.01), DD (r-knee, P = 0.01; r-hip; P = 0.01), and C (r-shoulder, P = 0.02).

Conclusions: Results suggest that a regular yoga practice may increase the flexibility and balance as well as whole body measures of male college athletes and therefore, may enhance athletic performances that require these characteristics."

Research Summary

High Intensity Stretch

Effect of 8-week High-intensity Stretching Training on Biceps Femoris Architecture (Freitas and Mil-Homens, 2015)

Background

Muscle architecture plays an important role in performance as it relates to length–tension and velocity–tension relationships. Resistance training is known to make alterations in muscle architecture, but the speculation that stretching might achieve this is still up for debate. One possible explanation is that stretching interventions tested to date may not have exposed subjects to high enough stretch intensities. Since range of motion (ROM) research results are dependent on duration, repetition, and frequency, perhaps architectural results are too.

Continued on next page

Continued from previous page

Purpose

This paper set out to establish if high-intensity passive static stretching could change biceps femoris muscle architecture in an 8-week protocol.

Methods

Ten men averaging 21.2 years of age were randomly assigned to either a stretching group or the control. Subjects were not to engage in any type of stretching or strengthening program, but were allowed to participate in activities of daily living. The stretching group received the intervention five times per week for 8 weeks. The intervention was described as a 450 second stretch (7.5 minutes) at the highest tolerable position, just short of painful. Every 90 seconds, the stretch was increased to a further position until the subjects could no longer tolerate a greater ROM. The fascicle length of the biceps femoris was recorded (using sonogram) in both groups before and after the study period.

Results

Adherence in the stretching group averaged 3.1 stretch protocols per week. Fascicle length increased by 13.6% and fascicle angle decreased by 15.1% for the stretching group. Additionally, ROM increased by 14.2 degrees over the course of the intervention, also for the stretching group.

Discussion

This research challenges the argument that stretching alone does not change muscle architecture. That said, it is important to note the details of the intervention. While we do stretch our hamstrings in yoga, sometimes for several minutes at a time, the postures are generally less aggressive. Imagine teaching your students to stretch as hard as they can to the point of pain for 7.5 continuous minutes! Moreover, I would guess adherence would be compromised and the students would likely "cheat" without you getting involved by pushing them into their highest tolerable stretch. As we will discover in the following section, eccentric training might be a more effective strategy to induce changes in muscle architecture (along with many other positive outcomes associated with strength training) than a passive stretching protocol. Finally, the small sample size (n = 5) and demographic (college-age men) is a major limitation in this study and a sweeping conclusion across populations should be cautioned against.

3 MECHANICAL BEHAVIOR

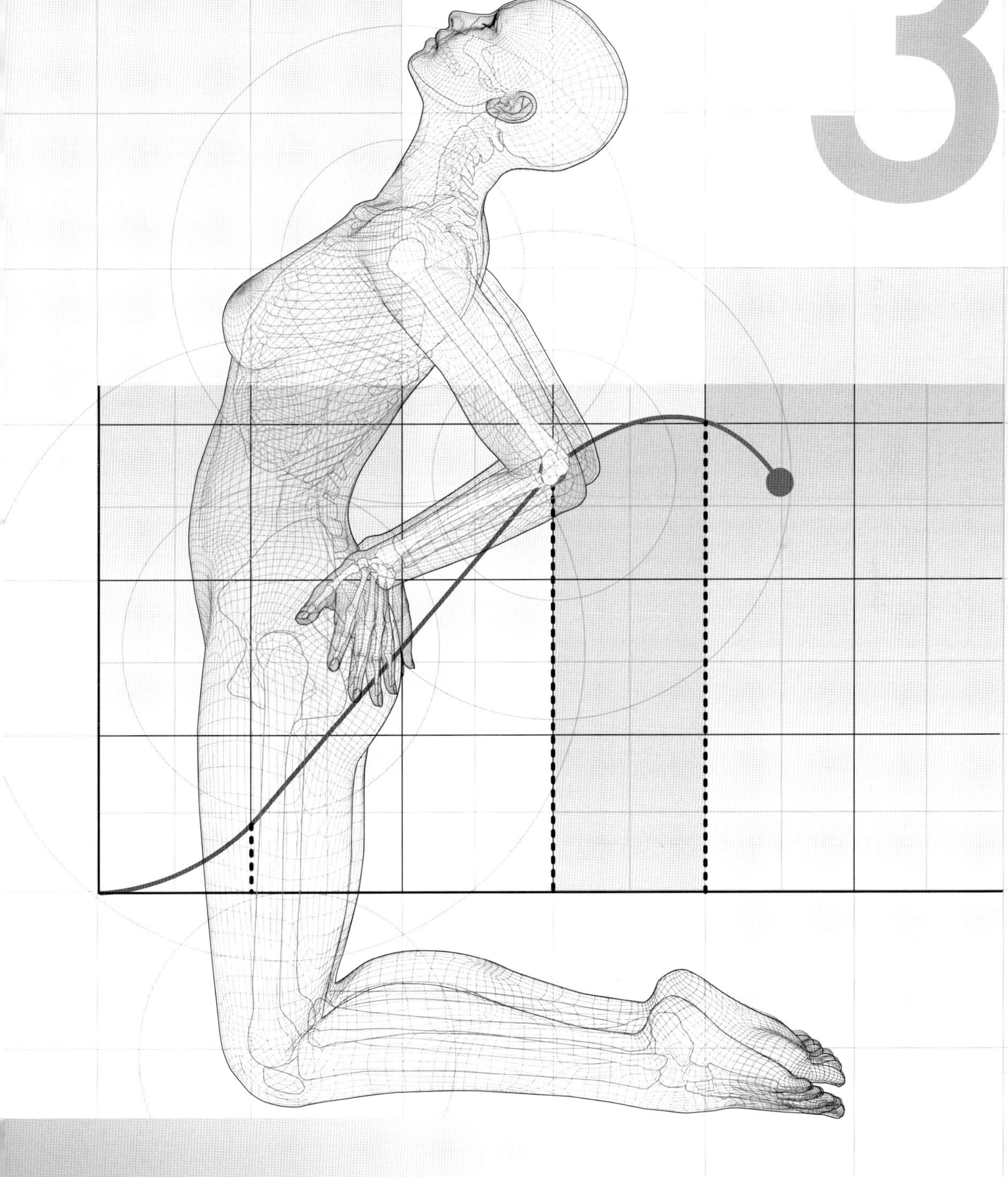

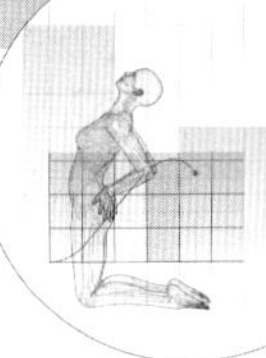

We will now shift the focus of study to connective tissue because it is central to the narrative of yoga and adaptation to tensile load. The study of the neuromuscular system would definitely carry more weight than the musculoskeletal and facial systems in the study of strength and conditioning, flexibility, and skill acquisition. That is not to say yoga is never assessed in the context of hypertrophy and strength gains, neuromechanics of flexibility, and motor learning/control, but these topics are not the primary focus here. Instead, we will examine how yoga might affect the mechanical properties of bones, joints, ligaments, and tendons.

Consider for a moment some of the common musculoskeletal afflictions you associate with yoga – they can be conditions you expect yoga to ease, or conditions you believe yoga might cause. Since we know the musculoskeletal system is always managing stress and adapting to load, the same condition might appear on either side of the cause/treatment spectrum. For example, a search of the literature returns a paper citing yoga as a cause of osteoporosis-related compression fractures (Sinaki, 2013) and another paper citing yoga as a treatment capable of reversing osteoporosis (Lu et al., 2016). This conundrum has appeared before in our discussion of optimal loading and will continue to appear throughout the book, and research in general.

Regardless, if you or someone you know has developed an ache or pain through the practice of yoga, or has relieved one, the process of identifying these musculoskeletal conditions establishes the importance of studying connective tissue properties. With the exception of non-specific chronic low back pain (NSCLBP), you may find that most conditions on your list reside in the connective tissue layers. Stress fractures, arthritis, ligament sprains, and tendinopathies all affect connective tissues such as bones, cartilage, ligaments, and tendons. A rotator cuff tear almost always refers to a tendon. A hamstring pull is usually at the proximal tendon and when it is in fact a muscle strain, it affects the myofascial layers of the muscle organ. Labral tears of the hip or shoulder, meniscal tears in the knee, or bulging discs all affect fibrocartilage. Many impingement syndromes affect various layers of connective tissue. Even some back pain researchers present arguments that the condition resides in the fascia. For the most part, however, NSCLBP is "non-specific" in that it cannot be assigned to a specific structure or cause. It's near impossible to identify a musculoskeletal condition that does not reside in the connective tissue layers.

While we are not yet discussing injuries in depth at this stage in the book, I mention them now because we can all agree that a responsible and professional yoga teacher would have a vested interest in doing her best to avoid practices that might cause injury. If most of these injuries are connective tissue injuries, it would be prudent to learn as much as possible about connective tissue properties. Moreover, if we know that connective tissues can increase their capacity to tolerate load through exposure to load, yoga teachers would want to learn about how to effectively promote such an adaptation. For these reasons my research on stretching evolved to focus less on range of motion (ROM), which is mostly devoid of the load conversation, and more on connective tissue mechanical properties, particularly in response to tensile loading.

The mechanical properties of connective tissues are determined by a combination of tissue composition, structure, and behavior, which are governed by both cellular and extra-cellular functions (Fig. 3.1). The present chapter focuses on the behavior of connective

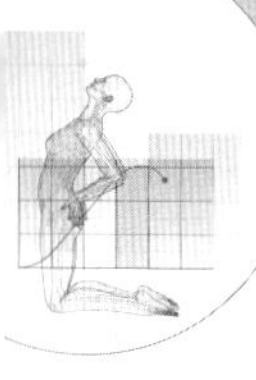

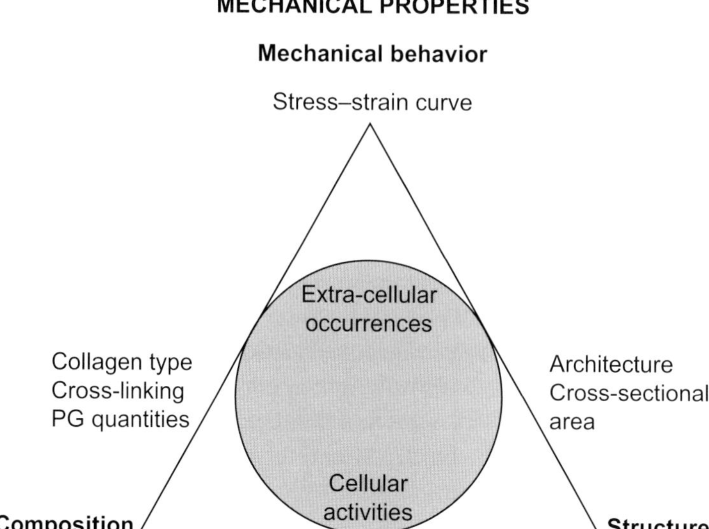

Fig. 3.1
Mechanical behavior, governed by non-cellular factors, is just one contributing factor to musculoskeletal tissue properties.

tissue which is determined mainly by the behavior of the **collagen** of which these tissues are made. How additional components and their architecture affect mechanical properties will be discussed in the following chapter. As with previous chapters the clear definition of mechanical terms is one of the most important aspects of studying tissue behavior. By understanding behavioral adaptations to mechanical load we can proceed in future chapters to a well-versed discussion of tissue capacity and injury.

Stress and Strain

The mechanical behavior of a material is expressed by its relationship to stress and **strain** (Fig. 3.2). When loaded, a material compresses, stretches, shears, bends or torques, depending on the direction in which the loads are applied. These deformations are referred to as strain, and the internal resistance is referred to as stress. We again encounter a word here that has a negative colloquial use. Strain often implies difficult to achieve, or requiring excessive effort. Even the use of the term "muscle strain" defines a muscle injury or what is often referred to as muscle tear – a deformation of muscle tissue beyond its capacity to withstand stress. Biomechanically speaking, strain is neither good nor bad, it is simply a measure of the units of deformation a material undergoes when exposed to load.

Materials with elastic properties exhibit strain during exposure to load but return to the previous resting shape when the load is no longer applied. Materials with plastic properties maintain the strain they exhibited during load even after it has been removed. Clay is a malleable material that exhibits plastic properties as it retains its new shape even after the forces that molded it have been removed. Plasticity in an elastic waistband,

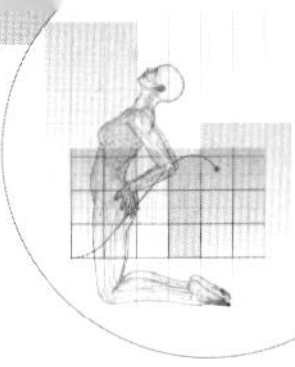

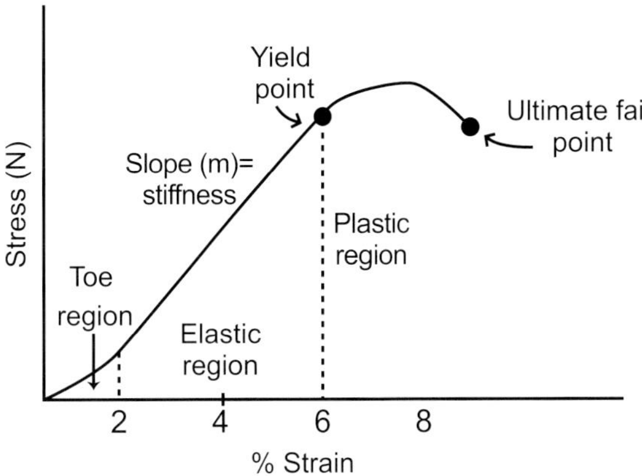

Fig. 3.2
The stress–strain curve. This particular graph depicts a hypothetical tissue for demonstrative purposes. The exact appearance of the stress–strain curve varies within tissues and among individuals.

however, occurs as *some* of the elastic fibers break, causing the waistband to "stretch out" and fail to return to its resting length. While in some materials, plastic deformations are the result of structural damage, the clay example tells us plasticity should not automatically have a negative connotation. A point of contention among both researchers and clinicians is to what degree connective tissue exhibits plastic behavior, like clay, and when/if structural damage occurs. We will continue to investigate the possibilities here.

For certain, materials do have a mechanical limit – the maximum amount of strain a material can exhibit before full failure or complete rupture. The stress a material can withstand is relative to the units of strain. Continue to apply a tensile load to the elastic waistband and eventually the strain would reach a length where all of its component parts would fail, and it would tear apart fully. In materials science this is called the ultimate fail point.

In human connective tissues under tension, strain is usually measured in millimeters, just as stress is commonly measured in newtons (N). The values for the units of stress relative to each unit of strain can be plotted on a graph, called the stress–strain curve. Sometimes named a load deformation curve, the graph visually expresses the mechanical behavior of tissues.

For those who have repressed high school algebra, let me explain. The horizontal plane (x-axis) represents the percentage of strain and the vertical plane (y-axis) represents the units of stress. An increase in strain resulting from an externally applied load is represented by plotting a point horizontally along the x-axis, and an increase in stress, the internal reaction to the strain, is plotted vertically, along the y-axis. In mathematics, the x-axis is the independent variable and the y-axis is the dependent variable. This rule makes strain a function of an applied load and stress dependent on the units of strain. Here, stress is technically a measure of resistance to strain, or the internal reaction attempting to restore original shape. Externally loading a tissue causes strain, which in turn causes internal stress. Moreover, because a load must act

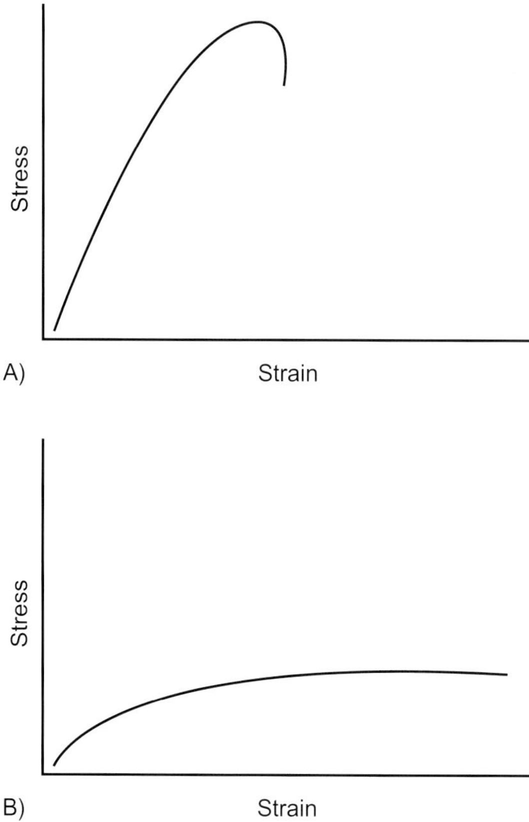

Fig. 3.3
Comparison of hypothetical stress–strain curves. (A) Brittle materials are represented by high stress and low strain. (B) Ductile materials are represented by high strain and low stress.

on a material in order for it to strain, the relationship is sometimes explained in the opposite direction. The scientist or mathematician might criticize me for this, but for the yoga teacher/student to conceptualize the relationship between stress and strain, it is sometimes easier to present mechanical behavior with strain being dependent on stress. For example, the graph of a brittle material like glass would have a very high value for y with a low value for x because it strains very little when stress is high (technically, when strained, the resisting/restoring stress increases greatly). Whereas a ductile material like copper would have a very large value for x and relatively low values for y because it strains easily when stress is low (technically, when strained at high levels, the resisting/restoring stress remains low). Regardless of how you choose to understand the relationship, human tissues clearly do not act in the same way as glass or copper (Fig. 3.3).

Under increasing strain, collagen, a primary component of human connective tissues, behaves elastically at first, then plastically, until reaching the ultimate fail point. The plastic region is the point of contention mentioned previously. Many assume stretching collagen will induce adaptive lengthening, or change, like clay, in spite of any good

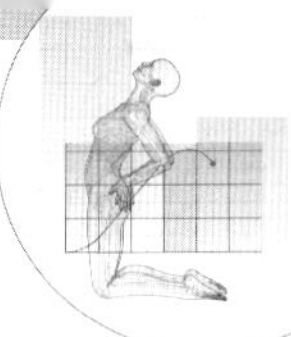

Table 3.1
Collagen Strain Capacities

Position on the x-axis	% Strain
Toe region	1–2%
Elastic region	3–4%
Yield point	≈4%
Plastic region	4–6%
Ultimate fail point	≈8–10%

evidence to support these types of plastic changes (remember, an increase in ROM does not automatically imply adaptive lengthening of tissue). Others assume stretching collagen will eventually be the cause of disrupted molecular bonds, or micro-tears, much like the failing fibers of the stretched out elastic waistband. Unlike the waistband, human tissue, has living components and is always remodeling. Since we know that muscle rebuilds in response to muscle damage, it would seem logical to conclude that connective tissue rebuilds in response to micro-failures. In spite of its widespread acceptance, the notion that stretching healthy connective tissue leads to "lengthened" or "stretched out" tissue ultimately causing joint laxity, is not something I have been able to confirm with the available research.

The stress–strain curve for collagen-based tissues is divided into three main regions graphically depicted by a linear slope and two non-linear curves (Table 3.1). The first region of strain is called the toe region. Collagen fibers at rest exhibit a crimped configuration and straighten upon initial strain. The toe region accounts for the first 1–2% of strain. In the second, elastic region, the straightened fibers yield, resulting in greater strain. This yield adds tension to the tissue which stores potential energy such that the reversibility of strain is largely a passive event, requiring minimal muscle force to produce. This elastic region accounts for 3–4% of collagen strain. The third region, beyond the yield point, is the plastic region and accounts, on average, for about 4–6% strain. Since fibrillar microfailures are a normal response to loading and our tissues are constantly in a state of both synthesis and degradation, this strain range does not necessarily imply injury, although it certainly could. The end of the plastic region is capped by the ultimate fail point, which happens around 8–10% of collagen strain. For context, during normal movements, tendons and ligaments strain between about 2% and 5%.

The differing shapes of the graphical regions exhibit an inconsistent response to strain. In the elastic region, the ratio of stress to strain (y:x) is positive and linear (i.e. a straight upwardly sloped line), meaning that for every unit of strain, an equally proportional unit of stress develops. In the plastic region, additional increases in strain result in smaller, albeit still increasing units of stress. As the ultimate fail point approaches, the non-linear plastic region might curve into a negative, decreasing slope as the compromised tissue loses its resistance/restoring stress capacity the more it strains.

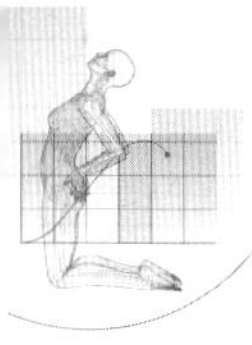

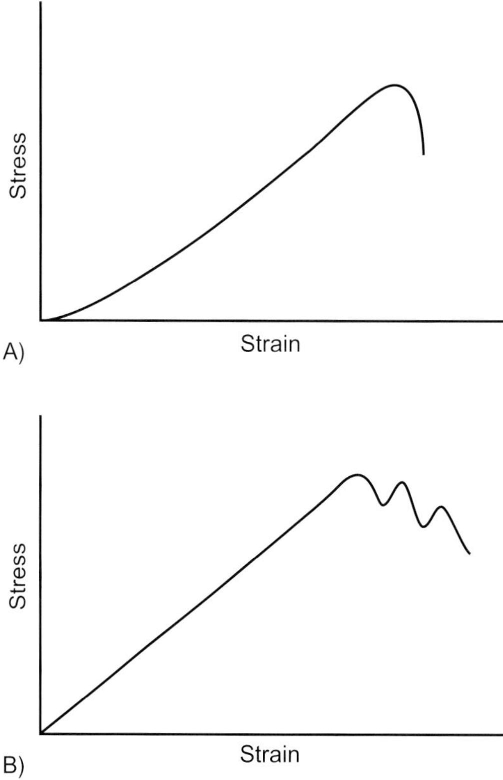

Fig. 3.4

In general, (A) ligaments withstand lower load than tendons and fail more suddenly while (B) tendons waver a bit more before failure. However, the Achilles tendon behaves more like a ligament and the anterior cruciate ligament (ACL) behaves more like a tendon, so the rule has exceptions. This is one reason why surgeons sometimes use a hamstring tendon graft to reconstruct the ACL.

In the non-linear toe region, the curve is inverted when compared to the plastic region; therefore, greater strain is met with lower increments of stress due to the straightening of crimp occurring prior to elastic yield. Crimp is essential for maintaining a homeostatic tension within the tissues as mechanical changes occur during activity. In fact, healthy tendons adjust crimp patterns by altering length and amplitude during repetitive loading and cyclical activities which may then induce alterations in mechanical behavior (Freedman et al., 2015; Lavagnino et al., 2017). In regard to adaptability, it is the dependent variable or stress along the y-axis that can change in response to loading (and time, as we will cover shortly). The independent variable, strain, is fixed, meaning the different regions do not move to the right or left along the x-axis (Fig. 3.4).

To use an analogy, we can reduce the behavior of individual collagen fibers to that of a rubber band. Strain the rubber band and it becomes stressed and stores energy. How much stress it can sustain, or tolerate, depends on how much you strain it; however, once you reach the material's mechanical limit, the structural integrity of the rubber band is

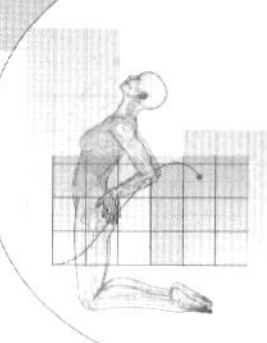

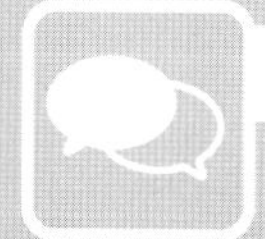

Thought Provoker

Stress and Strain in Yoga

Stress and strain are two different variables. Stress is load and strain is deformation or length of stretch. If you could lower all the way into the bottom of Garland Pose (Deep Squat) such that your knees were in maximum flexion, the anterior knee could not strain any further, correct? The only way to strain the anterior knee further would be to bend the knee further, but it is already in maximal flexion. If you wanted to increase the stress on the knee, you could add external load, like holding a 10 lb. sandbag overhead. In the absence of an external load, you could isometrically contract the muscles surrounding the knee at the bottom of the squat to provide an internally produced load. These are both examples where you can increase stress without increasing strain.

Looking at how you already teach, can you identify props and specific cues you could use to provide increased stress without increasing strain (i.e. not needing to push into end range of motion)?

compromised. It is possible that after you remove the straining force, a portion of the strain was irreversible, diminishing the tensile capacity of the rubber band. Stay within its mechanical limit and the rubber band retains its original capacity.

When a tissue made of bundles of collagen strains beyond the mechanical limit, its mechanical capabilities may weaken, and/or an adaptive response to repair and rebuild may trigger. In any case, continue to strain and eventually you will get total failure. Stay within the mechanical limit, and the tissue has the ability to increase its capacity to tolerate load. It will not, however, increase the capacity for individual collagen fibers to stretch farther than the fail point. Strain regions are fixed.

Where rubber bands fail as analogies is that rubber bands don't adapt to applied loads. If rubber bands behaved like human tissues, loading the rubber band would increase its tensional capacity and you could apply more load before reaching the mechanical threshold. Where rubber bands serve well as analogies is that a rubber band has a fixed strain capacity and it also works well to explain the details of elastic behavior.

Elasticity

Elasticity explains the tendency for a material to return to resting length after the tensile load is removed – like when releasing a slingshot. When the slingshot is retracted, recall that the stretched material stores energy, which we call potential energy. When the force holding tension on the material is removed, the potential energy becomes kinetic energy, and the release of energy is expressed through motion. This release of energy is passive, requiring no additional external force, or conscious thought for that matter, to unleash.

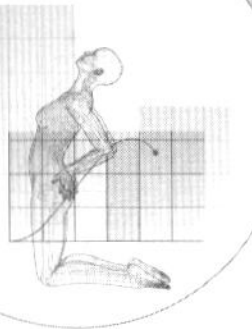

A spring is the standard example of elastic behavior, as defined by Hooke's Law, which can be generalized to say the strain of an elastic material is proportional to force applied. This statement reflects the linear relationship of the elastic region. For example, if you open a spring-loaded screen door, the spring lengthens proportionally to the amount of force you apply to the door. Energy is stored until you release the door and it slams behind you with no effort on your part. A perfect spring would be represented by a single linear stress strain curve (a straight upwardly sloped line). In human tissue, the stress strain curve represents Hookean behavior in the elastic region, but not beyond.

In explosive movements, an active stretch (eccentric contraction) is followed by active shortening (concentric contraction), referred to as the stretch shortening cycle (SSC). One of the proposed mechanisms of the SCC is the capture of elastic energy during the stretch phase to be released in conjunction with the concentric action. For example, when jumping from a standing position, by first flexing at the ankle, knee, and hip, one can utilize the stored potential energy captured by the stretch of the passive connective tissue components to then propel vertically into the air.

During cyclical movements such as walking and running, your connective tissues store and release energy to help propel the limbs, economizing the amount of force the muscles must produce. The elasticity of tendons is most apparent when comparing a single movement with the same movement followed by a counter movement. During a single movement such as dorsiflexion to plantar flexion (i.e. a single calf raise), the calf muscles shorten, and the tendon length remains mostly unchanged, suggesting movement occurs mostly as a result of the concentric muscle contraction. During reactive movements with a prior counter movement (i.e. repeated calf raises), however, the muscle length remains mostly unchanged and the tendon is lengthened and shortened, suggesting the movement occurs mostly as a result of tendon elasticity (Kawakami et al., 2002). Generally speaking, yoga is not a cyclical activity that utilizes tendon elasticity. Going back to the rules of specificity, how likely do you think it is for yoga to improve performance in a cyclical activity such as running?

It is important to note that the stress–strain curves presented thus far are hypothetical graphs used for instructional purposes. It is not an actual representation of any particular human tissue. Since tissue behavior will vary among individuals due to a variety of factors such as genetics, gender, age, loading history, and location of tissue, measurements using laboratory equipment would be needed to determine the exact behavior of a tissue. To determine the stress–strain curve of a specific tendon, for example, strain can be quantified utilizing ultrasound while the corresponding amount of force can be measured with a dynamometer. These values are used to establish a ratio of stress to strain, called **stiffness**.

Stiffness and Compliance

A significant misunderstanding around tissue behavior is caused by the colloquial uses of mechanical terms. Stiffness, a quality of which we typically attempt to rid ourselves, is nothing more than the ratio of stress to strain (Fig. 3.5). Stiffness is represented on the linear component of the stress–strain curve and is expressed by the slope of the line ($m=\Delta y/\Delta x$, where Δ represents the "change in"). The steeper the slope of the elastic region, the greater the stiffness – meaning for a certain amount of strain (x), the tissue resists with a

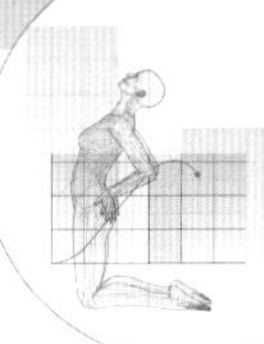

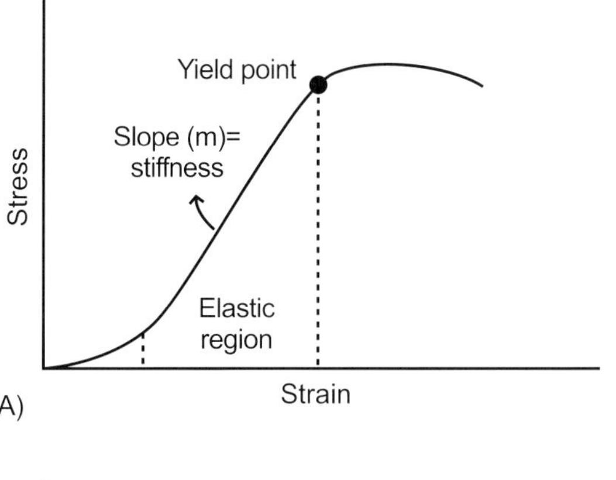

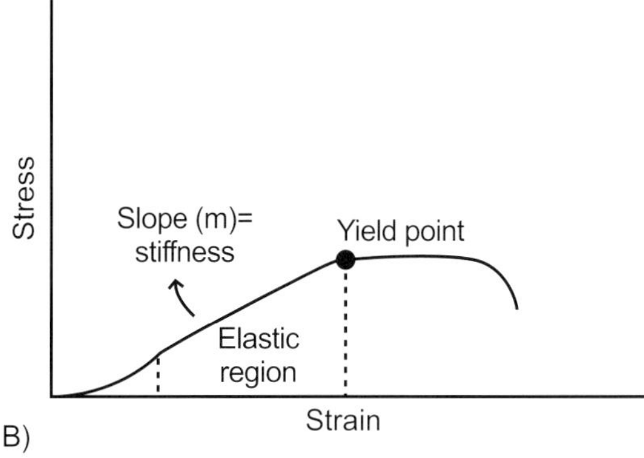

Fig. 3.5

Stiff versus compliant. (A) The greater the slope of the elastic region, the greater the stiffness. (B) The less the slope of the elastic region, the greater the compliance.

greater amount of stress (y). The more gradual the slope, the less stiffness, where a certain amount of strain is met with a lesser amount of resistant stress. The relationship is always positive; each additional unit of strain is met with some degree of greater stress.

In the elastic region of the stress–strain curve, the ratio of stress to strain is expressed by Young's modulus. Also referred to as the modulus of elasticity, it is derived from Hooke's Law (Fig. 3.6), which is expressed by F=kx (where F = force, of course, k = stiffness, x = displacement). Stainless steel is an extremely stiff material, as are tendons, whereas stretchy pants are not.

In materials science the reciprocal of stiffness is called compliance. Because the colloquial uses of the terms stiffness and **compliance** (otherwise known as flexibility) imply something else, it is worth the effort to define them biomechanically. First, since flexibility is so often equated with ROM, compliance is a better word to describe the mechanical behavior reciprocal to stiffness. Flexibility, as a measure of ROM, is not necessarily limited by the stiffness of the tissue. You can have stiff or compliant tissues, and still be plenty flexible or inflexible, respectively. In ROM testing, the greater one's ROM, the greater one's flexibility. The limit to one's flexibility could be mechanical or sensory, or more likely both. Stiff or compliant tendons, however, are not the sole determining factor.

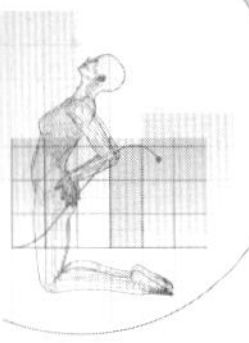

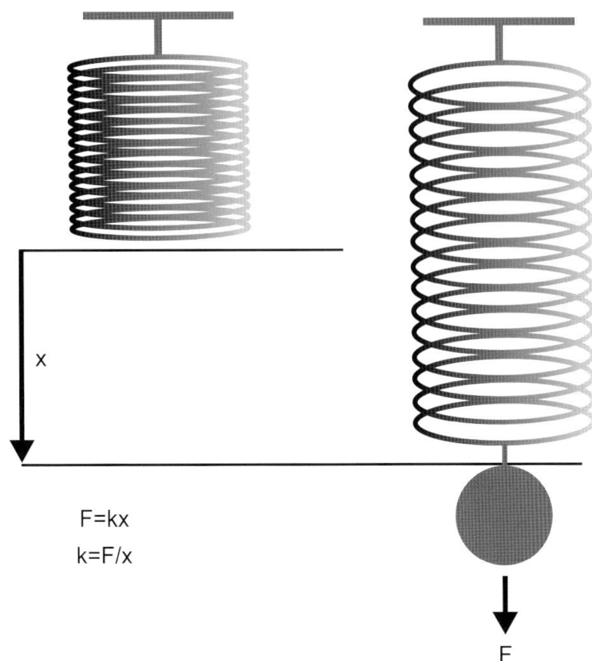

Fig. 3.6
Hooke's Law describes the relationship between applied force (stress) and displacement (strain) in terms of stiffness (k=F/x). It is the same mathematical relationship for stiffness derived from the stress–strain curve (m=y/x), where stress is described as the resisting/ restoring force instead of the applied force. The units of measurement are the same in both equations.

To visualize the behavior of a tendon, think of a stiff versus a compliant rubber band. The stiffer rubber band requires more force to strain than the compliant rubber band, but both will eventually strain at the limit of the composite material's mechanical range. The stiffer, more difficult to stretch rubber band will store the potential energy of the stress and more rapidly rebound when the load is removed. The compliant, more easily stretched rubber band will also store potential energy, and, because it yields more readily under light loads, the comparatively greater range releases more energy upon recoil, just not as rapidly.

Stiff tendons perform well in tasks utilizing smaller ROMs at both low and heavy loads. A stiff Achilles tendon would translate into economy of running for a distance runner who can take advantage of the stored energy from the dorsiflexed ankle and extended hip (i.e. stretched tendons) in the back leg and utilize the rapid release for toe-off in the swing phase. Less force production needed from the calf muscles and hip flexors means less metabolic expenditure for the runner. Here, stiffness might actually be desirable.

Compliant tendons perform well in tasks utilizing greater ROMs when the load is mostly small. A sprinter, who takes longer strides than a distance runner, may benefit from more compliant tendons because the amount of stored potential energy gained

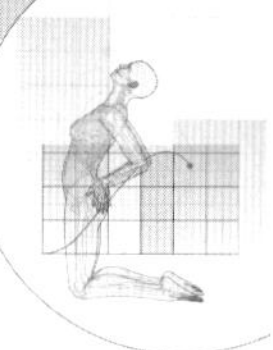

from the extra length is used to propel the leg forward, again reducing the metabolic expenditure of the muscles having to move the leg. Since the leg is relatively light, it does not require the high-speed force released by the stiffer tendons. Neither stiff nor compliant tendons determine an individual's flexibility, and neither has a value of "good" or "bad" for you.

As you can see, a stiff, less compliant material has the capacity to strain – it will just require more force. Tendons can be trained under certain loading parameters to improve stiffness. Whether or not tendons can be passively stretched into increased compliance is still not fully agreed upon – the literature suggests it might, but not definitively. A classic research paper studied the effects of a 3-week passive stretching intervention on tendon stiffness. Results showed no significant change despite a significant increase in flexibility (Kubo, Kanehisa and Fukunaga, 2002). As noted in the stretching chapter, passive resistance torque has been shown in some studies to decrease in response to acute stretching, but those results refer most often to changes in the muscle portion of the muscle-tendon unit (MTU).

Passive stiffness in the entire MTU has been shown to decrease by 31% throughout the passive ROM after a 4-week stretching intervention (i.e. 5 days per week, 4 stretching bouts per day, each consisting of 3 × 30 second repetitions) (Marshall, Cashman and Cheema, 2011). While this particular study design does not indicate in which tissue exactly the change occurs, the decrease in stiffness likely occurs in the muscle region. A recent review concluded that any increase in tendon compliance in response to passive, dynamic, or proprioceptive neuromuscular facilitation (PNF) stretching is trivial, even though a profound effect is commonly asserted (Freitas, Mendes and Andrade, 2017). The researchers reported maximum tolerable passive torque and muscle stiffness as the most common mechanisms of change, reiterating the role of both the sensory and the mechanical theories. Unsurprisingly, considering that for every study finding alterations in mechanical behavior another finds no change in muscle or tendon stiffness, attributing increased flexibility to increases in tolerance only (Konrad and Tilp, 2014), the evidence is said to be equivocal.

Tendons are designed to be particularly stiff given their location and function. Tendons are positioned to longitudinally transmit the force generated by muscle across a joint and to the bone. Greater force production by the muscle increases the tensile stress on tendons. This may lead one to assume one could increase compliance simply by choosing a sedentary lifestyle! It is more likely that one would train in a specific sport and compliant tendons would adapt in response to the demands placed on them. The principle of specificity still applies. Since there are also other factors in mechanical properties (e.g. structure and composition), we can safely reject the notion that inactivity leads to any favorable adaptation. Additionally, stiffness and compliance are only two of the many mechanical behaviors of tendons, so we still have many more terms to define before making any conclusions. For now, we will cover the research on how to adapt tendon stiffness.

Tendon stiffness is a favorable adaptation to high magnitude loading by which tendons increase their load-bearing capacity. Tendons respond particularly well to higher loads, requiring relatively strong muscle contractions. The greater the muscle force, the greater the tensile stress on the tendon, the stiffer they generally become. Colloquially, stiffness

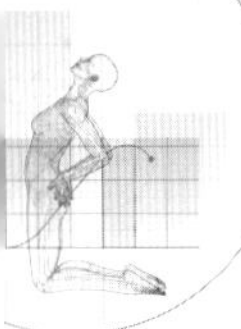

Scientific Literacy

Electromyography

Electromyography (EMG) is a method used to measure the contractile muscular response to an electrical impulse from the nervous system. EMG does not measure the strength, nor the force production of the muscle, but rather the neural drive which excites the muscle (called myoelectric activity) (Vigotsky et al., 2017).

Most EMG studies are conducted by applying sensors to the skin's surface over the target muscle (surface EMG). Less often, EMG is measured using a fine wire electrode inserted into the muscle by penetrating the skin with a needle. As this method is more invasive, garnering approval from the research ethics board is perceived to be more difficult, although I understand this is not necessarily true.

In maximum voluntary contractions (MVC) research, EMG amplitudes are measures of maximal isometric contractions. EMG sensors are applied to the target muscle and the subject is asked to maximally contract isometrically. The sensors are connected to a computer which provides an oscillating representation of the contraction. The highest amplitude represents 100%. Subjects then perform the exercises under investigation and the amplitudes are then divided into the MVC to identify a percentage of muscle activation.

In some cases the MVC in a certain exercise may exceed 100%. This is because the voluntary isometric contraction is not associated with a task and certain conditions of a given task may increase neural drive. For example, maximally contracting your hamstrings against fixed resistance may not produce as much force as trying to reach a personal record in your deadlift. Motivation goes a long way.

has taken on a negative connotation as it's thought to be a maladaptation caused by either too much tension or repetitive motion. Getting rid of stiffness by way of stretching then becomes idealized in spite of the evidence favoring the importance of mechanical loading for tendon adaptation.

Tendons, as with any other adaptable musculoskeletal tissue, follow the progressive overload principle. That is, loads need to be of a high enough magnitude to elicit the adaptive response, but not so high as to exceed capacity. Depending on the research you cite, loads need to be between 60% and 80% of 1 repetition maximum (RM). Recently, however, immense developments in tendon research have greatly improved our understanding of tendon behavior. According to a current comprehensive review on tendon adaptations, we can confidently state that 80% of 1 RM loads over 12 weeks are the preferred minimum load and also that tendons respond to all contraction types. Concentric, isometric, and eccentric contractions all impose enough stress on the tendons to sufficiently increase stiffness when compared to a control, with eccentric contractions

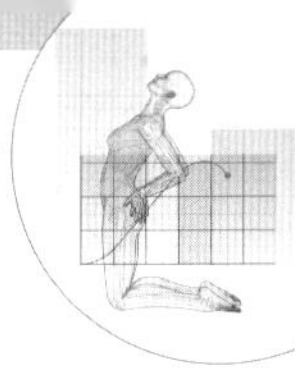

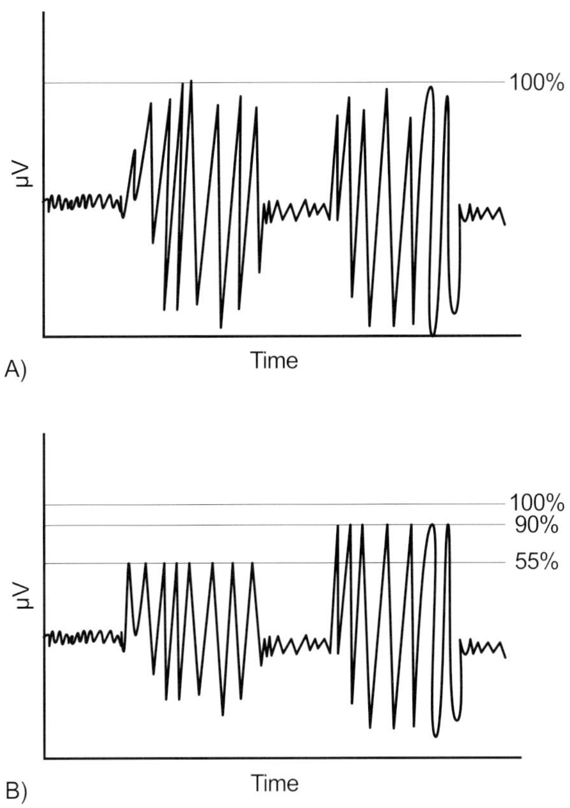

Fig. 3.7
EMG amplitudes. (A) Maximum voluntary contraction (MVC). (B) 55% and 90% MVC.

promoting the greatest adaptations (Malliaras et al., 2013). Isometric contractions will be discussed in more detail later.

A systematic review concluded that, overall, magnitude is more important than contraction type, but tendons also respond to diverse loading, such as variable rate and direction (Bohm, Mersmann and Arampatzis, 2015). Moreover, it has been shown that lighter loads, such as 55% maximum voluntary contraction (MVC), are insufficient when compared to 90% MVC repeated isometric contractions over 14 weeks (Arampatzis, Karamanidis and Albracht, 2007).

The term MVC may be unfamiliar so I will explain here. A 1 RM was explained in Chapter 1. If your 1 RM squat is 50 kg, your strength and conditioning program may then require you train for 8 repetitions (reps) at 80% (40 kg) or 10 reps at 75% (37.5 kg), for example. In yoga, we don't, for the most part, use external weights. We can use a value instead called MVC or maximum voluntary isometric contraction (MVIC). This is measured in a laboratory using electromyograph (EMG) equipment (Fig. 3.7). You would contract the target muscle maximally to measure the maximum value and then you could perform your exercises at 80% as indicated on the monitor. To get a general sense, contract your glutes at maximum effort and then reduce the effort to about 80%. In the beginning it may be easier to start at 10% and ramp up incrementally to 100% and

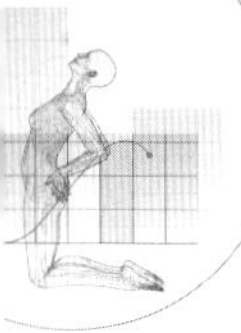

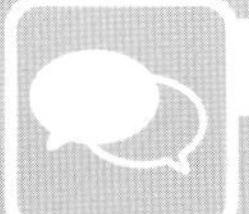

Thought Provoker

Terminology

We use a lot of words in yoga which have different technical definitions from the colloquial ones. The feeling of stiffness, for example, is something we might want to stretch away. Now that stiffness has a specific mechanical definition, it might seem less negative. Consider other terms we use in class: strengthening, toning, stretching, and releasing. Do you have clear mechanical definitions for each of them?

then decrease to 80% to get a feel for it. Of course, without lab equipment we would have no way of knowing if your sensations are accurate, but it does give you a general sense of how much effort is needed to reach loads that induce tendon adaptations.

Yoga Sutra 2:46 states, "*sthira sukham āsanam.*" Loosely translated it means the postures are balanced with steadiness and ease. While the notion is poetic and certainly provides a foundation for a practice rooted in history and tradition, it leaves us with compelling questions, and wanting more. We may choose to teach asana with language of steadiness and ease, but our understanding of biomechanical principles allows us to be more precise. When we choose to imply that yoga strengthens tendons and ligaments, through the tendon research we can now express particular conditions within a yoga practice that may satisfy those implications, and vice versa. Exactly how the contents of this book will influence your teaching is for you to discover. My role is to deliver the research, share with you how I have integrated it into my teaching, and expect you will synthesize the material with far more ingenuity.

Collagen behavior, we have determined, is mutable and adaptable, but to what extent? So far, we have shown that we can improve load-bearing capacity of tissue. Can we improve strain capacity? We shall explore.

Mechanical Range

Mechanical range, or the strain value along the x-axis, is a measure of collagen strain capacity. This limit is not considered to be adaptable; meaning the horizontal position of the ultimate fail point on the stress–strain curve does not migrate horizontally. The yield point is also fixed horizontally. Vertically, however, these positions do fluctuate in response to changes in stiffness (slope). This tells us that we can increase our capacity to withstand stress prior to reaching strain capacity, but strain capacity itself is mostly fixed. A subject to explore then is whether or not plastic changes resulting in longer, or shorter, tissues are possible.

In ROM research, we represent the relationship between force and range with the torque angle curve (Fig. 3.8). Two possible mechanisms for changes in ROM are often considered. First, the actual amount of available tissue could potentially increase in total length and would thereby display a torque angle curve that is entirely shifted along the horizontal axis. A shorter tissue would display a curve shifted to the left, and a longer tissue to the right. Second, the tissue could simply change its extensibility and would thereby display a curve with the same starting values for angle and torque but with a different trajectory. Extensibility (earlier referred to as "stretchability") is defined as a "change in joint angle with the application of a standardized torque" (Ben and Harvey, 2010). In stretching studies, when we do see extensibility changes we tend to see curves that are shifted neither left nor right. Therefore, we cannot confidently conclude tissue changes in length as a response to stretching.

Referring back to the anesthesia studies, the tissues appear to have enough length to achieve greater joint ROMs when the nervous system's control is diminished or blocked. If ROM were compromised by shortened tissue, one might expect the tissue to refuse to yield or, at the very worst, the tissue to be damaged/torn during the anesthetized stretch.

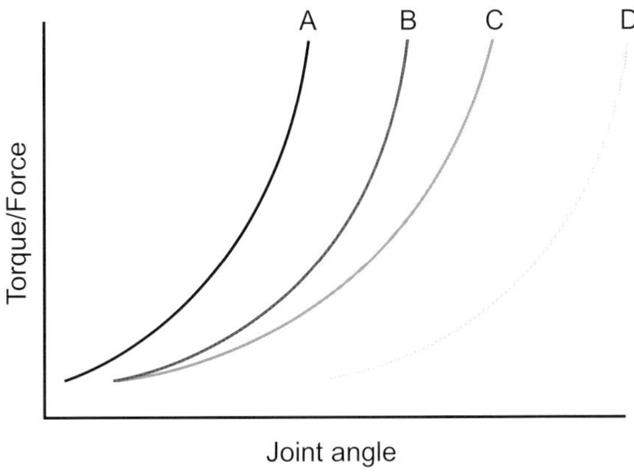

Fig. 3.8

Hypothetical relationship between varying tissue lengths at standardized resistance torque. (A) Shortened tissue. (B and C) "Normal" tissue length with lesser and greater extensibility. (D) Lengthened tissue.

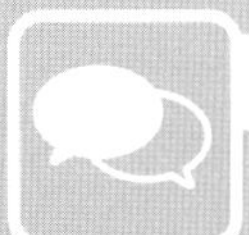

Thought Provoker

Tight Hamstrings

In the case of those infamously tight and unyielding hamstrings, it is far more likely that the feeling of tightness is the source of proprioceptive input provided by the muscle spindles (sensory receptors within muscles detecting changes in length) than by shortened tissue. This would explain the sensation associated with tightness and would further explain why anybody stretching will feel tight at their own end range of motion (ROM), including the very flexible. What is your position on the effects of tissue stretching on length? Can you stretch "normal" healthy tissue too much?

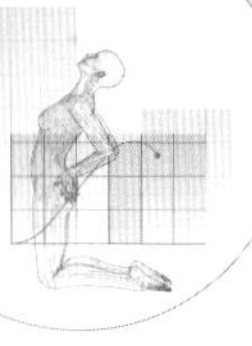

Conversely, if the stretched tissue adapted to become plastically longer, this adaptation could not possibly occur in a single anesthetized stretch.

ROM aside, just looking at the stress–strain curve, if plastic changes in length did occur over time, this would result in a change *in units* of the composite material (collagen) being stretched, not in the behavior of the collagen. Mechanical range, defined by the limit of its capacity for strain (i.e. ultimate fail point), is known to be about 8–10%. It has been found to decrease to 3% when insufficiently stretched or to increase to 20% when stretched often. This still leaves us with the question about plastic changes in tissue length.

Let us explore the concept of tightness. The colloquial use of the term "tight" often conjures up images of "shrunken" and shortened length of tissue. If the tight tissues were shortened, then reducing tightness would have to require tissue lengthening, but skeptics of fascial release techniques (e.g. static stretching, foam rolling, etc.) are not convinced they are effective for improving mechanical range or length. Scleroderma, also known as systemic sclerosis, is an autoimmune disease triggering an overproduction of collagen which results in hardened, thickened collagenous tissues marked by mechanical rigidity. If fascial release techniques lengthened tissue or altered mechanical range, we might have a known treatment for scleroderma, but to date, we do not. While popular fascial release techniques, in the general population, do often lead one to experience increases in flexibility outcomes and a decrease in the sensation of tightness, we simply do not have enough compelling evidence to suggest collagen actually increases in length.

Another common condition worth discussing is the **contracture**. The term also implies some sort or shortened tissue, but with the information we have discussed thus far we should be compelled to investigate further, beginning with the definition of a contracture. A review of the literature (Farmer and James, 2001; Fergusson, Hutton and Drodge, 2007) resulted in the following composite definition: Any orthopedic or neurological condition which may limit range of motion by affecting the joint capsule, ligaments, tendons, or muscles, skin and subcutaneous tissue, for which the epidemiological, etiological, biomechanical, biochemical, pathophysiological, and genetic factors are mostly unknown and uncertain. This tells us very little about the condition, or the cause for that matter, other than it is marked by limited ROM. In fact, individuals who present with contractures can have conditions ranging from spinal cord or brain injuries through strokes and burns to post-operative scarring and more. If contractures were caused solely by shortened joint capsules and ligaments, and stretching lengthened these tissues, one would expect stretching to reverse the contracture.

Pause and turn to page 106 for a summary of related research.

Now, let us explore the opposite of tightness, the concept of **laxity**. Laxity is another one of those terms that has developed an implied meaning that does not align with the definition found in the scientific literature. Yoga students are often warned against over-stretching, suggesting that too much stretching results in permanently loose, lengthened, and slackened tissues. In terms of changes to collagen, laxity is defined as the "percent change in nonrecoverable length" from pre to post loading and is a result of temporary morphological changes after loading and fatiguing. With rest, changes revert, and tension is reestablished (Freedman et al., 2015). Laxity is not defined by plastic changes in length and whatever changes do occur are temporary and recoverable with rest. It should be noted here that laxity is not referring to the loss of tensile strength that might result from a ligament injury due to a high-rate, high-magnitude force, or even surgery. Interestingly, injured ligaments were thought to be inert tissues with little to no capacity to recover their mechanical properties, but they are today recognized as highly active tissues that increase their recovery potential with early loading (Hauser et al., 2013). Finally, laxity is also not the same as hypermobility, which is a genetic condition marked by decreased collagen tension resulting from disruptions in collagen structure. Hypermobility will be discussed further in later chapters, once collagen structure has been explored.

Speaking of temporary changes, the time has arrived to discuss another series of mechanical behaviors which result in impermanent changes. Until this point we have reduced collagen to an elastic tissue, but connective tissues are not purely elastic because they exhibit additional behaviors not represented by the stress–strain curve. These behaviors are qualities of **viscoelasticity**, where the effect of time on mechanical properties reflects how viscous behaviors blend with elastic behavior.

Viscoelastic Phenomena

Viscoelasticity is the combination of viscosity and elasticity. Viscosity is the measure of a material's (usually a fluid) resistance to shear when strained. Similarly to elasticity, when a force is applied the behavior of a viscous substance is measured by its resistance stress, a result of the internal friction of the substance. Honey, when compared with water, is an example of a more viscous fluid. A teaspoon of honey resists shear when poured off the spoon, more than a teaspoon of water. As we have established, elasticity describes a solid material's ability to return to resting length. A rubber band is an example of an elastic

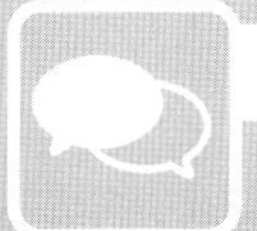

Thought Provoker

Gummy Worms

Gummy worms, made of hydrolyzed collagen, are excellent examples of viscoelastic materials and demonstrate the behavior of connective tissue quite well. I bring gummy worms to my live courses to provide tactile experience of creep and stress relaxation. One weekend I taught at a vegan studio and they would not allow me to bring the gummy worms. Instead, they bought me vegan gummy worms, made of a plant-based thickening agent. My demonstration did not work, which proved to be a useful lesson in itself.

As you read through the following section on viscoelasticity, you may want to stretch a non-vegan gummy worm with the described parameters to witness the behaviors.

material which returns to resting length when the load is removed. Honey, however, is not elastic; if it were, upon up-righting the spoon, the honey would recoil back into the spoon. To envision a viscoelastic material, combine the qualities of a rubber band with the qualities of honey where the honey slows the strain of the rubber band and the rubber band aids the honey in returning to resting length. Human connective tissue, as well as the individual collagen fibrils of which it is composed, exhibit this viscoelastic behavior (Svensson et al., 2010).

Viscoelastic phenomena are time and temperature dependent, where strain patterns and the resulting stress are conditional to variables such as rate, duration, or °C. As noted in the stress–strain curve, elastic behavior is a positive, linear relationship between stress and strain. Viscoelastic materials, like collagen, do not quite behave linearly as the internal friction does not remain constant. In order to express connective tissue behavior more specifically, we must consider additional relationships.

Creep and Recovery

Creep is the viscoelastic phenomenon explained by the relationship between strain and time (Fig. 3.9). A material that creeps is characterized by an initially rapid increase in strain followed by a slower increase in strain over time, where stress is held constant. If you were to pull on the two opposite ends of a viscoelastic material (e.g. a gummy worm) at a constant force, following the immediate change in length, the material will continue to strain, albeit at a slower rate. In the human muscle–tendon unit, the greatest strain has been measured to occur within the first 15–20 seconds, after which the strain slows considerably (Ryan et al., 2010).

When human connective tissues creep, they become temporarily lengthened. Creep is not a plastic response, nor an elastic response, but a viscoelastic response. Upon unloading, the tissue recovers and returns to its resting length, although at a slower rate than an elastic material. Even in the case of prolonged, progressive creep, the tissue recovers. Additionally, creep is not damaging to the collagen fibers as perhaps an abrupt, forceful

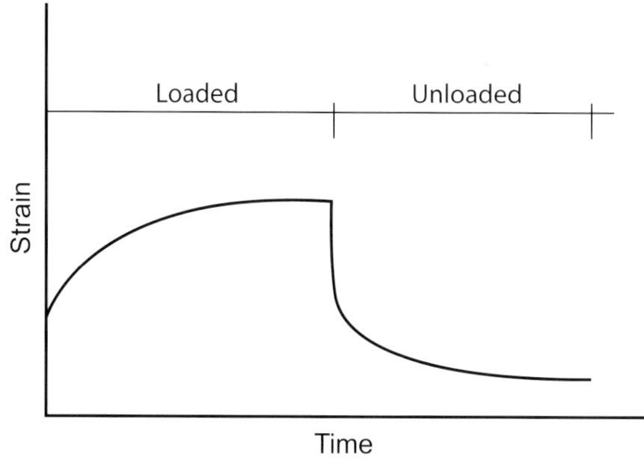

Fig. 3.9
Creep and recovery. Under a constant load, viscoelastic tissues strain quickly at first and then at a slowing rate over time. When the load is removed the tissue recovers.

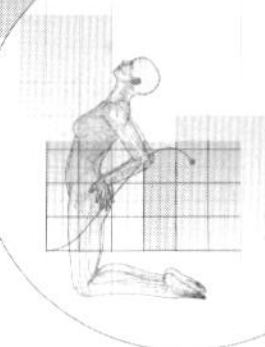

stretch might be. Viscoelastic phenomena occur due to temporary changes in molecular arrangement, not due to structural damage or micro tears. Analogies such as gummy worms or taffy are therefore imperfect, especially when we creep these analogous materials long enough to fail. The human body is a closed system and tissues, therefore, do not creep to failure with everyday, normal movements, including long stretches or excessive bouts of immobility. If that were the case, the average office worker who constantly sits on the job might find her lumbodorsal fascia dragging behind her on the floor at the end of a long workday. Since creep is a recoverable phenomenon, it is neither a concern for damage nor for long-term weakening via plastic adaptations.

In the immediate moment of creep, however, there will be decrease in stiffness and elasticity. Doug Richards, a kinesiology professor at the University of Toronto, tells the story of how the Toronto airport was able to reduce the amount of back injuries that were occurring while passengers were retrieving their luggage by redesigning the airport to include a longer walk between the gates and baggage claim. After hours of sitting on a plane, the lumbodorsal fascia and spinal ligaments creep and the diminished stiffness means there is less elasticity available to assist in lifting a heavy load, placing greater demand on the mechanically disadvantaged spinal muscles. The long walk through the terminal is sufficient time for the tissues to recover, stiffness and elasticity are restored, and the connective tissue is again able to share the workload with the back muscles.

Scientific Literacy

Inflated Conclusions

It can be tempting at times to make inflated conclusions when interpreting research. The catchy phrase "sitting is the new smoking" is an example of an inflated conclusion. We do have evidence that a sedentary life has its health risks. We also have evidence that isolated bouts of exercise may not be enough to counteract an otherwise sedentary life. Of course, we have evidence that exercise has health benefits. Combined, these do not imply that sitting has a mortality rate similar to smoking. Such a statement has resulted in the rise of standing desks. Assuming that standing at a work station is better than sitting at a work station all day is another inflated conclusion. Just because sitting for extended periods of time may be harmful, it does not automatically imply standing for extended periods of time is beneficial.

Inflated conclusions are dramatic and attention grabbing. This is why consumer media inflate conclusions when reporting on research. Interpreting research with integrity can be dry, mundane and unsatisfying. Certainty is much more appealing than uncertainty. It's far more interesting to know that coffee will kill you or that red wine will save your life, than it is to consider the dosage and all the other variables that might play a role in your life expectancy. It is advisable to always read the original research paper when possible.

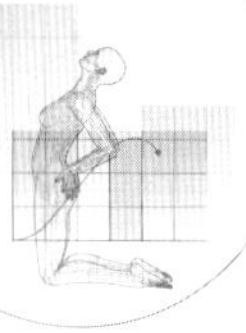

Likewise, creep should not be assumed to be beneficial for increasing capacity. In order to increase load-bearing capacity, we must increase loading parameters. Yes, duration is one of those parameters, but within a framework of progressive magnitude, direction, and rate. It is possible that passive stretch and creep would induce adaptation in drastically untrained tissues, or perhaps in the early stages of rehabilitation post injury, but it is unlikely at later stages of training. Creep is the measure of the change in strain over time at a constant load, not a progressive load. If passively creeping your tissues was an effective application of progressive overload, the office worker would develop tremendous load-bearing capacity from hours of creeping while sitting at her desk! Everything we know about exercise and adaptation tells us this is not the case, and substantial adaptation requires the input of higher intensity stressors.

Some yoga practices consist of passive stretches held for approximately 3–5 minutes. The purpose of these long-held stretches varies from a quieting of the nervous system to a stressing of the connective tissue, depending on the instructor. Biomechanics is our focus here, and our interest lies in uncovering a quantifiable effect on connective tissue during such stretches. If you recall, the ACSM guidelines for flexibility training are in the 30–60 second range, therefore most of the stretching research observes the shorter durations and measures outcomes that we discussed in Chapter 2, such as injury and performance. The few published studies that look at longer holds measure muscle architecture, passive resistance torque, changes in tissue behavior and cellular activities (we will cover those not yet examined later).

Creep is frequently studied in terms of function, pain, and load transfer. Creep may also play a role in the prevention of "overstretching" ligaments, protecting the tissue by altering crimp patterns and inducing temporary laxity (Hauser et al., 2013). It is possible that the long passive stretches some of us warn against to prevent "overstretching" are exactly the mechanism by which we prevent it! To date, however, I am not aware of any studies measuring the short- or long-term positive adaptive responses to stretching interventions of passive 3–5 minute holds resembling those of a yoga class, where creep is the mechanism of action central to the study design.

What we do know is that creep is a measure of strain over time. We also know that

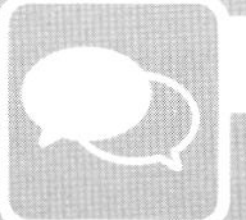

Thought Provoker

Stretching Ligaments

A lot is said about stretching connective tissue. Some say stretching tendons and/or ligaments is useful, some say it is dangerous. As usual, the answer probably lies somewhere in the middle and will depend on the individual. Can you identify what you have learned, what you believe, what you have dismissed, and if the information presented thus far has challenged you to reconsider what you may have heard?

increasing load-bearing capacity requires progressive loading. Increased strain that occurs as a function of a creep is a function of time, not progressive loading (remember, load is constant), and is also recoverable. Therefore, without further evidence it is prudent to conclude that creep does not sufficiently stress connective tissue to permanently alter the stress–strain curve. Some very recent interesting developments in our understanding of the microbiology of stretching, however, suggest there is much to learn. I would expect future studies to influence our current conclusions about low load, passive stretching effects on connective tissue. We will explore these themes further in the following chapter on histology.

Stress Relaxation

Stress relaxation is the viscoelastic phenomenon explained by the relationship between stress and time (Fig. 3.10). To measure stress relaxation, strain remains constant and the change in stress over time is examined, whereas with creep, the load is constant and the change in strain over time is measured. This phenomenon is characterized by an initially high stress that decreases over time while maintaining the initial strain. If you were to pull on the two opposite ends of a viscoelastic material (e.g. a gummy worm, again) until you reached a specific length and held this length constant, you would find that over time the effort required to hold the position would decrease. In other words, it would require less force over time to maintain a constant

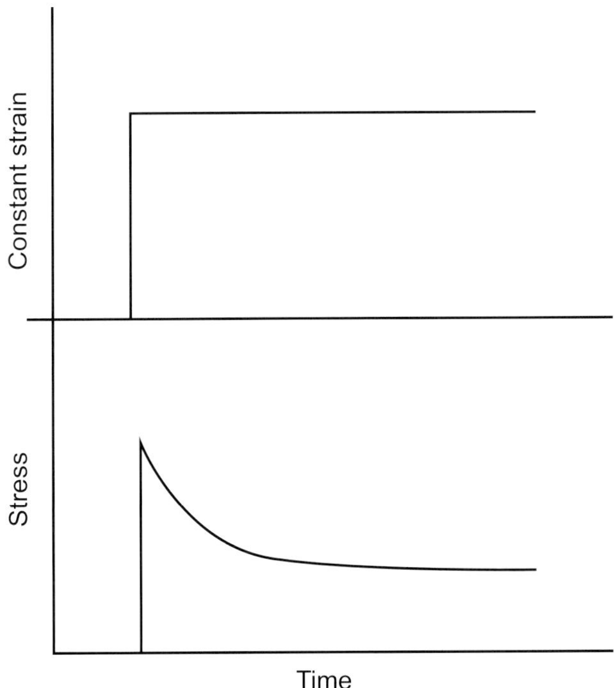

Fig. 3.10

Stress relaxation. Under a constant strain, the initial stress in viscoelastic tissues is high at first and then decreases at a slowing rate over time.

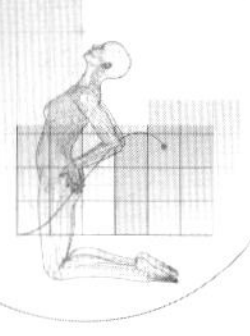

strain and, concurrently, the resistance to shear would also decrease. As with creep, this is a function of temporary changes in molecular arrangement and decreases in internal friction, not permanent ones.

Stress relaxation contributes to the reduction in passive resistance torque during static stretching. While it is not the only factor to consider in this change in behavior, it certainly helps to explain why a stretch may feel like it encounters less resistance as time in the pose increases. The sensation of less resistance over time could be purely sensory or could be the result of an actual shift in the mechanical state. The purpose here is not to review the details of the abundance of stretching data again, but to highlight the behavior of our connective tissue so we may have a greater understanding of the variables at play during a stretch. When we perceive connective tissue to behave in an absolute and finite manner, we lose sight of its complexity. When we reduce viscoelastic connective tissues to elastic analogies like rubber bands and therabands, we get an incomplete picture. Tissue behavior modifies continually, even within the same individual during a given stretch, based simply on time in the position.

With regards to restorative yoga and 3–5 minute passive stretches, we can learn a lot from creep and stress relaxation as a theory, even without proficiency in the specific research on the topic. Our biggest lesson here may be in the language we use when teaching these postures. You now understand that an overall feeling of looseness and improved flexibility after a yoga class may be due to temporary viscoelastic changes, rather than evidence of permanent changes in tissue length. Ultimately, we may choose to make fewer claims about the effects of yoga on flexibility as the role of creep and stress relaxation have not, as of yet, been studied in the context of yoga.

Hysteresis

The study of **hysteresis** requires we return to the stress–strain curve and Hooke's Law. Hysteresis defines the before and after behavior of the elastic region of the stress–strain curve (Fig. 3.11). The dependence on time, however, is not measured by duration, as in

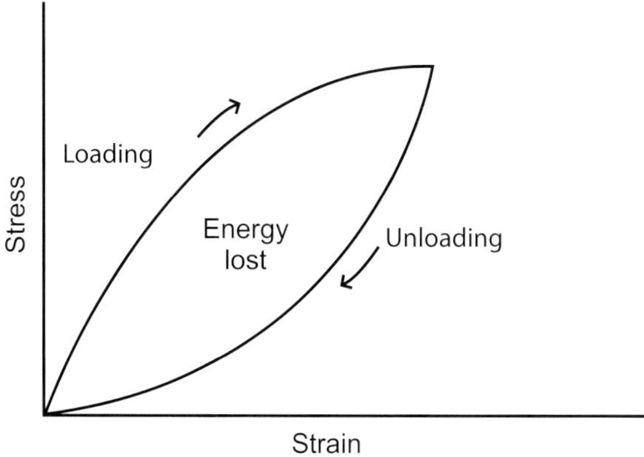

Fig. 3.11
Hysteresis. The hysteresis loop represents the energy lost between loading and unloading.

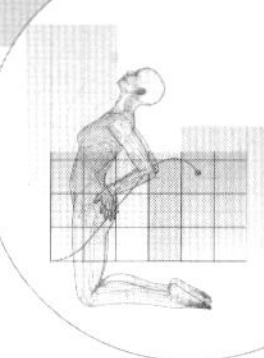

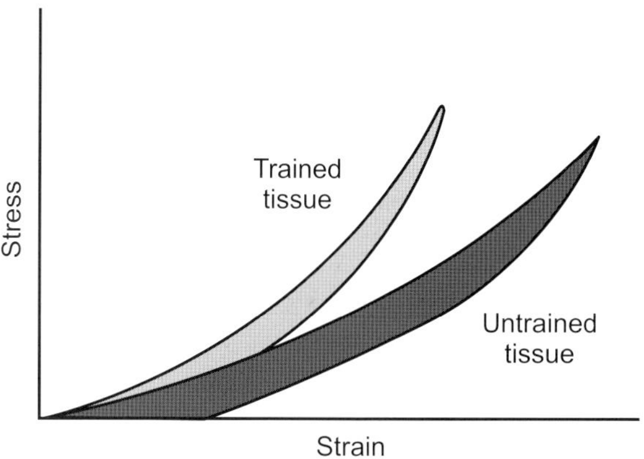

Fig. 3.12
Comparison of hysteresis curves. Training can increase the energy storage capacity of tissues. Illustration modified after Schleip et al. (2012).

the case of creep and stress relaxation, but rather represents behavior as a reliance on the preceding event. A purely elastic material, when stretched, stores 100% of the energy as potential energy. When the load is removed, zero energy is lost and the return to resting length follows the same linear pathway during both loading and unloading. The amount of energy stored when the band is stretched determines the amount of energy released; the latter relies on the former. As you may recall, this proportional relationship (Hooke's Law), which explains the behavior of a perfect spring where 100% of the applied force is captured, stored, and released, does not adequately explain tissue behavior (nor any other material for that matter), because some energy is technically always lost.

In viscoelastic materials, the stress to strain ratio changes between loading and unloading. If a tendon is stretched, the stress is less during unloading than during loading. Graphically, the result is a loading curve, followed by an unloading curve positionally dependent on the previous curve. The potential energy stored during the stretch that does not convert to kinetic energy when the tissue is unloaded changes form and becomes thermal energy. This transformed energy is expressed by the area in between the two curves which represents energy "lost" and dissipated as heat (as energy cannot be created or destroyed, therefore it must go somewhere).

The less the area between the curves, the more efficient the tissue. The greater the area between the curves, the less efficient the tissue. Tendons with smaller hysteresis values display greater qualities of elasticity and have greater capacity to store energy. Tendons with larger hysteresis values display lesser qualities of elasticity and have diminished capacity to store energy. Additionally, as with other mechanical behaviors within the elastic region, hysteresis is also adaptable (Fig. 3.12). Training in activities that require greater storage capacity will result in tissues that develop lower hysteresis values (i.e. capacity to store more potential energy). One could say a larger hysteresis value, perhaps as an effect of untrained or deconditioned tissue, displays a dampening effect.

Another imperfect but satisfactory analogy which serves to explain a dampening effect is a screen door that has been affixed with an external source of friction, known actually as a dampener. The spring alone is subject to Hooke's Law, therefore, no energy should be lost between the loading and unloading phase. When we let go of the screen door, it would slam shut. A dampener can be installed, however, to absorb some of that stored energy so there is less force remaining when you let go (i.e. unloading). The energy absorbed by the dampener allows for softer closure of the screen door. In the case of hysteresis, no external dampener is applied, and the mechanism is built into the mechanical behavior of the tissue.

In terms of human performance, the dampening effect is generally an undesirable quality. In cyclical activities such as running, the less energy lost (i.e. a lower hysteresis value), the more efficiently your body will move. Rather than producing muscle force to generate each joint position through the gait cycle, energy is stored and reused to create springiness. For example, an arbitrary tendon hysteresis value of 20% translates into a remaining 80% of potential energy available for returning the tendon to its resting length. This translates into decreased metabolic fatigue and increased running economy.

As we already know, static stretching may have a detrimental effect on stiffness in the short term. We may, therefore, conclude that static stretching has little advantage for a runner, particularly before a run. Interestingly, however, static stretching decreases hysteresis. In a study of eight male subjects who statically stretched the medial gastrocnemius three times per day over a 3-week period (each session consisted of five static stretches, each held for 45 seconds) tendon hysteresis decreased from 19.9% to 12.5%. That translates into an additional 7.4% increase in reusable energy. Such a stretching protocol may increase running economy and be advantageous after all (Kubo, Kanehisa and Fukunaga, 2002).

Additionally, the same research team found that after a single held 10-minute long stretch of the same muscle, hysteresis decreased similarly (Kubo et al., 2001). Since these papers did not actually measure running outcomes, we cannot claim an effect either way. It does, however, demand we consider the possibility. Maybe a pre-run stretch is not as bad as much of the performance research has concluded.

Thought Provoker

Strain Rate Sensitivity

For a tactile experience of strain rate sensitivity try making a dense paste using cornstarch and water. Prepare this mixture in small bowl by adding cornstarch slowly and mixing well before adding more. The mixture is ready once the paste is relatively firm (appearing to be solid with no fluid-like areas). Slowly press the pad of your thumb into the surface and feel your finger sink into the mixture. Now rapidly press your thumb onto the surface and notice the mixture does not yield to you.

Are there any other materials you can think of that exhibit strain rate sensitivity? How much do you think strain rate sensitivity influences yoga *āsana*?

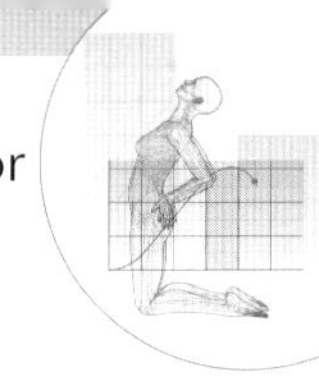

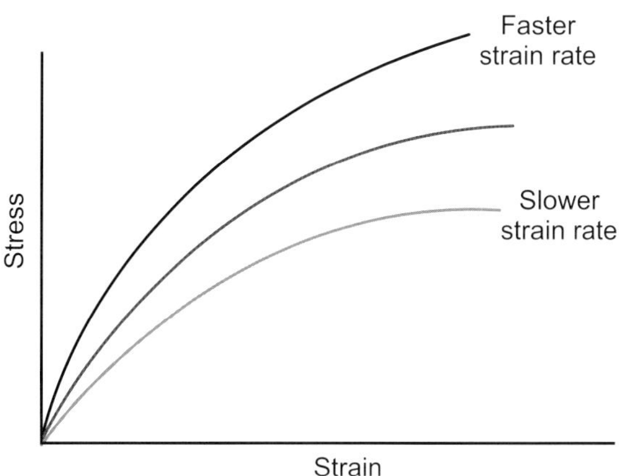

Fig. 3.13
Strain rate sensitivity. The ratio of stress to strain is rate dependent.

Strain Rate Sensitivity

Generally, but not always, a slow *rate of strain* will resist less than a rapid rate of strain (Fig. 3.13). For example, imagine pushing honey through a syringe at different rates. The slower rate will be met with the least resistance and the faster rate will be met with the greatest resistance. This mechanical behavior is referred to as the strain rate and is displayed by human connective tissues. Bones loaded at a faster rate behave with greater stiffness than those loaded at a slower rate, exhibiting strain rate sensitivity. Thankfully, bones are excellent at absorbing forces at high rates, enabling us to perform a variety of physical feats, but as we know, bones have their limits.

Scientific Literacy

Rater Reliability

Reliability refers to the consistency by which data are collected. The data collectors are referred to as "raters" because they assess and rate one or more variables. For example, when measuring range of motion (ROM) before and after a 6-week stretching intervention, the data collector must identically position the participant, determine the precise location of her anatomical landmarks, and then accurately place the goniometer to read the resulting joint angle. Any number of factors could compromise a reliable rating: different clothing worn by the participant, using a different model goniometer between trials, poor rater training, etc.

Inter-rater reliability refers to the consistency across multiple data collectors and intra-rater reliability refers to the consistency across a single data collector. Variability among and within human raters serves as a potential source of error and can

Continued on next page

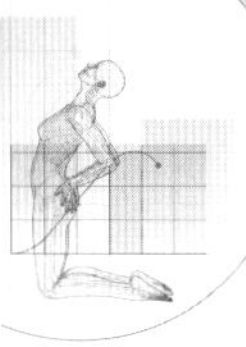

Continued from previous page

be detrimental for the overall confidence and accuracy of a study. It is rare to find perfect agreement among raters, and therefore studies often try to minimize variability through training. Statistical tests then analyze the differences between raters and within raters to determine effectiveness of training and reliability of the methods employed during data collection.

As a non-scientific, but fun, real-world example where rater reliability is crucial, I'll refer back to my years as a bartender. Each month, the liquor inventory was always done between closing on the 31st and opening on the 1st of every month (New Year's Day was never fun). One bartender picked up each bottle individually, looked at its contents and rated it on its fullness on a scale of 1 to 10; an almost empty bottle was rated with a 1, a bottle half full was rated with a 5, and so on. Another bartender had a clipboard and a list of the liquors and would write the number next to the corresponding brand/type. The number one rule was to be consistent with our duties. We never changed roles, or the inventory would be erratic because my 7 might be another bartender's 8. Expand that margin of error to a nightclub with more than 10 points of sale and hundreds of bottles of open liquor, projecting profits and loss with any level of accuracy would be impossible.

Strain rate is considered in regard to the anterior cruciate ligament (ACL), a ligament that is often injured because it is frequently subjected to sudden changes in direction or speed (high rate loads). Earlier, it was mentioned that hamstring tendons and patellar tendons are often grafted to repair a torn ACL, this is partially because they have similar strain rate sensitivities and therefore suitably replicate ACL behavior.

Strain rate sensitivity is also taken into account when researching stretching. If you have a pool of subjects stretching their calves, and one subject unknowingly dorsiflexes at a faster rate than another subject, any differences in stiffness measures may be due to failure to control for strain rate sensitivity. This would be considered a poor study design. More often, you will find experiments account for this phenomenon by indicating in the methods section the velocity at which the subjects were passively stretched and how many degrees of joint rotation were administered. For example, Kubo et al. (2001), measured the stiffness of the medial gastrocnemius tendon after a 10-minute passive stretch, and noted that each of the seven male participants was moved from 0 to 35 degrees of dorsiflexion at a constant velocity of 5 degrees per second. You can imagine that 7 seconds to dorsiflexion is relatively slow when compared to how people normally stretch their calves. This was likely intentional, so as not to be met with increased resistance to stretch due to rapid loading.

Whether or not strain-rate sensitivity dictates how we should perform postures is up for discussion. On one hand, the velocity at which we enter a pose may affect ROM due to strain-rate sensitivity. It's hard to know if that difference is distinguishable by sensation or appearance (not requiring lab equipment to measure). If so, perhaps our ubiquitous "letting go" instruction could simply be achieved by

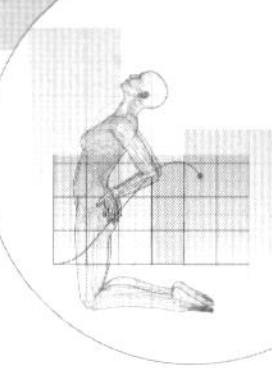

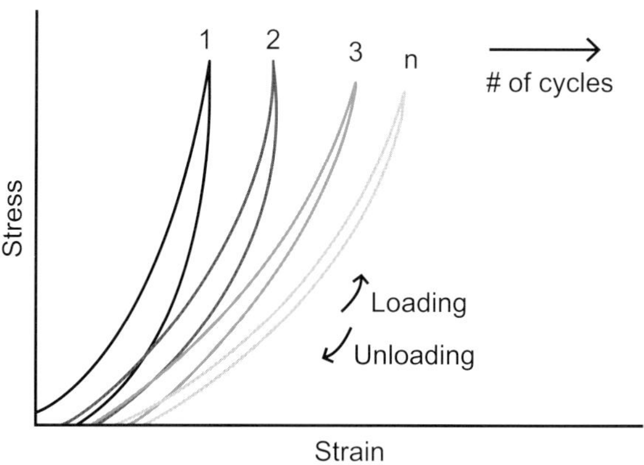

Fig. 3.14
Cycle effect – hysteresis. Storage capacity increases with consecutive loading.

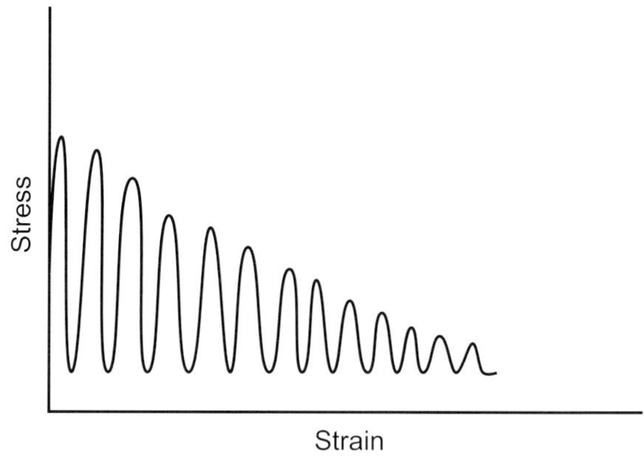

Fig. 3.15
Cycle effect – stress relaxation. Stress decreases with consecutive loading.

slowing things down a bit in the transitions rather than trying to relax muscles once in the pose. On the other hand, moving into poses quickly might create conditions promoting elasticity. Neither one is better, and the selection should be determined by intended outcomes.

Cycle Effect

Finally, some viscoelastic phenomena, such as hysteresis and stress relaxation, are further defined by their behavior over repetitions. Called the **cycle effect**, each consecutive stress measure is dependent on the previous stress measure.

During hysteresis (Fig. 3.14), each time the tissue is placed under tension, the stored potential energy lost (area inside the loading and unloading curves) decreases. The storage capacity increases as the number of cycles increases. During repetitive jumping (i.e. the Achilles tendon is stretched and released) the amount of muscle force needed to create the movement will decrease with each subsequent jump and the economy of the movement will be more efficient.

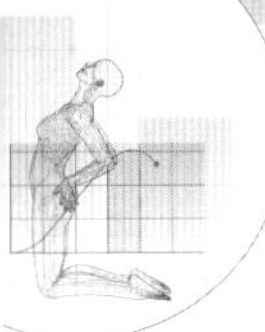

Correspondingly, during stress-relaxation (Fig. 3.15), for each subsequent strain repetition, stress decreases. Ballistic stretching, where one bounces in a stretched position, may be met with less resistance for each subsequent bounce as the tissues undergo stress relaxation. I'm speculating here, but perhaps it was once thought that the decreasing resistance in response to repetitive stretching was cause for potential risk of tissue damage, and that is why ballistic stretching fell out fashion for some time. Knowing what we know today, however, such an assumption now seems misinformed. Recently, ballistic stretching has, in fact, been capitalized on as method of fascia training complete with teaching certifications (Schleip and Müller, 2013). It seems that the safety recommendations to avoid load have been replaced with the protective effects of load exposure.

Temperature

Another variable, in addition to load and time, which influences tissues and gets its fair share of judgment on opposing sides is temperature. Most viscoelastic materials exhibit less internal friction when warm, meaning they are easier to strain. While everyone can hopefully agree that warm-ups are beneficial in preparing the body for the greater intensity load parameters to follow, there are some disagreements about temperature.

Concerning a standard warm-up as suggested by the ACSM, some light cardio and/or dynamic movements effectively brings blood flow to the muscles and warms up the tissue. If stretching is part of the warm-up, ACSM suggests dynamic stretching except in circumstances where static stretching is specific to the sport, such as ballet dancing (Garber et al., 2011). In terms of mechanical behavior, the increase in temperature changes connective tissue viscoelasticity by reducing the internal friction, theoretically reducing the risk of injury. Honey pours more easily when warm than cold; it is easier to add honey from a spoon to a hot cup of tea than to add the honey to a glass of iced tea. Movement is met with less resistance and greater ease when the musculoskeletal tissues are warm than when they are cold.

The effect of temperature on tissues, however, is not as straightforward as simply warming-up since temperature is not consistent throughout the body or across all populations. The gastrointestinal tract has a higher temperature than the brain and spinal cord, which in turn have a higher temperature than the skin. This design allows for transfer and dissipation of heat away from the higher temperature areas to maintain thermal homeostasis. Joints lacking dense surrounding musculature, such as the knee and ankle, tend to remain cooler after a warm-up. Women, during certain phases of their menstrual cycle exhibit cooler overall body temperatures, a time which has been associated with greater incidence of ACL tears. Cooler, minimally insulated distal joints have been shown to require more force to passively move through an ROM than after the use of an externally applied heat source such as a heat wrap (Petrofsky, Laymon and Lee, 2013). The conclusion here may be that practicing yoga in a hot room is beneficial to distal joints and will reduce injury. There is much concern about hot yoga as it is often practiced in highly humid rooms over 40°C (104°F).

In this environment sweating cannot function as well to cool the body and maintain thermal homeostasis. Thus core temperatures rise along with a proposed risk for heat injury or heat stroke. Another common argument for the risks of hot yoga is that stretching in these elevated temperatures can cause injury to connective tissue, as the heat causes a decrease in internal friction and weakens its resistance via viscoelastic phenomena. Collagen may be more susceptible to failure at lower strain percentages when reaching temperatures upwards of 40°C (104°F). The internal body temperature, however, is remarkably stable due to homeostatic efficiency. If our internal temperatures fluctuated easily in response to our external environment, we would experience impaired function of most systems in the body on a hot summer day or a cold winter night. Regardless, the presumption here contradicts the previous one by concluding yoga practiced in a hot room might be dangerous to the joints rather than beneficial.

The effect of hot yoga on connective tissue viscoelastic behavior has not, to my knowledge, been studied directly. Recently, however, a published study set out to measure core temperatures in students practicing hot yoga via an ingestible body temperature sensor. The results averaged 103.2°F in men and 102.0°F in women, temperature thresholds at which the risk for heat-related complications increases substantially (Quandt et al., 2015). Although there was no control group, these

Pause and turn to page 107 for a summary of related research.

levels are certainly alarming (and would be for any type of exercise), resulting in an online objection about the particular study design instigated by another researcher whose team used the same type of sensor but normalized the data collected at far more frequent intervals and found average temperatures to remain in the safe zone of 100.3°F (Fritz et al., 2014). The conflicting data reflect core temperatures and not those of surface tissues, therefore, we cannot conclude that collagen structure around the distal joints has been impaired. My suggestion is we find some middle ground. Hot yoga may pose some risks at extreme exertion levels, but whether those risks include greater susceptibility to stretch-related injuries cannot be concluded based on the available evidence.

Mechanical Properties

Post undergraduate school I spent some time pursuing a second degree in civil engineering, and therefore had a decent amount of exposure to materials science. When I first studied connective tissue mechanics, I could not believe that the same graphs, equations, and mechanical terminology I had studied during my years in engineering school existed for the human body. I don't know why I never considered this information would be available for human tissue. Obviously, after my first graduate level biomechanics course, I knew I had finally found the field of study which would answer the many questions that had gone unanswered over the years.

Admittedly, I was too quick to jump to conclusions. My eagerness, along with a strong bias that yoga caused a host of soft tissue stretching injuries, resulted in a narrow view of mechanical behavior on tissue properties. I saw the stress–strain as an absolute

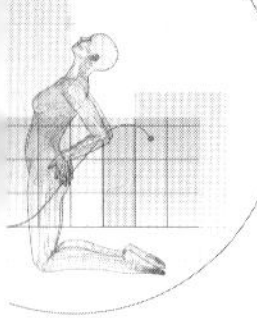

model: stay within the elastic region, you are safe; venture into the plastic region, you are asking for trouble. What further study revealed to me is that mechanical properties are not only governed by behavior, but also by structure and composition. Unfortunately this required a commitment to the study of microbiology, which my math and engineering mind wanted to reject. Fortunately, a detailed and complex study of the microscopic cellular and extra-cellular aspects of tissue is not necessary to gain an appreciation of its role in mechanical properties. An overview of both structure and composition will suffice.

Research Summary

Cochrane Review on Stretching

Stretch for the Treatment and Prevention of Contracture: An Abridged Republication of a Cochrane Systematic Review (Harvey et al., 2017)

Background

Contractures impair range of motion (ROM) and negatively affect function and quality of life. Stretching is currently the preferred treatment for contractures of both orthopedic and neurological origins.

Purpose

The review sets out to determine the short-term effects (within 1 week after the intervention) on ROM in subjects with contractures.

Methods

Databases were searched for papers that fit several criteria. The subjects could be any age and either had a contracture or were predisposed to developing a contracture. Stretch interventions had be administered for at least 20 seconds more than once and had to be compared against a control. Stretch application included body positions, splints, casting, and manual therapy. Active or passive mobility of a synovial joint was measured in degrees, passive torque, or a linear distance between two body parts. After screening, 28 papers on neurological cases and 21 on orthopedic cases were included, containing 898 subjects and 1237 subjects respectively.

Results

The neurological cases averaged a 2 degree change in ROM and the orthopedic cases a 1 degree change, both ranging largely between 0 and 3 degrees. In both cases, the researchers deemed the results clinically insignificant since a maximum improvement in joint mobility appears to be just 3 degrees. In all studies, the interventions lasted no longer than 7 months, most lasting between 4 and 12 weeks. The shortest

Continued on next page

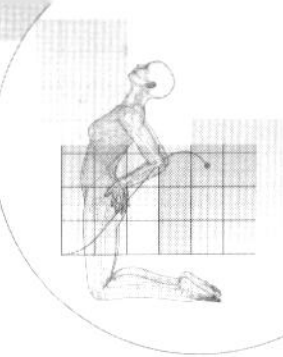

Continued from previous page

duration was 1.7 hours of stretch over 2 weeks, the longest was 1512 hours of stretch over 9 weeks (24 hours per day in a splint). Another dozen studies included more than 500 hours of stretching, some of which were over 1000 hours. The paper concluded "stretch does not have clinically important effects on joint mobility" in subjects diagnosed with contracture and highlights that this evidence contradicts common treatment protocols. The researchers point out that, as 7 months was the maximum duration, we cannot know what outcomes years of stretching would bring.

Discussion

In terms of its aim, this paper is pretty straightforward. I review it here in an effort to shed light on some common assumptions. First, there is an assumption that joint contracture is a connective tissue shortening or densification, limiting its mechanical range. Second, there is an assumption that stretching it would restore the tissue length or mechanical range. Third, there is an assumption that in healthy subjects, limited ROM must therefore also be a product of connective tissue length or mechanical range and that stretching would cause plastic changes to length or behavior. While some of these assumptions are certainly possible, the evidence is lacking and the conclusions of this paper demand we strongly consider other mechanisms.

Research Summary

Hot Yoga

Heart Rate and Core Temperature Responses to Bikram Yoga (Quandt et al., 2015)

Background

Hot yoga has become increasingly popular in the mainstream. Bikram yoga is practiced in a 105°F room set at 40% humidity. A single session typically lasts 90 minutes and includes 26 postures and two breathing practices. Previous research suggests benefits of Bikram include increased strength, flexibility, and balance, and decreases in metabolic risk factors and perceived stress. The risks associated with hot yoga practiced in these conditions are unknown.

Purpose

This paper set out to determine if core temperatures (CT) and heart rate (HR) while practicing yoga in such an environment reached hazardous levels in regular Bikram students who were assumed to be acclimatized to the conditions of heat and humidity.

Continued on next page

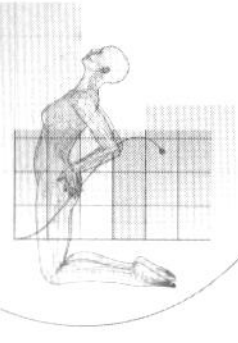

Continued from previous page

Methods

Seven men and thirteen women between the ages of 28 and 67 volunteered to participate in a Bikram yoga session wearing a heart rate monitor and ingesting a core temperature sensor. HR data were collected every 60 seconds and CT data were collected every 10 minutes (including prior to practice at 0 minutes). There was no control group not practicing yoga but still present in the heated room.

Results

For the men, the average HR was 80% and peak was 92% of predicted maximum HR. For the women, the average HR was 72% and peak was 85% of predicted maximum HR. For the men, average peak CT was 103.2 +/- .78°F, and for the women, average peak CT was 102.0 +/- .92°F. The highest overall recorded CT was at the end of the class and reached 104.1°F in a male. It was further noted that 35% of the subjects recorded CT of at least 103°F. None of the participants demonstrated or reported any signs of heat-related illness.

Discussion

The American Council on Exercise (ACE) fitness magazine published a summary of this paper written in a manner suitable for public consumption (Green, 2015). In light of the social media controversy this version created, I thought it was worth reviewing here. The original researchers recommended Bikram instructors be educated on heat-related illness and called for future research, whereas the ACE paper indicated there were risks associated with Bikram yoga and suggested shortening class time, minimizing the extreme environmental conditions, and promoting hydration. It is the selection of inflated conclusions in the ACE paper that caused the turmoil online.

A researcher from the Department of Health and Exercise Science at Colorado State University, Brian Tracy, who has published research on Bikram yoga was particularly vocal, and rightfully so. His rebuttal came in the form of an unofficial, unpublished document noting all of the study design flaws. His biggest complaint was in the CT data-collection process. His team had collected data at one time using the same equipment and had found CT averaged 100.3°F, a result clearly within the safe zone for exercise. They took measurements every 15 seconds then smoothed the data (a process which is used for drawing out patterns within a set). He argued that collecting data every 10 minutes does not provide an accurate insight into the elevating core temperatures as an outlying value could be recorded that is not indicative of overall and true CT. Unfortunately, at the time of this writing, he has not published that research and all I could find was an abstract from a conference presentation (Fritz et al., 2014). In a race to declare hot yoga safe, or unsafe, once and for all, it seems a lot of conclusions are being made on weak data. We simply need more high-quality, peer-reviewed, and published research.

STRUCTURE AND COMPOSITION

4

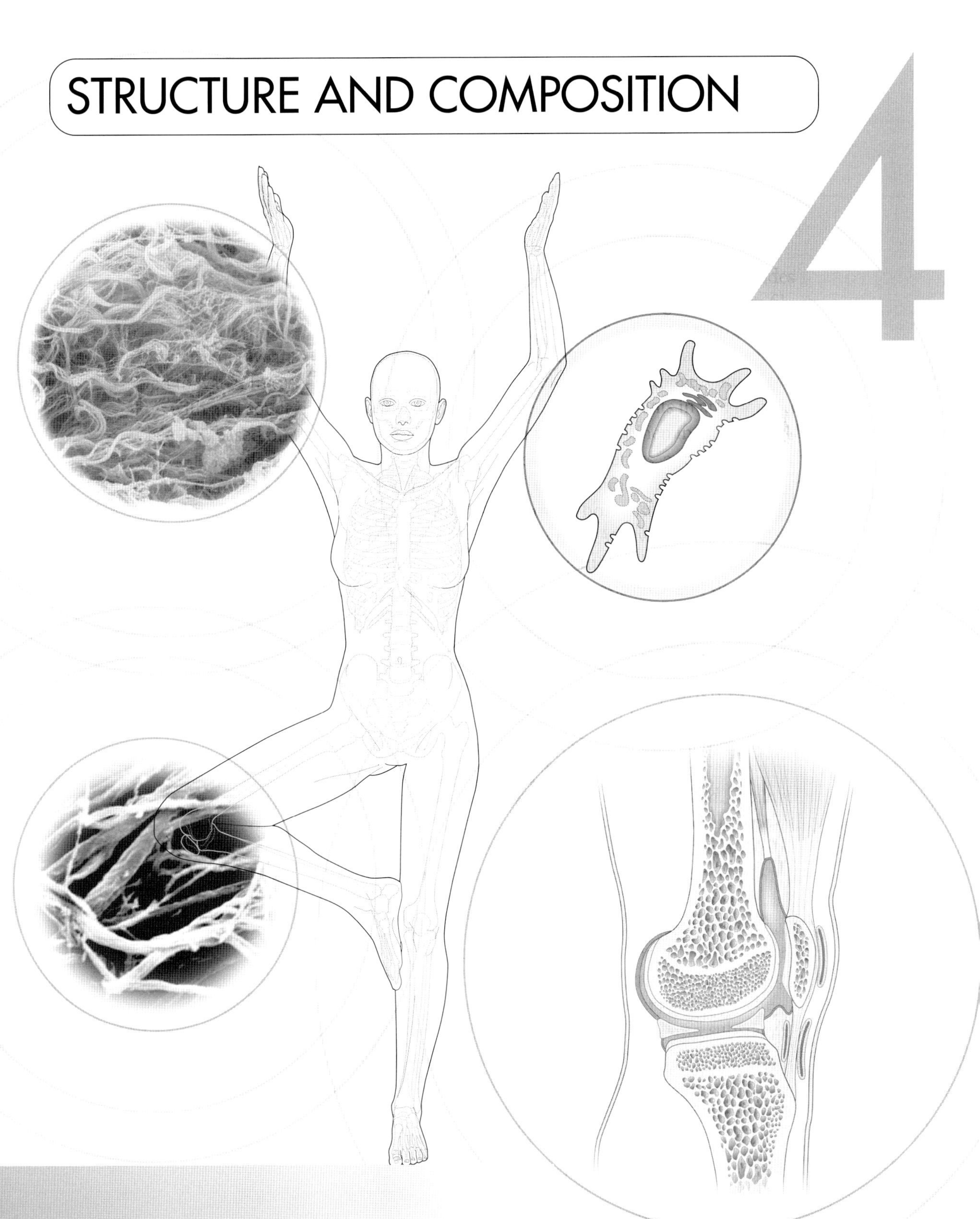

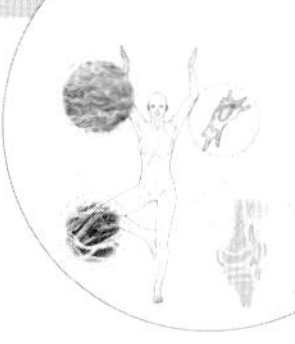

Gross anatomy is the study of macroscopic anatomy: what we can see with our eyes. In the anatomy lab, we learn through looking, touching, separating, and dissecting the fabrics of the human body. Through these observations we can make discoveries about form, function, and sometimes mechanical properties. A cadaver, however, is just another analogy, albeit a more sophisticated one. From what you've read here so far about collagen behavior, you may have interpreted the iliotibial band (ITB), for example, first to behave like a rubber band, then a gummy worm, but when you see, touch, and try to stretch an ITB postmortem, the inadequacies of these analogies become clear. You may, instead, choose to compare the ITB to a steel cable, as I did my first time. All of these comparisons, however, are in the macroscopic realm.

Histology is the study of the microscopic structures of biological tissues. These structures must be studied through a lens strong enough to amplify them, and they do not lend themselves well to manual exploration. In many cases, the tissues are dyed, then backlit, which during a magnification process, provides distinguishable textures, colors, and shapes. These representations are yet another analogy, offering another, but different partial view into the tissues. Just as engineers must consider the structure and composition of construction materials, the study of histology helps us understand how the structure and composition of connective tissues contribute to their mechanical properties, and this is the focus of this chapter.

Biological Tissues

Tissue is what we call the biological fabric, or composite material, made up of a collection of cells and other various molecular compounds serving a common purpose. The arrangement of these components determines the structure, or architecture of the tissue. In biology (and microbiology) form follows function and its purpose is expressed by design. A brief discussion of the types of tissue our body has will provide context for the further investigation of connective tissues.

The body is made up of four different types of tissue (Table 4.1). Most organs and systems are a combination of all of them. Each type of tissue is further classified by its form

Table 4.1
Types of Tissue

Type	Description
Epithelial	Tissues that secrete, absorb, and protect (e.g. glands are made of epithelium)
Connective	Connective tissues support, connect, separate, pervade the entire body, and sheath structures within all systems
Muscular	Muscular tissues are contractile and generate movement, including locomotion of the musculoskeletal system, cardiac pulsation of the cardiovascular system, or peristaltic waves of the digestive system
Nervous	Nervous tissues transmit, support, and protect. The brain, spinal cord, and peripheral nerves consist of nervous tissue

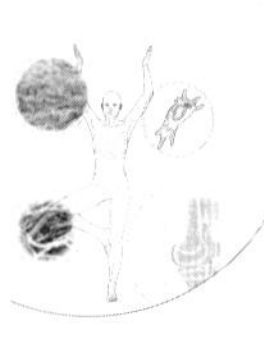

and function, the study of which could fill an entire textbook. Because our focus is on how biomechanics, mainly tissue mechanics, can inform a safe and sustainable practice, the present chapter will include only the types of connective tissues within the musculoskeletal system that we have already discussed leading up to this point.

In our study of the behavior of collagen in human connective tissue, we learned about stress, strain, and viscoelastic phenomena. Since collagen is not the only component of connective tissue, a more complete histological examination will reveal greater behavioral complexities and adaptive potentials. In addition to mechanical behaviors and adaptations, biological tissues also exhibit chemical behaviors and adaptations as the cells respond to mechanical inputs. Together, these processes known as mechanobiology will be the focus of our histological review.

Identifying Connective Tissue

As is often the case with anatomy in general, and when it comes to connective tissue specifically, how many classes there are depends on the authority. It is not uncommon to find authors who identify two, three, and even four types of connective tissue. For our purposes, we will discuss three types (Table 4.2) and support this position with an approach that connective tissue does not require collagen, but rather a structural framework containing cells.

All connective tissue is characterized by the presence of an **extra-cellular matrix** (ECM) made up of non-living compounds to provide structure and specialized cells to perform vital functions. In *supportive* and *proper* types, the collagen-based ECM is able to withstand high levels of tension and absorb forces to a degree that are unique to connective tissues. The cells, housed within the matrix, are the living component and function to regulate tissue synthesis, repair, and degradation. In blood and lymph, plasma is the fluid ECM which provides the structure to carry blood cells. Structurally, the composition of the matrix and attributes of the cells vary widely and exhibit properties reflecting local mechanical demands. Supportive connective tissues can function as struts (bones) or gliding surfaces (cartilage), and connective tissue proper can function as protective packing material (serous membranes) or suspension cables (tendons, ligaments).

Table 4.2
Classes of Connective Tissue

Type	Description
Supportive	Connective tissues like bone and cartilage that are hard and firm, but pliable and make up our skeleton
Proper	Connective tissue proper is a softer texture and includes joint capsules, ligaments, tendons, and deep fascia. Thicker striations of connective tissue are found in the adipose layer just beneath the dermis, called superficial fascia. Thinner, sometimes film-like connective tissues are also found in and around all organs and organ systems, often referred to as the visceral fascia
Fluid	Some connective tissues, such as blood and lymph, are fluid

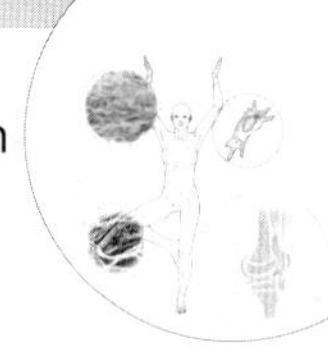

Connective tissue, by name, implies continuity and connectivity. The web of connective tissue proper is literally everywhere; it covers the entire body, surrounds each muscle and muscle fiber, all bones, organs and systems. It is entirely continuous with no demarcated beginning or end. As one tissue transitions into another, the structure and composition change based on mechanical demand (form follows function). This evolutionary perspective, where human structures adapted based on our progressions in motility (e.g. bipedal locomotion, long distance running) fits very well in the biomechanical narrative where human tissues have the ability to adapt.

Regarding the continuity of tissue, I must make a point to mention **fascia** here. Fascia has earned recent notoriety, but will not be in the spotlight here. For the sake of identifying it as a connective tissue, I will offer a few words now. In recent years, the surge of fascia research has led to a greater understanding of this once ignored structure while simultaneously elevating its status in our industry to become a targeted tissue to train. The idea that fascia can become more fit, more pliable, or less restrictive in response to certain methods of movement or massage is most usually met with either blind acceptance or staunch skepticism. If we accept the adaptive potential of connective tissue, we must embrace some sort of change over time is possible when loading fascia. Fascia is globally present, yet takes many forms, and so we can't expect all fascia to adapt identically. The arrangement and composition of myofascia would have a different form and function from the arrangement and composition of a neural sheath or the pericardium. Which raises the question, "What is the definition of fascia?"

Table 4.3
Fascia Nomenclature. Modified after Langevin and Huijing (2009)

Fascial Tissue	Description
Dense connective tissue	Densely packed, aligned in various directions
Areolar connective tissue	Sparsely packed, aligned in various directions
Superficial fascia	Subcutaneous
Deep fascia	Surrounding muscular system
Intermuscular septa	Between muscle compartments
Interosseous membrane	Membrane between adjacent bones
Periosteum	Surrounding bones
Neurovascular tract	Surrounding nerves and vasculature
Epimysium	Surrounding muscle organ
Intra- and extra-muscular aponeurosis	Tendinous sheets of fascia
Perimysium	Surrounding muscle fascicles
Endomysium	Surrounding muscle fibers

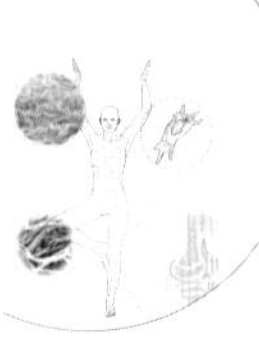

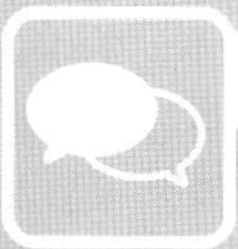

Thought Provoker

Fascia

Fascia, in light of its growing notoriety, has become a somewhat controversial topic. Skeptics insist the research to date is not compelling enough to make any drastic changes to the way we practice both manual and movement therapies, or to how we develop exercise programming. Enthusiasts promote fascia as the tissue of interest in their respective modality, attributing faulty movement patterns, dysfunction, and pain, as well as improvements thereof to it. Some teachers of certain styles of yoga even claim their yoga targets the fascia specifically, while suggesting other yoga targets the muscles. Where do you stand on the fascia spectrum? What is the mechanism of action, if any, by which fascia could be isolated? Could this mechanism of action be replicated with a different stylistic preference?

In recent years, scientists have been in collaboration to establish an international standard nomenclature to reflect the surge of research on different fascial structures (Table 4.3). As you can imagine this process is slow and not without debate. In 2009 fascia scientists proposed a recommended language and naming of connective tissue proper that included 12 categories of fascia, including aponeuroses (broad flat sheets of tendon-like tissue), interosseous membranes (a connective tissue membrane between two bones such as ulna and radius), and the periosteum (connective tissue membrane surrounding bone) but excluding tendons, ligaments, and joint capsules (Langevin and Huijing, 2009).

In 2016, the committee published a paper with a proposed definition of fascia: "A fascia is a sheath, a sheet or any other dissectible aggregation of connective tissue to attach, enclose and separate muscles, bones, organs, blood vessels and nerves, etc." (Adstrum et al., 2016). Note that a fascia refers to a general category of tissue but not all fasciae (the plural of fascia) have the same behavior or function. Therefore, when speaking of a specific fascia, it is worth mentioning the category from the above table.

Moreover, if we have many fasciae with specific functions, we can assemble them all to create a system. For example, if we include the heart, arteries, capillaries, and veins, we have a cardiovascular system. Thus, the committee concurrently published a definition for a fascial system, different from a fascial tissue. Paraphrased and abbreviated for simplicity here, the definition explains that the fascial system encompasses all soft connective tissues to establish the all-pervasive web as a coordinated and holistically functioning unit while integrating with and enabling all other systems (Adstrum et al., 2016). One could argue the same of the cardiovascular system, or any other system for that matter. The continuity of the arteries and veins to the heart could imply they are the heart, just as the periosteum and an aponeurosis are both fascia. Moreover, the cardiovascular system is an independent system with its own function to transport blood, but it also integrates with and enables all other systems. When was the last time you saw a fully functioning human with a non-functioning cardiovascular system?

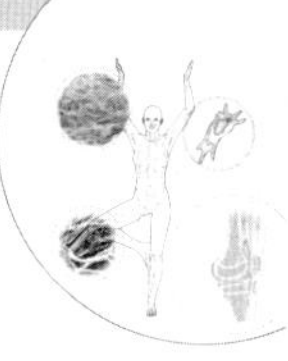

Shortly after publication, a rebuttal to the Adstrum (2016) paper presented the idea that fascia does not literally separate any structure. Body parts only separate through the act of dissection; therefore, fascia does not separate itself, we separate it. The author proposed this alternative definition: "A fascia is a sheath, a sheet or any other dissectible aggregation of connective tissue that attaches, encloses and delineates muscles, bones, organs, blood vessels and nerves, etc." (Scarr, 2016). After additional expert contributions, the original team slightly altered the wording in their fascial system definition but maintained the wording for the fascia definition pending feedback from the Federative International Committee on Anatomical Terminology (Stecco et al., 2018). I present this information here to highlight the conflict and collaboration of the process and that semantics in anatomy do matter greatly. Until standard nomenclature is accepted, we can play our professional part by using clear and concise terminology and descriptions whenever possible.

I will follow my own advice immediately and highlight which tissues we will be investigating in the present chapter. Our histological review will primarily cover tendons, ligaments, and joint capsules, but not fascia, for two primary reasons. First, these are the tissues primarily researched in exercise science. The explosion of tendon research in recent years has revealed much about the adaptable nature of these tissues during exercise as well as injury prevention and management. A thorough understanding of this body of literature will provide greater competency when participating in the injury and asana conversation coming later. Second, the tissues we will cover are histologically similar so that we may examine the commonalities between these tissues, rather than the differences. When differences are relevant, as in the case of cartilage or bone, I will be clear to which tissue I am referring to. Otherwise, the use of the phrase "connective tissue," refers to the dense musculoskeletal connective tissue proper including tendons, ligaments, and joint capsules.

Connectivity and Continuity

One of the first things we learn when studying basic anatomy is that tendons connect muscle to bone and ligaments connect bone to bone. This is easy to remember but, as with all separating and naming of parts, memorizing this fact teaches us little about their integrated function. Moreover, it is rare to study joint capsules as they are usually cut away in anatomy books to make identifying the ligaments clearer. Tendons are usually drawn as extensions of muscle organs, but little thought is given to their relationship with the endo-, peri-, and epimysium. Finally, tendons and ligaments are presented as distinct tissues with distinct functions.

This distinction by anatomy is correct but incomplete. One could certainly argue that tendons transmit muscle force to bone to create movement and that ligaments act as joint stabilizers. From a gross anatomy perspective, this is true, but from a histological perspective, the tendons and ligaments have much more in common. They share similar structures, have many of the same components and emerge from the same embryonic tissue. Thus, studying connective tissue proper includes far more than learning an anatomical name, and our comprehension improves when we explore its continuity.

It is easy to mentally separate bone from a ligament as their structures are quite different. Bones are hard, ligaments are soft, but if you start studying bone in more detail, you discover it is sheathed in a soft tissue fascial layer called the periosteum. In dissection, you can take a blade and some tweezers to the surface of the femur bone and start to lift

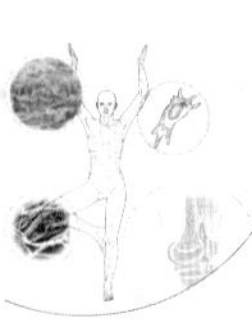

a multi-dimensional but incredibly thin layer of soft tissue. As you continue to reflect the soft layers, it seems there is always a bit more periosteum you can lift off. Until there is none left, at which point it seems you've penetrated the ossified tissue.

Joint capsules, which encapsulate the entire joint space, blend into this periosteum layer eventually becoming hard bone. The inner layer of the joint capsule is the synovial layer, which secretes synovial fluid into the joint space. The outer layer is a fibrous layer that is similar to the fibrous structure of ligaments. In fact many ligaments are no more than a thickened area of the joint capsule. The knee joint is a good example to use. In the text books, the knee is said to have four ligaments – two forming a cross inside the joint space and one running longitudinally on the medial and lateral sides of the joint. The joint capsule is most always cut away to reveal these two structures and the two within joint space. In vivo, actually, a fibrous band covers the entire joint space, containing the synovial fluid within. Neither the lateral nor medial collateral ligament is separate from the fibrous layer of the joint capsule. Only a very sharp blade and a judgment call by the individual wielding that blade can dissect and identify these "individual" ligaments.

One could say such ligaments are not distinct from joint capsules, but rather emerge from them (Fig. 4.1). To illustrate, imagine the fibrous joint capsule looked something like thick packing tape with parallel threads running through it. If somewhere along

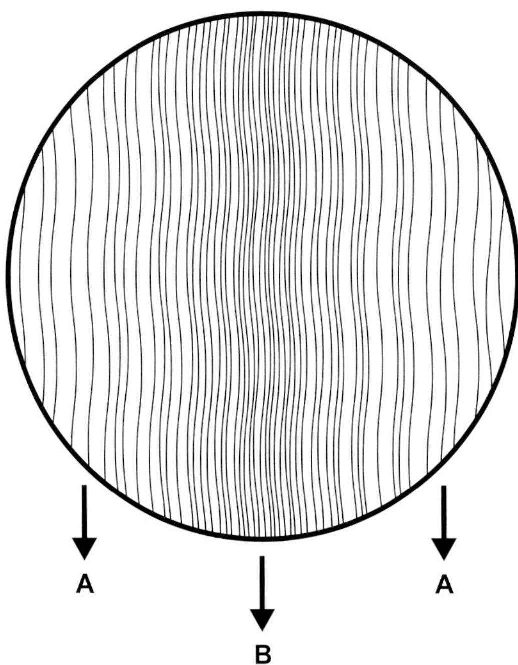

Fig. 4.1
Packing tape analogy. When one histologically similar tissue emerges from another the delineation is not always distinctly clear. Tissue A is clearly less dense than tissue B, but the exact line of separation between them is uncertain.

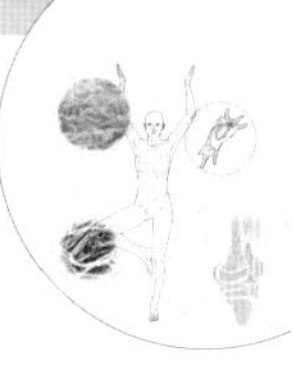

the width of the tape, the threads become more densely packed, you could compare the distance between threads to determine the area of greatest concentration to call that a ligament. Another individual, however, may have judged that area to a millimeter wider. You would both be correct, the distinction is not always that obvious, and that is how similar the structures are. You will see how connective tissue proper, based on its histology, and for the purposes of loading it in yoga, can be generalized as one type of tissue spread throughout different specific anatomical regions (i.e. the tendons, ligaments, and joint capsules of the lateral ankle).

Many times, the distinction is obvious. In the example of the knee ligaments above, the anterior cruciate ligament (ACL) and the posterior cruciate ligament (PCL) are inside the joint space, completely separate from the external joint capsule. Tendons, especially long tendons, are also quite distinct, until they approach a joint capsule where they blend into the ligamentous capsule which blends into the periosteum. Some tendons, like the long head of the biceps, travel inside the joint capsule and attach to the periosteum instead of the capsule, claiming their own identity. However, if you travel the other way along the tendon, toward the muscle, you will discover the tendon becomes the ECM of the skeletal muscle, organized into the three connecting layers known as the *epimysium*, *perimysium*, and *endomysium*.

Embedded within and throughout are the muscle proteins actin, myosin, and titin configured into fascicles and then fibers. The components of the muscle ECM resemble the ECM of the tendon, not the components of the contractile muscle tissue. Therefore, histologically, one could say a tendon-like tissue runs the entire length of the muscle organ but presents more conspicuously at the end points than it does in the belly of the muscle. This perspective allows for inclusion of muscle organs into the connective tissue system as the "container" in which muscle proteins are held and by which they are shaped is connective tissue.

In my younger years, I was a nightclub bartender. There were a few cocktails that required layering of the liqueurs, which was achievable if you knew their densities. As long as you poured the heavier liqueur first, you could distinctly "float" the lighter one on top, providing you gently poured it along the inside edge of the glass. If you poured the lighter liqueur first, the layer effect was lost. Sure, the denser liqueur would still sink to the bottom, but there would be a muddled effect in the middle versus a clean line between the layers. Our tissues are often muddled in the transition areas. We are not assembled together with different substances, rather our tissues evolved out of a single zygote which differentiated over time through programmed biological processes influenced by mechanical inputs.

The Extra-Cellular Matrix

The ECM, appropriately named, describes the environment around which cells perform their functions (Fig. 4.2). The ECM of cartilage and bone appears in different structural configurations based on location (and physical demand, of course). Articular cartilage of the joints, made of hyaline cartilage, is irregularly packed and is especially well-designed for resisting compressive forces. The densely packed amorphous ECM of cartilage leaves little to no interstitial space (i.e. fluid-filled space surrounding cells) but is marked by small cavities, called lacunae, which house clusters of cells. Fibrocartilage incorporates densely and regularly arranged fibers, similar to those found in tendons and ligaments,

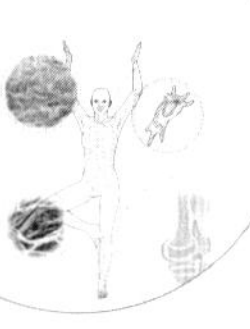

into its cartilaginous structure, enabling it to resist both compression and tension quite well. Fibrocartilage is therefore located in highly exposed areas particularly tolerant to load, such as the intervertebral discs and menisci. The osseous tissue (i.e. bone) matrix shares a similar structure to cartilage, but with a greater quantity of collagen fibers and the addition of calcium salts. The ECM of bone also has lacunae for cells but has additional spaces around which the matrix circularly forms to provide channels for nerves and blood vessels. Bone architecture is not congruous throughout the body as cortical bone tends to be more compact than trabecular (spongy) bone. The specific composition and deliberate structure of the ECM all play a role in the staggeringly complex biochemical relationships between the cells and their environment.

We have established that an ECM, a network comprising mostly carbohydrates and proteins of varying molecular configurations and water, is critical to the classification of connective tissue. Some authorities further require the composition of the ECM to consist of fibers, or long threads that form the fabric, and hence the debate about whether or not a fluid is a connective tissue. Whereas the presence of fibers is somewhat intuitive when studying tendons and ligaments, the matrix of bone, in addition to mineral salts, such as calcium, for hardness, also contains mostly fibers. These fibers are made of proteins that when arranged together withstand very high levels of tension (more than stainless steel when compared size for size). These proteins are collagen and elastin.

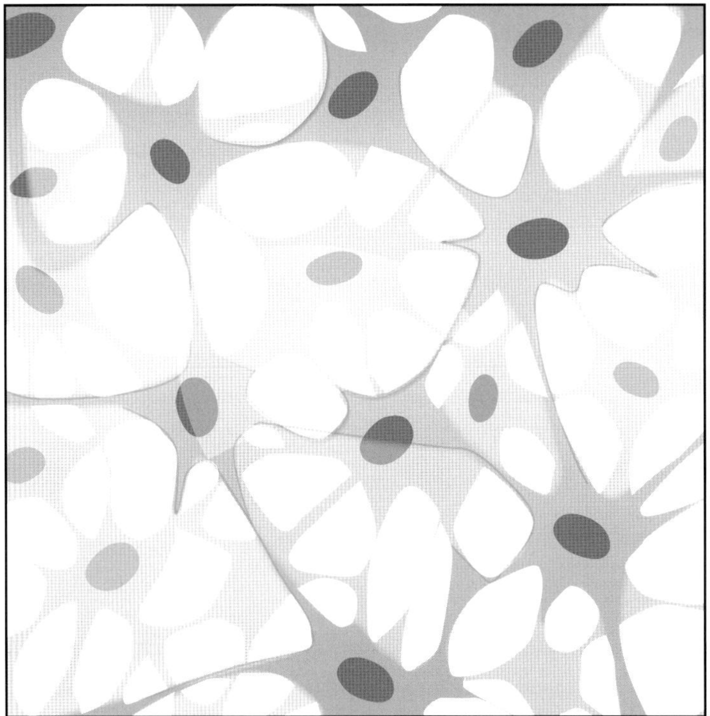

Fig. 4.2
Extra-cellular matrix. The connective tissue network that provides the cells with structural and chemical environment.

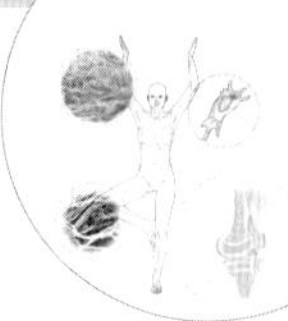

Collagen

Collagen is the most abundant protein in the body, making up not just our tendons, ligaments, cartilage and bones, but also our skin, intervertebral discs, blood vessels, and more. Type I collagen, in addition to types II, III, IV, and VI represent approximately 95% of the 28 types identified to date, all differing in molecular structure depending on function (Kadler et al., 2007). Collagen type I is the most common, making up 80% of this 95%. Types I, III, and V appear in long strands. In general, type I collagen is the most abundant type present in ligaments and tendons, followed by type III. *Articular cartilage* is made primarily of type II collagen and bone contains type I, with a scant amount of type V. Tendons and ligaments get their tensile capacity because of the presence of collagen, mainly collagen type I. Previously injured connective tissues have been shown to contain greater quantities of type III collagen, which is characterized by lesser tensile capacity than type I (Hauser et al., 2013).

Cartilage and bone, in addition to withstanding compression, also withstand immense tension due to the presence of collagen fibers in the ECM. Cartilage maintains greater flexibility than bone largely due to its higher water content. The hardness and rigidity of bone is credited to the presence of calcium salts within the matrix. Aging cartilage lends itself to calcification and eventually ossification (the hardening associated with bone formation), a factor in degenerative osteoarthritis (degraded articular cartilage and underlying bone). Articular cartilage, made of *hyaline cartilage*, covers bone within joint surfaces. Hyaline cartilage has a glassy appearance and a pliable but springy texture in spite of the large collagen fiber content. This appearance differs from that of fibrocartilage, which is found in areas exposed to higher pressures such as the intervertebral discs and menisci of the knee. *Fibrocartilage* has a more fibrous, ossified appearance as it is comprised of rows of collagen fibers which become progressively mineralized as it approaches neighboring bone. Both cartilage and bone are further sheathed in additional layers of fibrous connective tissue called the perichondrium and periosteum, respectively.

As with all other proteins, collagen is made up of molecules called *amino acids*. When these molecules arrange together to form a long chain, it becomes a *polypeptide*. Collagen is formed by three such polypeptide chains wound together in a triple helix configuration (Fig. 4.3). Hydrogen bonds form between the chains, providing the collagen fibril with its tensile capacity, which can be further increased by molecular cross-linking (bonding) with other components. Finally, the collagen fibrils bundle together to form the thicker fibers. Genetic variants in these molecular configurations and spontaneous organization will affect tissue capacity. The hypermobility condition Ehlers-Danlos syndrome and the frail bone disease osteogenesis imperfecta are the result of such collagen mutations (Brodsky and Persikov, 2005).

Collagen turnover refers to the ongoing process of collagen synthesis and degradation. Collagen is presently known to have a half-life of approximately 300–500 days, meaning that this is roughly how long it will take for collagen to degrade to half its content. Simultaneously, collagen is constantly synthesizing, with the overall net turnover being influenced by mechanical loading. Conventional wisdom is that ligaments in particular, as well as tendons to some degree, are relatively inert tissues. Collagen turnover suggests otherwise, as does the discovery that tendons can hypertrophy

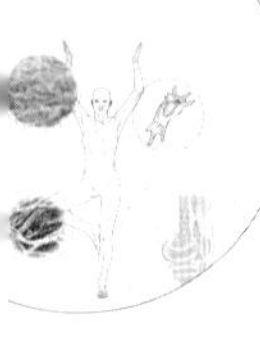

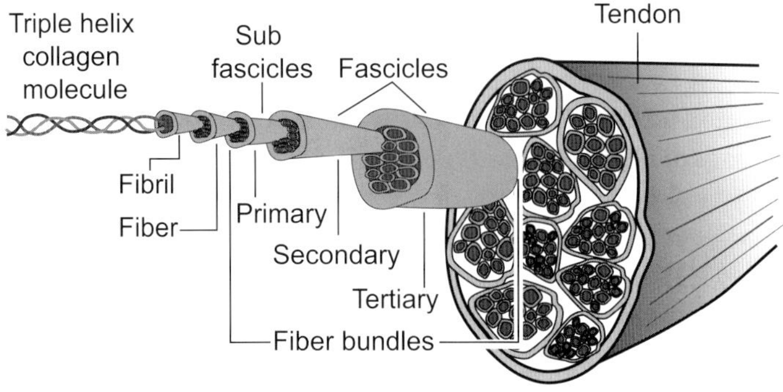

Fig. 4.3
Tendon structure. Collagen molecules are arranged in a triple helix configuration that bundle together in a hierarchical structure.

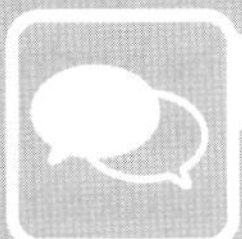

Thought Provoker

Hypermobility

Hypermobility is a condition defined by a genetic variant in the molecular structure of collagen. Historically, hypermobility has received little attention and the amount of available research reflects this obscurity. Recently, however, the condition has garnered some increased awareness. As with many trends in the fitness, yoga, and similar industries, along with the increased attention comes an assertive pendulum swing in the other direction. At the time of this writing, I personally do not believe the yoga community, as a whole, has swung the pendulum even close to the center and more attention is still needed. If you are a teacher, how might you raise awareness of hypermobility without diagnosing your students (beyond your scope), while simultaneously being cautious to avoid encouraging a self-diagnosis? Do you think students who do not have the genetic variant need to be concerned with "overstretching" in a yoga class?

(i.e. enlargen). Where it may be accepted that these tissues are very much mechanically sensitive and active tissues with an adaptable nature, much is still unknown. How and if rapidly synthesized collagen gets integrated into the slowly adapting, more stable collagen containing structures is still being investigated (Magnusson, Heinemeier and Kjaer, 2016). With collagaen turnover in mind, the narrative about protecting tissue evolves somewhat. The concern for overuse and the prevention of "wear and tear" shifts to a concern for underuse and the promotion of exposure and repair.

Elastin

Elastin is another fibrous protein component of the extra-cellular matrix. Hydrophobic amino acids provide elastin with its durability, and its recoil capabilities make it the perfect component for tissues undergoing repeated strain, such as tendons and ligaments (Halper and Kjaer, 2014). Its name might lead you to believe its presence makes a tissue less stiff or more "elastic." While elastin is in fact capable of greater strain than collagen, elasticity refers to a material's ability to return to its resting shape, not the ease by which its shape deforms. This goes against the common sense description of elasticity but, fortunately, we have properly defined elasticity in the mechanical sense. To illustrate, if you were to compare a steel marble with a rubber ball, common sense might lead you to assume the steel marble is less elastic because you can't visibly deform it with your bare hands. If you were to drop the two, however, the steel marble would bounce higher because when both are dropped, they compress slightly, but the steel marble restores its shape more rapidly and, therefore, is more elastic than rubber. The steel marble is stiffer, and the rubber ball is more compliant, but it can be easily forgotten that elasticity is an expression of recoil, not malleability.

Despite elastin displaying a greater strain capacity than collagen, it makes up only a small part of connective tissue (roughly 2–5%). For reasons unknown, the ligamenta nuchae and flava of the head and spine are made up of considerably more elastin fibers even though the remainder of the spine is thoroughly braced and surrounded by much stiffer, collagen dominant ligaments. It has been speculated that the increased presence of elastin creates a more extensible tissue, capable of greater strain, but any presence of collagen would likely limit the overall tissue behavior. Imagine building a suspension bridge with rubber ropes intertwined with the steel cables. Would not the steel limit the extensibility and strain of the structure?

Inquisitive minds have questioned the role of elastin and suggested it plays a major role in healing, holding the ECM together during tissue tears until the clotting and early stages of collagen production can repair the wound (Zorn, 2007). Perhaps its role is less about its individual mechanical behavior and more about its contribution to the ECM as a whole. Its hydrophobic structure, in conjunction with neighboring hydrophilic components, is known to regulate tissue hydration via hydrogen bonding (Halper and Kjaer, 2014). Such considerations further highlight the role that structure and composition have in overall mechanical properties and reveal that biochemistry and biomechanics are not mutually exclusive.

Fiber Arrangement

The mechanical properties of human tissues are affected not just by the mechanical behavior of the substance of which it is made, but also by the architecture of that substance. Using a non-biological material as an example, a length of yarn exhibits certain mechanical behavior, but a sweater knit of yarn will exhibit a different behavior based on the type of stitch used. A looser knit sweater may stretch more easily than a tightly knit sweater made with the same yarn, thereby being easier to pull on, because the structure of the final product influences its properties. The same can be said of human connective tissue.

Connective tissue matrix arrangements are classified by *density* and *regularity* (Fig. 4.4). Density is measured on a scale of loosely to densely arranged fibers, somewhat analogous to a loosely or tightly woven fabric. Regularity is measured on a scale of irregular to regular, where regularity reflects uniformity and irregularly arranged

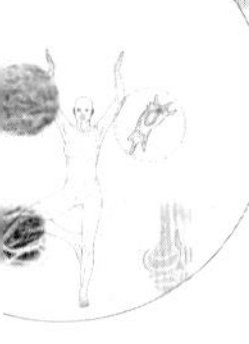

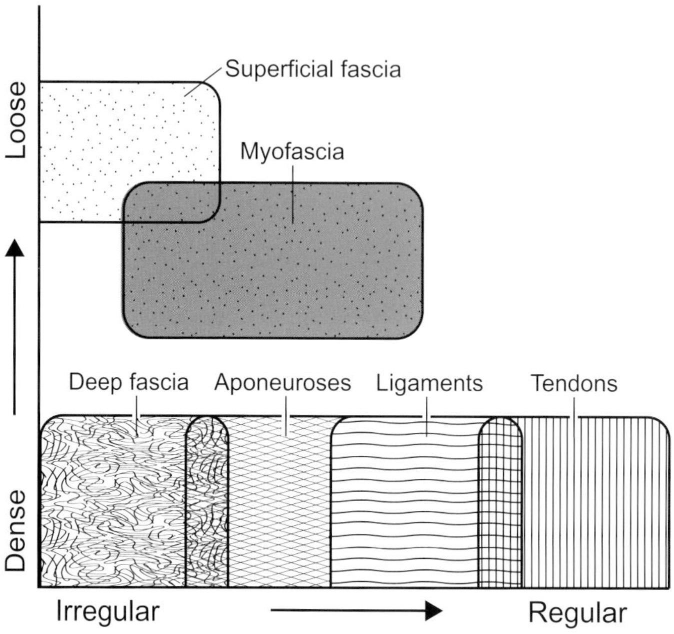

Fig. 4.4
Fiber arrangement. Regularity increases from left right. Density decreases from bottom to top. Note the tissues overlap as arrangement is a continuum. Illustration modified after Schleip et al. (2012).

fibers are multi-directional. If form follows function, then density and regularity are the result of the loading parameters to which the tissue has been exposed.

The density scale reflects how collagen fibers arrange spatially from closely packed to loosely packed. The deep fascial layer, which surrounds muscle organs, as well as other types of connective tissue proper, is closely packed, whereas superficial fascia is loosely arranged. Loose, however, does not imply structurally weak. Remember, superficial fascia is still made of collagen and thus maintains its tremendous tensile strength. Nevertheless, density, being a structural aspect, does play a role in overall mechanical properties. Musculoskeletal connective tissues are dense on the scale because of their primary role in transmitting great amounts of force over sustained periods of tension. Loosely packed fibers have a greater amount of interstitial space than closely packed fibers leaving more room for vessels, nerves, additional fluids, lipids, and other molecular compounds and substances characteristic of loosely arranged fascia.

The term density should not be conflated with the thickening or scarring of connective tissue, called fibrosis (i.e. disordered or abnormal fibers) resulting in faulty mechanical properties. While fibrotic tissue is defined by increased collagen density, more collagen dense tissue is not necessarily fibrotic. This distinction is important during discussions about dense connective tissue developing due to optimal loading or repetitive loading and overuse, with the former simply being a standard structural identifier and the latter implying pathology.

The regularity scale reflects how collagen fibers are arranged from multidirectional to unidirectional. This arrangement is largely a result of the directionality of the loads applied. On the far right of the scale, the most uniform arrangement is seen in tendons. Tendons longitudinally receive and transmit force from muscle to bone. Therefore, the fibers are, for the most part, unidirectional or linear. Ligament fibers are almost linear but develop a slightly less regular arrangement to reflect the number of directions in which motion can occur (i.e. degrees of freedom) around the joint they serve. Aponeuroses have wider and more diverse attachments than tendons or ligaments, thus developing a lattice pattern. The specific angles formed by the fiber arrangement optimizes the transmission of force for that tissue's purpose. Finally, on the far left we see collagen fibers with a highly irregular, felt-like pattern. This irregular arrangement is deliberate and is found in other connective tissue layers as well.

Just as density can be confused with fibrosis, so can regularity. Scar tissue is often characterized by disorganized collagen which may appear to be the same as irregularly arranged collagen. After all, they both appear to have multidirectionally aligned fibers. Histologically, however, they are quite different. Irregularly arranged fibers reflect a healthy tissue, deliberately configured based on function; form following function. Disorganized fibers (Fig. 4.5) reflect an abnormal, potentially pathological arrangement often due to inadequate loading, insufficient movement, injury, surgery,

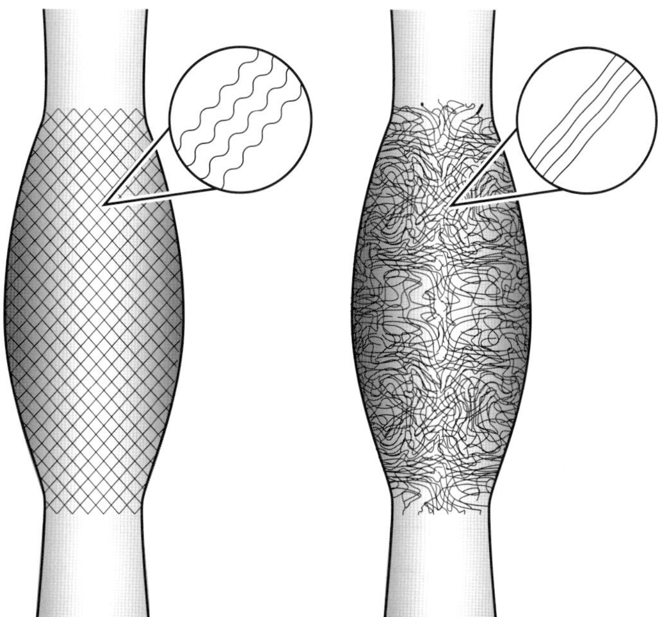

Fig. 4.5
Organized vs disorganized tissue. The tissue on the left is organized and maintains crimp. The tissue on the right is the same as the tissue on the left, only it is disorganized and has lost its crimp. Organization differs from arrangement in that a disorganized tissue is abnormal, but an irregular tissue is normal. Illustration modified after Schleip et al. (2012).

trauma or collagen accumulation; form following dysfuntion. In short, collagen fibers can be well organized albeit in an irregular configuration.

A mechanical property of connective tissue dependent upon fiber arrangement is called **anisotropy** (Fig. 4.6). Bones, for example are *anisotropic*, meaning their behavior is directionally dictated. Bones respond differently to a longitudinal load than to transverse or oblique loads, largely due to the direction in which bones most often receive load. An *isotropic* material, on the other hand, does not exhibit a directional behavior bias. A theraband is an isotropic material as longitudinally, laterally, or obliquely applied loads result in identical units of strain. The mathematics behind the anisotropic behaviors of human connective tissue get very complicated very fast, yet are currently being investigated by biomechanists searching for some clinical wisdom regarding force transmission in manual and movement therapies. The aforementioned aponeurotic angles fall under such research (Chaudhry et al., 2012).

Another structural aspect that influences mechanical properties is the thickness of the tissues, measured by its cross-sectional area (CSA). The CSA reflects changes in fibrillar quantity and diameter, rather than density or regularity. Increases in tendon CSA, also called tendon hypertrophy, occur in response to high magnitude loading. Similar to the research on tendon stiffness, CSA appears to increase in response to loading and decrease in response to underloading. Increases in CSA should not be confused with tendon thickening associated with tendon pathologies (tendinopathy). Increases in CSA are positive physiological adaptations to the collagen structure in response to optimal mechanical loading. Tendon and ligament thickening pathologies occur as maladaptive responses which might be caused by abnormal loading or overloading, and can be characterized by disorganized collagen accumulation, excess water, or elevated levels of an additional matrix component called **ground substance**.

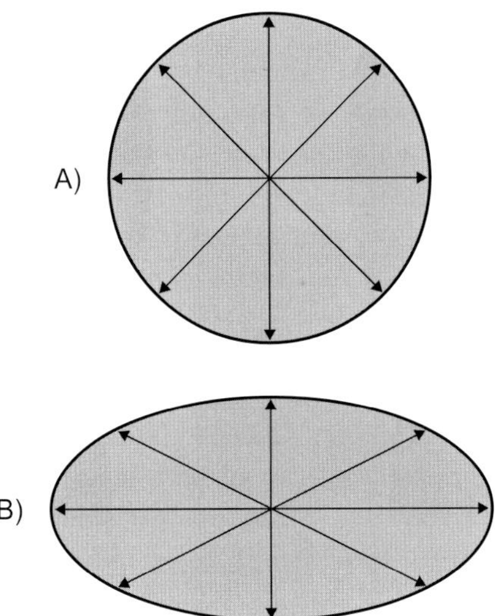

Fig. 4.6
(A) Isotropic materials behave identically regardless of direction. (B) Anisotropic materials behave differently depending on direction.

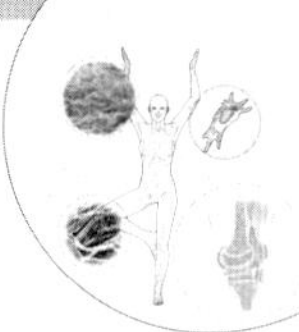

Ground Substance

The extra-cellular matrix, in addition to the fibrous network, contains an interfibrillar component in which the collagen and elastin are embedded, referred to as ground substance. This rich chemical environment is composed of water, glycoproteins (a protein attached to a carbohydrate), and a variety of molecules and compounds classified as hormones, enzymes, and antibodies. These additional components regulate the interstitial space through chemical reactions and molecular bonds while also regulating cellular functions. Ground substance attracts and binds with large proportions of water to form a sticky and gel-like viscous environment that functions as a stabilizer by absorbing compressive forces.

Ground substance further consists of proteoglycans (PGs). PGs are polysaccharides (carbohydrates) bound to proteins that aid with the frictionless sliding of collagen fibers, add density to the interstitial space, and protect cells from harmful penetrating bacteria. Glycosaminoglycans (GAGs), the carbohydrate portion of the PGs, are especially attracted to water. In essence, connective tissue is somewhat like a sponge, endlessly swelling with and squeezing out water, transporting essential nutrients in and nonessential waste out, based on the mechanical demands of movement. When interstitial fluid flow slows, PGs risk dehydration, increasing the glue-like properties, and decreasing the sliding and transporting abilities. Rather than shuttling undesirable waste out, waste may remain trapped within the ECM, disrupting histochemical homeostasis.

As with other components of connective tissue, PGs and GAGs vary by location and environment. A GAG you may be familiar with is the long molecular chain *chondroitin sulfate*. Abundant in cartilage, it contributes to compression resistance and simultaneously increases in response to compression. It is sold over-the-counter in capsule form along with glucosamine in an attempt to reverse or prevent osteoarthritis. It is thought that ingesting chondroitin sulfate adds density to the degenerating cartilage, since it is an essential component. Unfortunately, the mechanism by which dietary GAGs would find their way to the knee joint, for example, is not readily understood. It is improbable for the molecular structure of a GAG to remain intact after a trip through the gastrointestinal tract. Not unsurprisingly, the research supporting its efficacy is lacking.

Another GAG you may be familiar with is *hyaluronan*, or *hyaluronic acid*. Hyaluronan is a primary component in loose connective tissue and synovial fluid. In synovial fluid, when hyaluronan binds (through a process called cross-linking) to another glycoprotein, lubricin, the resulting network supplies the surrounding cartilage with lubricating properties that prevent wear under certain loading conditions that it cannot achieve in its unbound state (Greene et al., 2011). If we expand our view of synovial fluid beyond just an inert substance that "greases the wheels" to include how it fluctuates to best manage the mechanical demand, we can appreciate the value of chemical bonds within the ground substance on mechanical properties of connective tissue.

I've chosen these two simple examples to highlight the role of ground substance on biomechanical and biochemical properties because they are familiar topics to most people. In actuality an in-depth discussion on the complex role of ground substance in connective tissue is far beyond the focus of this book. What does warrant further discussion, regarding the extra-cellular matrix, is how the sum of its components

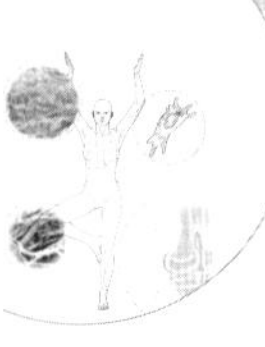

interact with the cellular component of connective tissue in collagen synthesis processes and tissue adaptation.

Cells

In connective tissue, the extra-cellular matrix is named as such because it refers to the structural network, or matrix, outside of, or "extra to," the cell. Within, lies the interstitial space filled with interstitial fluid, where the cells also reside. To use architecture as an analogy, you are the cell, your house is the ECM and the space inside the walls is the interstitial space (absent of fluid, obviously). The cells secrete their own environment, like a spider does its web, literally producing the ECM. We already know that bones increase density and tendons become stiffer when exposed to adequate load parameters. By studying the cells, we will learn about the mechanism by which this occurs.

Fibroblasts are unspecialized cells that produce collagen in connective tissue proper. Fibroblasts specialize in their response to mechanical forces to produce different types of connective tissues. Specialized fibroblasts take on a new name becoming tenocytes to make tendons and desmocytes to make ligaments and joint capsules. Fibroblasts may also become osteoblasts and chondroblasts, producing bone and cartilage, respectively. Generally speaking, a cell ending in -blast is a less mature but more metabolically active version of a cell ending in -cyte. Fibroblast specialization may occur in both directions, secreting higher levels of collagen or slowing production when necessary. Fibroblasts are also able to specialize across connective tissue types, such as when tension-preferring tendon cells start producing an ECM resembling cartilage after sufficient exposure to compressive forces. This mutability of fibroblasts tells us that at a histological level connective tissues are more similar than they are distinct.

One's connective tissue is a recording of one's loading history. It morphs over time through activity and exercise, or the absence thereof. Connective tissue is always changing because collagen is always in some state of turnover. In bone, collagen resorption is regulated by a cell called the osteoclast. Osteoclasts remove, or degrade, bone while osteoblasts add, or synthesize, bone. During youth, osteoblast activity is greater than osteoclast activity, therefore, bones grow and increase in density. As we age osteoblast activity slows, which may eventually lead to the condition osteopenia, and eventually osteoporosis. Fortunately, although within limit, we can stimulate osteoblast activity to outweigh osteoclast activity, thereby increasing bone density through compressive forces, such as high-impact sports.

Cartilage turnover is less prolific than in bone. After adolescence, when chondroblasts become chondrocytes, the mature cells become separated by the dense structure of the ECM and cluster in the cave-like structures called lacunae. The avascular quality of cartilage fails to provide nutrients to these pockets and the cell's function is diminished. As we age, cartilage often becomes ossified, further compromising the health of these cells. Injury, inflammation, and genetics further challenge the cellular environment, promoting catabolism beyond repair. In osteoarthritis cartilage degenerates or calcifies and is unable to recover like bone. Essentially, an osteoporotic joint is a failing joint and is an exception to the general rule that load stimulates collagen synthesis (Goldring, 2012; Heinemeier et al., 2016).

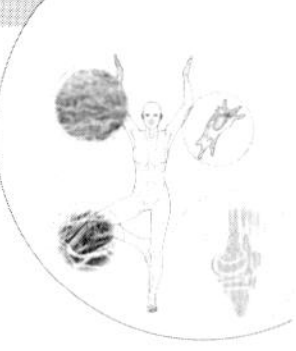

The collagen turnover process of tendons and ligaments is both a chronic and an acute process. Over long periods of time, collagen degrades through a half-life phenomenon. There is no -clast cell to degrade tendons and ligaments that we know of; it simply happens over time. Simultaneously, fibroblasts are secreting collagen and synthesizing new tissue. In the acute phase, after bouts of high-intensity exercise (i.e. 3-hour run), collagen synthesis peaks after approximately 24 hours and continues for another 2 or 3 days. Degradation peaks and subsides sooner than synthesis, resulting in a cumulative degradation during the first 24 hours, followed by synthesis, reaching an equilibrium at about 72 hours after exercise (Fig. 4.7) (Magnusson, Langberg and Kjaer, 2010). It has been proposed that over-use injuries may occur as a result of matrix degradation due to insufficient rest periods. As with the study of any pathogenesis, over-use injuries are more complex than a simple time line and it should not be interpreted as suggesting a daily yoga practice automatically results in injury. Tendons are mostly considered to be highly stable, yet still adaptable tissues and that turnover varies across and within tissues and is influenced by CSA, hormones, and age (Magnusson, Heinemeier and Kjaer, 2016).

The process by which fibroblasts are signaled to secrete collagen is largely mechanical in nature. As the tissue is stressed, the mechanosensitive cells sense the load parameters and behave accordingly, providing the intelligence to build a suitably responsive environment. Fibroblasts receive this communication of forces via the physical attachment to the ECM called cell-matrix adhesions. If each cell is "adhered" to the continuous connective tissue matrix, this allows for communication among cells spanning distal

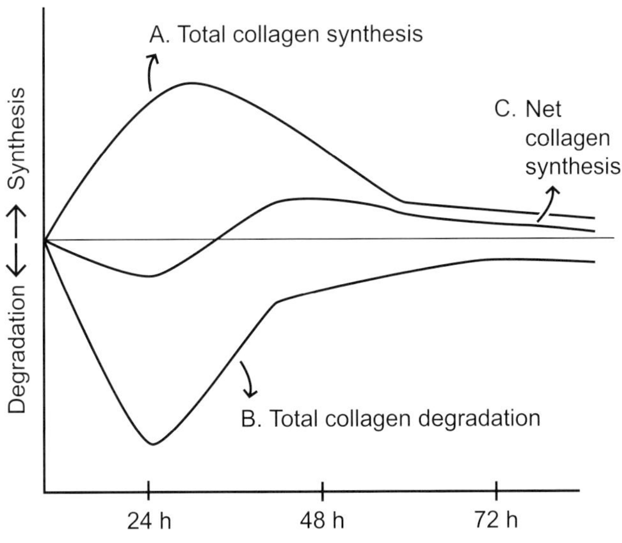

Fig. 4.7

Acute collagen turnover in tendons after high-intensity exercise. (A) Collagen synthesizes. (B) Collagen concurrently degrades. (C) Combined, net collagen is degraded after 24 hours and synthesized at 48 hours after exercise. Equilibrium is reached at about 72 hours post exercise. Illustration modified after Magnusson, Langberg and Kjaer (2010).

Scientific Literacy

Efficacy vs Effectiveness

Efficacy refers to the internal validity of a study; meaning, how well do the study design and execution result in an accurate measurement of the true relationships between well-controlled independent and dependent variables.

Effectiveness refers to the external validity; meaning how well can the results be generalized to the world outside the lab.

In drug research, the efficacy of a blood pressure drug, for example, is examined to determine how well it does what it is intended to do. Beta-blockers treat hypertension by slowing down your heart rate and preventing the heart from pumping too hard. In turn, blood flows through the vessels with less force. The efficacy of beta-blockers is determined by how well the drugs achieve this effect. The effectiveness of beta-blockers, however, is determined by how effectively they save lives.

In the last decade, researchers have produced interesting results on fibroblast activity after stretching. The cell bodies appear to enlarge after a low-magnitude, high-duration stretch spurring a variety of cellular processes including collagen production. The efficacy of stretching on connective tissue modeling will be determined as future research replicates and validates such findings. The effectiveness of low-magnitude, high-duration stretching in the prevention of tendon tears in recreational athletes due to such modeling effects has yet to be determined.

locations within the tissue. It is this cell signaling which allows for chemical and structural responses between fibroblasts and the ECM, called **mechanotransduction.**

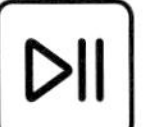

Pause and turn to page 130 for a summary of related research.

Cell matrix-adhesions (Fig. 4.8) are created by cell adhesion proteins such as *fibronectin*, *integrins*, and *laminins*. Fibronectin is an extra-cellular protein that has the ability to bind collagen fibers to cell membrane proteins called integrins. Integrins are receptors that attach to the cytoskeleton within the cell and fibronectin outside the cell, sensing applied loads and transmitting the force through the cell membrane and into the fibroblast. The cell is sensitive to its shape because of its cytoskeleton. Cells are no longer thought to be fluid-filled bags, but rather a microcosm of the larger organism with an internal skeleton-like structure (i.e. the cytoskeleton) and an external stretchy container (i.e. the cell membrane) under tension. There is more on this in Chapter 6. Laminins are extra-cellular proteins that also bind to integrins and modulate the cell's normal functions including influencing specialization and resisting apoptosis (programmed cell death).

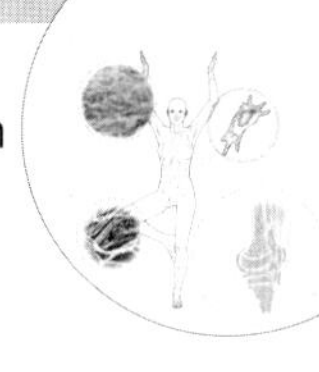

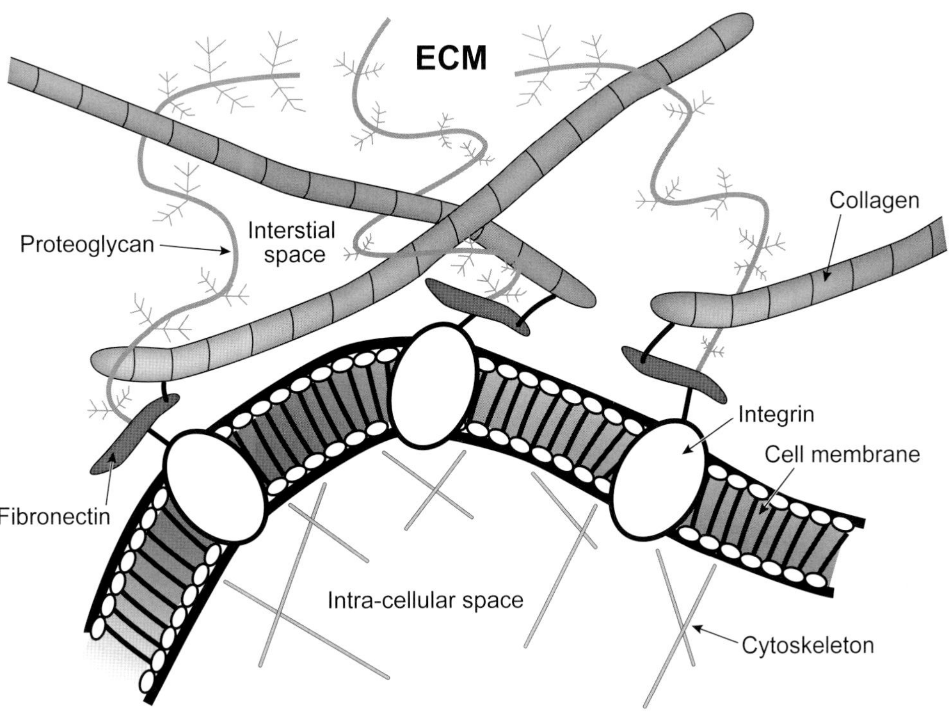

Fig. 4.8
Cell matrix-adhesion illustrates how collagen fibers of the extra-cellular matrix bind to the cell membrane.

The current question we should be asking is how exactly does all this (i.e. observation of, or research on, controlled mechanical inputs in laboratory settings) translate to yoga? When highly controlled experiments result in fibroblast signaling and increases in collagen synthesis and tissue repair, it might be enticing to casually assume clinical relevance. When laboratory experiments can regulate inflammation and modulate the presence of enzymes and growth hormones, it might be enticing to casually assume these results can be replicated in a clinical setting (including a yoga studio). When fibroblasts implanted into a bioengineered tissue heal a wound through a controlled stretch, can we really assume a restorative yoga pose will heal an injury in a student? While the notion is attractive, we must stop and appreciate the complexity of connective tissue properties thus far and consider how behavior, structure, and composition all play an important role. This question leads us into a more detailed examination of tissue adaptation, tissue injury, and tissue repair.

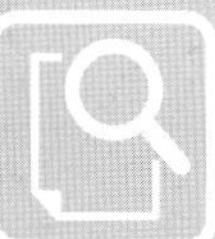

Research Summary

Stretching and Tissue Repair

Duration and Magnitude of Myofascial Release in 3-Dimensional Bioengineered Tendons: Effects on Wound Healing (Cao et al., 2015)

Background

Myofascial release (an applied external load that stretches collagen) is commonly used to treat musculoskeletal pathologies, decrease pain, and improve range of motion. Because fibroblasts regulate collagen synthesis and they are sensitive to strain, it may be possible to identify the strain conditions most favorable to tissue repair. The researchers had previously conducted experiments on a 2-dimensional matrix with favorable results and set out to improve upon their model with a 3-dimensional one.

Purpose

The study set out to determine the correlation between strain and the promotion of wound healing.

Methods

Bioengineered tendons incubated with human dermal fibroblasts were wounded with a steel blade and then stretched and observed. The effect of duration was studied in one group by stretching the tissue to a constant 6% strain for 0, 1, 2, 3, 4, and 5 minutes. The effect of magnitude was studied in another group by stretching the tissue for a constant of 90 seconds at 0%, 3%, 6%, 9%, and 12% strain. In both groups, the 0 strain was the control. Measurements of the wound were taken before the interventions and at 3, 18, 24, and 48 hours after.

Results

The magnitude group reduced the wound size with statistical significance by 24 hours after a 3% strain and by 48 hours after a 6% and 9% strain. Yet at 48 hours, the 3% and 6% improved the most and the control (0%) outcome was similar to the 9% strain group. The 12% strain made it worse immediately and up to 18 hours after the intervention, recovering somewhat by 48 hours but the wound was still larger than baseline.

The duration group shrunk the wound with statistical significance at 1 minute after 48 hours, at 3 minutes in 18 hours, and at 5 minutes in 3 hours. The 1-minute strain was equally as effective as the control (0 minutes) and the 3, 4, and 5 minute groups result in observable wound size reduction in as little as 3 hours after the intervention.

Continued on next page

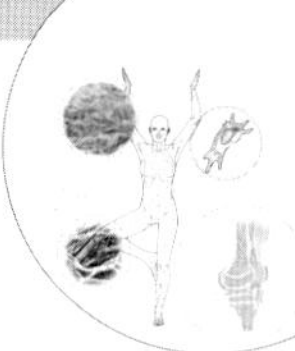

Continued from previous page

Discussion

Fibroblasts are highly responsive to differences in strain magnitude and duration. It appears that low magnitude and long duration is most effective for tissue repair. This research on engineered tissue is considered high quality but the process is very expensive, therefore replicating these results will take time and funding. Additionally, even if the results are replicated, it cannot be safely assumed that the in vitro conditions can be replicated in vivo, especially in the uncontrolled environment of a yoga studio or therapist's office. This does not make the research any less exciting, however, as studies like this pave the way for future researchers to develop study designs.

TISSUE ADAPTATION

5

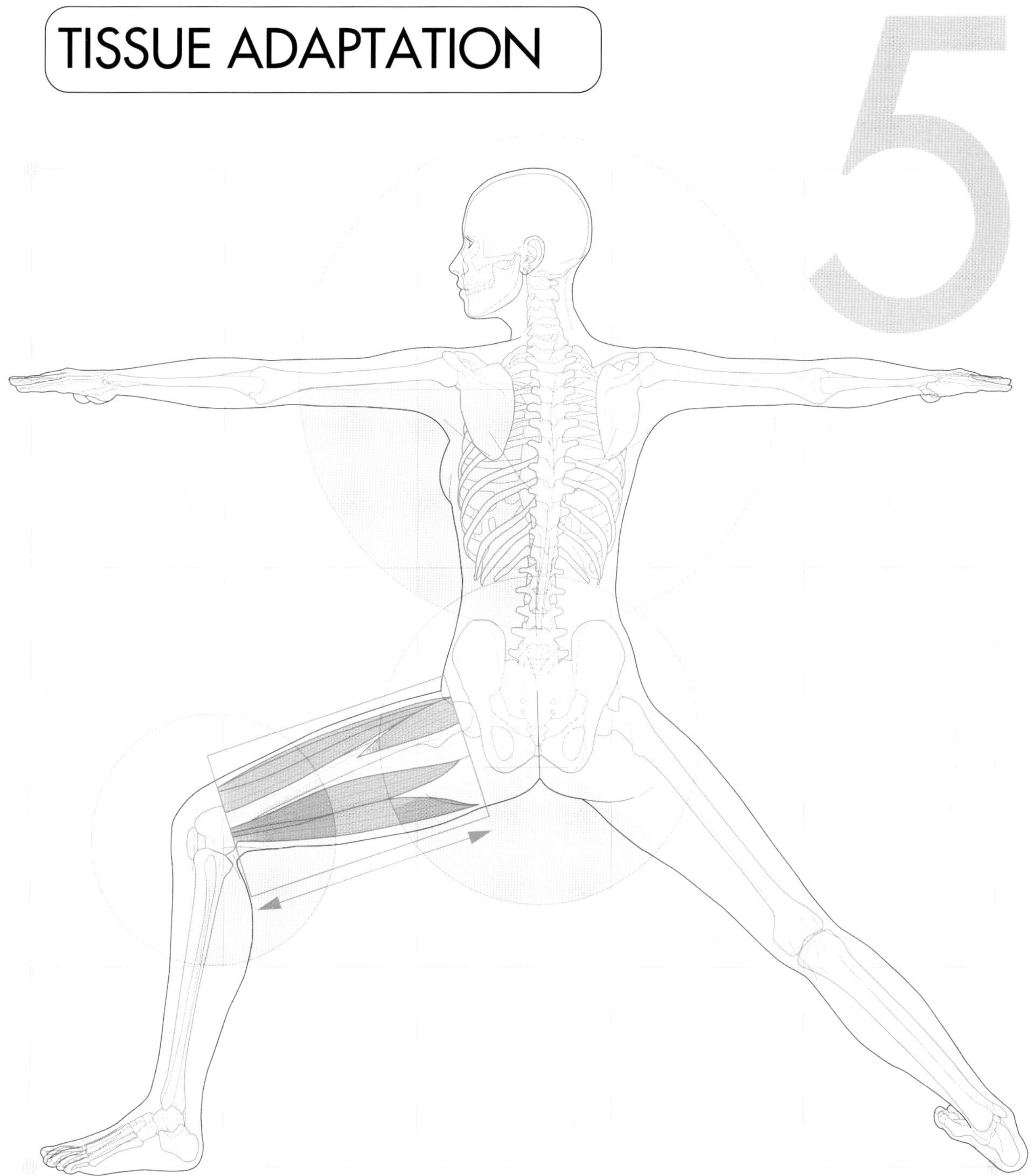

Subsequent to the review of stretching and discussion of connective tissue properties is the exploration of how, and if, stretching influences connective tissue properties, and how that relates to yoga. Although some may argue that yoga is not stretching, it would be difficult to deny that yoga exposes tissue to tensile loads. In my attempt to redefine stretching as it relates to yoga, this distinction is crucial. Conventional stretching promotes flexibility and range of motion (ROM) whereas tensile loading considers force and biology. By moving conventional stretching to the background and tensile loading to the foreground, yoga asana moves aesthetics to the background and brings tissue adaptation to the foreground.

It should be overwhelmingly clear at this point that connective tissue is anything but inert. It is a living, changing, adapting tissue whose mechanical properties are the effect of mutable characteristics including behavior, structure, and composition. Earlier we defined tissue behavior as the capacity to resist and surrender to deformation. Later we examined how this behavior, or capacity to bear load, is adaptable through certain loading parameters, just as the absence of sufficient mechanical inputs can result in maladaptation. Now, with the discussion of structure and composition more complete, we can explore tissue adaptation in greater depth, including how injuries may occur and heal, and how it all relates to a yoga practice. The investigation is timely because, at the time of writing, there has been a lot of talk about the importance of safety in yoga. What exactly constitutes a safe practice? If safe is defined as being protected against injury or risk, then being very clear on what constitutes injury must follow.

Capacity

Thus far, we have used the term capacity purely in the context of mechanical properties; of course, this is a biomechanics book. It might be easy to assume that load-bearing capacity is purely a function of mechanical properties, because in non-living materials it is. The load-bearing capacity of the suspension bridge depends on the structure of the nylon rope (i.e. the condition of its fibers) and how well it functions (i.e. behavior of the material). Where this definition falls short is in its failure to consider the whole person, and focusing only on the tissue. When discussing the capacity of tissues within a human, pain is an additional variable to consider. While increasing the capacity of any given tissue to bear load is most certainly a sound goal to pursue, the term capacity must be expanded to include structure, function, and pain (Fig. 5.1).

Structure is the most intuitive and easy to grasp variable of the three. As with most things related to the human body, the seemingly logical conclusion is often later discovered to be incomplete. Beginning in roughly the 1970s, the notion that structure was delicate and collagen fibers were easily frayed or torn was introduced and readily accepted. Even in the present day, it is still commonly assumed that if the loads applied are beyond the tissue's capacity the result will be structural degeneration, or overstretching. Researchers now understand that most structural damage to, or tearing of tendons is not mid-substance, but rather it occurs at the insertion point (i.e. an avulsion, where the tissue is torn off the bone) or at the muscular junction where the extra-cellular matrix (ECM) structure and composition changes. The belly of the tendon is remarkably resilient due to the incredible tensile strength of collagen, and therefore we must consider some other contributing factors when determining capacity.

Function is a tricky word to use. It has become a popular marketing term, and rightfully so. Don't we all want mobility, movement, and exercise to be functional? In this context, however, the term "function" refers mostly to mechanical behavior. Tendons are elastic and should have a spring-like function. When tendons are underloaded, their function as a spring diminishes, as does their capacity to bear load. When tendons do present with degenerated structure, their function, and their capacity, also diminish. As you can see, the variables intertwine and are often not mutually exclusive.

The third variable, pain, is where capacity gets complicated. Often, when poor structure and function are present, so is pain. This is the intuitive and easy-to-grasp situation. Sometimes, however, there is no pain and the tendon may still be degenerative, poorly functioning, or both. Even harder to embrace may be the fact that in some situations, there can be pain without any compromise in structure and function, and where there is only pain, capacity can still be limited. Imagine if the suspension bridge experienced pain. Its capacity to carry people across to the other side might be negatively affected. In humans, if loading a tendon causes pain, even if their structure and function are intact, *capacity* to bear load is likely reduced.

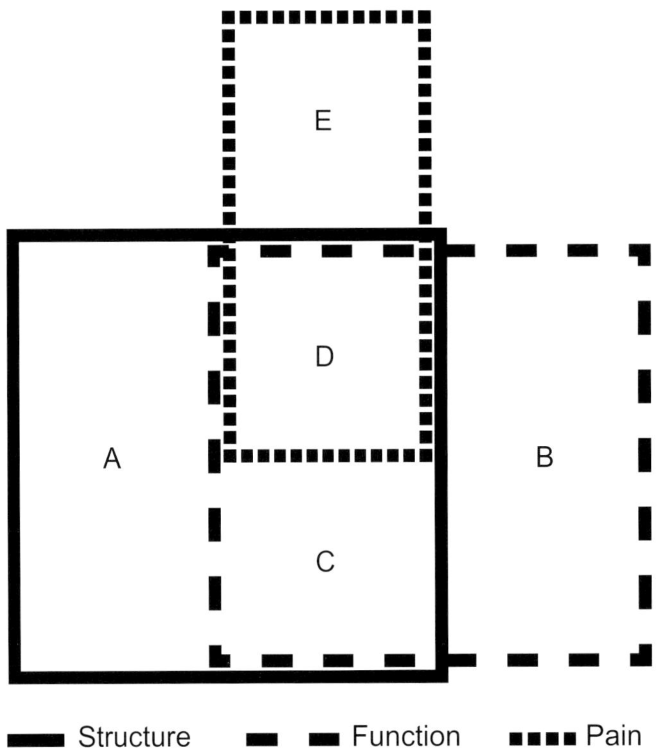

Fig. 5.1

Capacity as a function of structure, function, and pain. (A) Painless degenerative tendon prone to structural damage. (B) Underloaded painless tendon prone to overloading. (C) Painless, underloaded, and degenerative tendon. (D) Painful, underloaded and degenerative tendon. (E) Rare, but painful tendon with good structure and function. Illustration modified after Cook et al. (2016).

Moving forward, the concept of tissue adaptation and increasing/decreasing capacity must consider structure, function, and pain. In the literature, the formal definition reads: "A tissue is at full capacity when the individual is able to perform functional movements at the volume and frequency required without exacerbating symptoms or causing tissue injury" (Cook and Docking, 2015). Is this not what yoga teachers wish for their students? We wish for students to practice asana at full capacity without injury or pain. When Sun Salutations start aggravating the proximal hamstring tendon, or irritating the anterior shoulder, we must, by the above definition, admit capacity has been diminished. What is it about the yoga practice that might reduce capacity? Are we overstretching, underloading, both, or neither? These are the inquiries we will pursue in the present chapter, because if our aim is to teach and practice in a sustainable manner, we must understand the mechanisms that make for a sustainable yoga practice.

Pathology

As we know, connective tissues are adaptive and maladaptive in response to loading conditions and parameters. Concerning healthy tissue and yoga, the study of optimal loading and capacity provides insight into positive adaptation and sustainability. The opposite side of the same coin is to study tissue pathology and capacity in order to provide insight into the prevention of maladaptation.

Pathology is the study of disease. As a medical specialty its scope might include an analysis of origin/cause (i.e. etiology), diagnostic criteria, mode of contagion, prevention, treatment, morbidity, and mortality (i.e. epidemiology). Yoga therapy claims the territory of pathology and is commonly promoted as a complementary intervention to formal medical treatment for various types of diseases and conditions. Yoga therapy, in my experience, tends to focus less on musculoskeletal conditions than on diseases of the other systems of the body (e.g. cardiovascular, endocrine, etc.). Perhaps this is because the emphasis of yoga asana on the musculoskeletal system already encompasses adaptation and maladaptation of connective tissues, thereby including etiology and prevention in its scope. It is safe to say that teaching yoga with safety in mind requires some understanding of pathology and how to best mitigate it.

The growing acceptance that capacity is not solely determined by structure has resulted in an evolution of nomenclature around soft tissue injury. In recent years, the suffix "-opathy," as in tendinopathy or fasciopathy has been adopted by the scientific community, replacing those of the past. The suffix "-itis," as in Achilles tendonitis or plantar fasciitis, has previously been used to denote inflammation while the suffix "-osis," as in lateral elbow tendinosis (i.e. tennis elbow), has been used to denote degradation, or failure to heal, directing the focus away from inflammation. Chronic inflammation, however, creates an environment not conducive to healing, and therefore degradation is often present with inflammation. Moreover, -itis and/or -osis diagnosis requires a histological examination. Classifying the tissue as pathological (e.g. tendinopathy) allows for licensed healthcare professionals to cast a wide net over the condition to allow for multiple diagnostic conditions, many of which we are still trying to understand. The suffix -opathy, reflects advances in our current understanding of pain and injury by encompassing a spectrum of conditions which all seem to be provoked by loading (Scott, Backman and Speed, 2015).

In this vein, some research utilizes an even more simplified, identifying title that only indicates the region and the presence of pain. Plantar heel pain, for example, replaces plantar fasciopathy (formerly plantar fasciitis) because it is difficult to determine if the plantar fascia is the aggravating culprit, even when histological examination may suggest the possibility (Riel et al., 2017). Such a shift in nomenclature has both positive and negative potential with patient outcomes. One benefit is that the non-medicalized language may reduce fear and catastrophizing. A patient might feel less fragile and be willing to see if modifying load can modify symptoms if they aren't led to believe their tissue is damaged and fragile. A drawback is that patients might not feel they are being heard. Someone suffering from anterior knee pain may feel greater validation for their pain with a diagnosis of patellofemoral syndrome than an unceremonious acknowledgment and agreement of the presence of anterior knee pain, especially when there is a charge for this lack of formal medical diagnosis.

It may appear that such details about nomenclature are only relevant to researchers and clinicians, but I argue that yoga teachers could learn from these discussions. In many cases, yoga teachers are the first line of defense when non-serious but uncomfortable musculoskeletal conditions arise. Some students develop non-debilitating "aches and pains," come to class anyway, and then mention it to their teachers – often before they have determined whether or not they will schedule an orthopedic examination. Sometimes, the discomfort subsides and sometimes it progresses. While it is well beyond the scope of practice for a yoga teacher to diagnose and treat a pathology, yoga teachers do load tissues and aim to increase capacity; therefore they load tissues that sometimes have an existing, albeit temporary diminished capacity.

Tissues that become sensitive to loading are often referred to as "overused." Overuse, or repetitive stress, injuries have mostly been assumed to be structural in nature. In light of advances in research, one of the top tendon researchers, Jill Cook (Cook and Purdam, 2009), proposed a continuum model of tendon pathology. This model defines pathology as a collection of collagen structure abnormalities, inflammation, and tenocyte activity; it encompasses structure and composition. In the years since the model was introduced, however, the lack of correlation between tissue structure and pain has become increas-

Thought Provoker

Injury Status

Injury status is complex and multifaceted. While yoga teachers do not diagnose and treat injuries, they are very much involved in the injury conversation. Yoga teachers are tasked with protecting students from developing an injury in class. Also, yoga teachers often teach students who are recovering from an injury but have been cleared by their rehab specialist to return to yoga and other recreational activities. What is your position on injury within the context of capacity and pathology? Do these distinctions make you feel more or less qualified to provide safe instruction?

ingly evident; thus, she and her team revisited the continuum (Cook et al., 2016). They opened a dialog about symptoms, asking essential questions about complex interactions between pain, structure, and function. By including function with structure, underuse and underloading are now valid capacity considerations and not only overuse and overloading. By including sensitivity to loading with structure and function, symptoms are now also valid capacity considerations. While the complexities of pain science are not our focus here, it is impossible to discuss tissue pathology without some mention of painful symptoms. We will revisit these concepts as needed, but in order to further our inquiry into pathology we will first complete our understanding of the mutability of tissue and the microbiological processes that are associated with it.

Biochemistry of Repair

The histological processes by which a pathic tissue works to repair itself are mind bogglingly complex. Exhaustive comprehension of the many steps would be greatly facilitated by an advanced degree in chemistry and based on the assumption that most yoga teachers are not in possession of such a degree, I have done my best to simplify the process without reducing value. Please note that most of the section has been extracted from the tendon research, although an occasional reference to ligament research is included. In the past, ligaments were thought to be inert structures, with limited cellular activity, but today we understand them to share many of the complex processes we find in tendons (Hauser et al., 2013). Once again, for our purposes, we are exploring the commonality of these histologically similar tissues so that we can appreciate and encompass all of connective tissue proper. Even if the only thing that captures your interest in this section is the overwhelming sense of awe at the vastness of microscopic tissue activity, I will consider that a success.

Connective tissue is capable of healing as long as the functioning cells, regulatory hormones and enzymes, and signaling proteins are present. Vascularity is also important, as this is the pathway by which nutrients and waste are delivered to, and removed from, the wound site, respectively. Tendons and ligaments are minimally vascularized, relative to bone or muscle, and therefore injured tendons and ligaments rely on the more prolific blood flow from these neighboring tissues. The blood from muscle only reaches a short distance into the length of a tendon, and blood sourced from bone extends an even shorter distance, not much past the insertion point. Thus, the stages of healing are inconsistent and vary among individuals, tissues, and even the location of the wound. Regardless, we can summarize the healing process with a timeline highlighting the relevant events and identifiable stages.

Depending on the authority, connective tissue heals in three or four distinct phases. I have chosen to present a three-stage model (Table 5.1), which began as essentially a four-stage model, but the final two stages are combined. Each of the three phases is uniquely named, defined by a general time frame, and set apart by a multitude of microscopic, and distinct, albeit overlapping events. The first phase is marked by an immediate fibrotic scar which closes and seals the wound. Subsequent phases are essential for restoring tissue structure and function, although a remodeled tissue post injury is currently not thought to return to its pre-injured state.

Table 5.1
Repair Phases

Repair Phase	Duration	Processes
Phase I: Inflammatory response	Begins immediately post injury and lasts 3–7 days	Pain, redness, swelling, temperature increase Vasodilation and hematoma Inflammatory mediators regulate Mast cells and macrophages arrive Coagulum initiates repair process Mesenchymal stem cells (undifferentiated cells) Fibroelastic scar builds groundwork for collagen Type III collagen peaks (signals next phase)
Phase II: Repair and proliferation	Begins days 3–7 and lasts 4–6 weeks	Cytokines released Increase in GAGs High water content Mast cells and macrophages leave Collagen fibrils bundle into fibers
Phase III: Remodeling and maturation	Begins around 4–6 weeks and lasts 1–3 years	Type I collagen replaces weaker type III collagen Decrease vascularity Cell death ceases excess collagen production Collagen organizes, aligns with axis of loading

Phase I, the inflammatory phase, begins immediately after the adverse event and continues over the following 3 to 7 days. Following an initial and immediate vasoconstriction, vasodilation floods the area with red blood cells (RBCs) and white blood cells (WBCs) from outlying sources. The blood coagulates as a temporary patch until tenocytes proliferate and initiate a fibroelastic scar, binding the wounded area. Mast cells release granules such as histamines and heparin (i.e. anticoagulants that regulate a blood clot) and protect against pathogens (i.e. infectious microorganisms). Histamines increase permeability to the injury site, which is a benefit of inflammation, allowing for transportation of inflammatory mediators, cells, proteins, hormones, other materials needed for healing. Mesenchymal stem cells (MSCs) aid in repair by differentiating into tenocyte-like cells (as fibroblasts arise from MSCs). Macrophages, large phagocytic cells, clean up and digest material waste caused by the healing response. Type-III collagen, the thinner and weaker collagen, begins forming, which marks the peak and the end of phase I.

It is important to note that inflammation is a normal, essential part of the healing process. Inflammation involves the complex biological processes needed to create the necessary biological environment for repair. Likewise, an inflammatory environment, is also one indicator of a pathology (Abate et al., 2009). Chronic inflammation only exacerbates the harmful environmental conditions. Imagine you were remodeling your house and all the contractors and construction crews arrived with their materials to do their job but failed to remove any of the debris after completing their repairs. You would have a refurbished structure made of new and old materials, but a disorganized, poorly functioning home filled with materials, waste, and maybe even a few remaining crew members! The inflammatory stage delivers the cells and nutrients to complete the job but must eventually come to an end, so the tissue can become an organized, functional structure.

This is not to say that applications such as ice and compression should be avoided. Ice, in particular, may serve to reduce the heat, redness, and painful swelling during the inflammatory phase, and is an excellent nonpharmacologic analgesic. Whether or not it actually retards the inflammatory process is not certain. I do not wish to debate the harmful or harmless applications of ice here, as it is a heated topic. I only bring it up in the context of inflammation, and to highlight that the evidence for the common remedy known as RICE (i.e. rest, ice, compression, and elevation) is not compelling enough to categorically reject it or unconditionally advocate for it (van den Bekerom et al., 2012). During my years in graduate school, we learned that the term MEAT (i.e. mobilization, exercise, analgesics, and treatment) should replace RICE. The literature now seems to currently support POLICE (i.e. protection, optimal loading [Glasgow, Phillips and Bleakley, 2015], ice, compression, elevation). Rest appears to have fallen out of favor as an essential component to healing; in fact, anyone who has had a hip replacement knows the first thing they are asked to do after surgery is to walk, thereby loading the new hip. Yoga teachers may choose to defer an ice recommendation to licensed therapists and, instead, encourage light active or passive mobilization (if tolerable) to move inflammation through the affected area.

Phase II, the repair and proliferation phase, lasts roughly 4–8 weeks and continues with elevated collagen type III synthesis (increased levels of type III collagen is also another indicator of pathology). The macrophages deposit the transforming growth factor ß1 (TGF-ß1), which promotes collagen production. As collagen content increases, mechanical capacity improves, allowing for low loads to mechanically signal directional fiber alignment. The increase in fibroblast activity causes an increase in the release of cytokines, which are a collection of proteins that signal cells to differentiate, produce, and eventually terminate through apoptosis. Cytokines include a broad category of mediators such as interleukins (ILs), proteins such as matrix metalloproteinases (MMPs) and their inhibitors (TIMPs), and several additional growth factors (GFs). Glycosaminoglycans (GAGs; ground substance) and water are in abundance, simultaneously binding and unbinding, regulating molecular and cellular movement within the wound site. Collagen fibers bundle together, increasing thickness and diameter, and arrange longitudinally. The associated increase in tissue strength marks the transition into the next phase.

If you recall, load is the input essential to mechanotransduction, the process by which cells convert mechanical stimuli to biochemical responses within the ECM. Mechanotherapy refers to the process of using exercise to stimulate the healing response (Khan and Scott, 2009). Traditionally, the protocol for healing and repair involved rest, even immobilization at times, during the early phases. This came from a time when the prevailing thought was to give tissues time to heal in order to avoid further damage to a compromised tissue. Today, there is an increasing emphasis on the fibroblast's response in pathic tissues (Cook et al., 2016). A revolutionary study on Achilles and patellar tendons in 91 subjects determined that the area of structural abnormality was, not surprisingly, greater in pathological tendons than in a normal tendon, but what was surprising was that the cross-sectional area (CSA) of structural normality was also greater in pathological tendons than in normal tendons (Docking and Cook, 2016). This changes the narrative quite a bit; thickened tissues may not be a cause of pathology, but rather

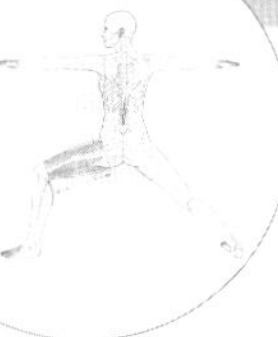

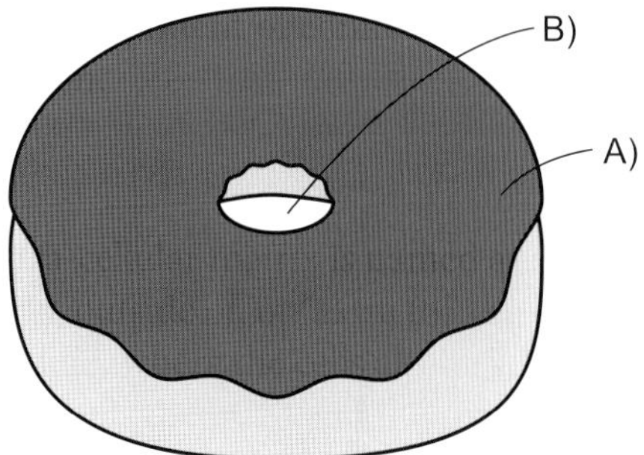

Fig. 5.2
The donut analogy of tendons. (A) Loading affects the healthy tissue, the donut. (B) The abnormal tissue, the donut hole, is protected by the surrounding healthy tissue, the donut.

a positive adaptive response to pathology. In this case, loading pathic tissues, versus resting them, may have the greater protective effect (Fig. 5.2). We already know this to be true for bone and it is only now we are beginning to understand its implication in tendons and, potentially, other connective tissues. Of course, this is not a carte blanche to load with reckless abandon. Excessive stress or strain during phase II has the potential to reignite the inflammatory response, causing a cycle of recurring inflammation and fibrosis referred to as smoldering fibrogenesis (Thornton and Hart, 2011). The result is a disorganized, weakened collagen matrix, unable to advance to the final phase of healing.

Phase III, the final and longest phase of healing, is defined by the remodeling and maturation of collagen fibers. This 2- to 3-year-long process is first marked by an increase in fibroblast volume as the resilient collagen type I replaces the weaker type III. After fiber production peaks, fibroblast volume reduces by apoptosis, and the collagen matrix forms cross-links to increase tensile capacity. Over time, the collagen fibers organize to align along the axis of loading. A decline in vascularity marks the later stage of phase III. Mechanical demands during this phase are essential for collagen organization.

Arguably, the timeline of phase III is most informative for yoga practitioners with an interest in the capacity and/or concern about the safety of individuals with past injuries. In the US, most insurance-based physical therapy treatment courses span about 4–6 weeks. At this point, if function is generally restored, and pain has diminished somewhat, the patient transitions from rehabilitation to resuming daily activities, including yoga (i.e. they are no longer classified as a patient, but as a client, or student). These students/clients are ready to continue to increase mechanical demands to promote mechanotransduction. Yet, they are far from fully rehabbed and optimal loading principles still, and always will, apply (i.e. specificity, adequate progression, and variability). In fact, loads during the phase III may very much resemble rehab loads during phase II, only the parameters should continue to progress. Finally, a yoga practitioner concerned with avoiding injuries in yoga altogether will benefit from a deeper inquiry into injury and how it is defined.

Injury Classification

Injury, precipitated by the prevailing tissue tearing model, dominates the literature to date as the primary mechanism or cause. This model explains that mechanical overload leading to injury occurs by one of two mechanisms: a single abrupt impact exceeding tissue capacity and resulting in a tear or lesser, albeit repeated, loads that cause "wear and tear" over time. Acute mechanical overload injuries are generally sustained as a result of a sudden, rapid, and unstoppable incident, such as a torn anterior cruciate ligament (ACL) resulting from a skiing accident. The alternative is an injury sustained slowly and over time, such as the development of a hamstring tendinopathy in a yoga practitioner. Often referred to as a repetitive stress injury, repetitive strain injury, or even overuse syndrome, the naming of a slowly developing injury in this way implies that repeated loading inevitably leads to tissue "wear and tear." A more suitable name might include underuse, or even under preparedness, in addition to overuse to account for poorly managed exposure to loads. Perhaps that yoga practitioner's hamstring tendon might properly have sustained the low load repetition if her training protocol included variable magnitudes, rates, and directions of loading with the intent to increase capacity.

We can look to osteoarthritis to further expand on the assumptions about repetitive loading. Knee osteoarthritis is widely believed to be a result of the "wear and tear" of the joint over time. This rationale would reflect that given the tissue remained the same, and didn't positively adapt over time, the older and the heavier we get, the more at risk we are for osteoarthritis. The diagnosis of arthritis has doubled in the last century, supporting this suggested correlation, since we live longer and are getting heavier. Yet, when age and body mass index were controlled for, we still find double the cases of arthritis compared to previous generations. Since nobody is claiming that our society is currently moving and exercising more than we should (in fact, it is quite the opposite), some other biological or mechanical factor is contributing (Wallace et al., 2017). This is just another example of why simplified mechanical analogies for the human body can tempt us into making false logical assumptions, and poorly chosen cues.

Injured tissues, historically defined by structural damage, are classified by three grades (Table 5.2). Some authorities classify injuries into four grades instead of three and with multiple subclassifications (Mueller-Wohlfahrt et al., 2013). For our purposes, the three-grade classification system will suffice. Grades I and II are tissue traumas identified as micro-damage, ranging from a few torn fibers (grade I) to a partial tear (grade II). Often, the tissue is still functional, and capacity or performance is unlikely to be compromised. Today, we relate partial tendon tears to tendinopathies because exactly how much of the injury is structural is unclear. A grade III injury is a full tear, or rupture, at the macroscopic level, rendering the tissue malfunctional. For tendons, such ruptures are quite uncommon, occurring mainly in the tendons of the rotator cuff, Achilles, and distal biceps brachii. In a landmark paper examining 891 subjects who experienced spontaneous tendon ruptures, 97% presented with an underlying pathology (Kannus and Jozsa, 1991), suggesting that full tears do not frequently occur in healthy tendons. With grade III injuries, performance relies on the recruitment of neighboring structures and capacity of the overall region is likely, but not guaranteed, to be substantially compromised. It seems reasonable to assume complete performance failure after such an injury; however, the human body shows us time and time again that it does not adhere to reason and logic. It is not uncommon to hear of cases where grade III tears have gone untreated – as in a torn ACL or rotator cuff – and where the neighboring structures are able to keep the joint operational and symptom free.

Table 5.2
Injury Classification

Injury Classification	Characteristics
Grade I	A few damaged fibers
Grade II	Partial tear
Grade III	Full tear

Here, then, we arrive at the inevitable discussion about the correlation (or lack thereof) between structural damage and pain. One must wonder how many tissue "abnormalities" go undetected. In the absence of pain, after all, structural degeneration is likely to go undetected since positively identifying any grade injury generally requires radiographic evidence (although imaging has its limitations), which tends only to be issued after a complaint of pain or discomfort. In the landmark study above, 80% of the subjects with an underlying pathology expressed no pain prior to rupture (Kannus and Jozsa, 1991). Cases where full rotator cuff tears are asymptomatic are not uncommon, whereas fully intact rotator cuff tendons can be highly symptomatic. The data on osteoarthritis, in particular, reveal discordance between symptoms and radiographic reports (Finan et al., 2013). Pain responses not only vary greatly among individuals, they even vary within the same individual. We all know someone with arthritis who has "good" days and "bad" days or complains the arthritis is "acting up" when it rains. The cartilage has not degenerated and regenerated on a daily basis – it was the symptom that fluctuated.

Undeniably, pain and tissue damage are poorly correlated. The data supporting this conclusion are not new, yet for most, such a statement still requires a robust list of citations. A brief literature search immediately displayed a half dozen reports of abnormal findings in asymptomatic populations. In 51 shoulder scans of men ages 40–70, 96% had some sort of abnormality including tendon tears, arthritis, bursal thickening, etc. (Girish et al., 2011). In 53 adults, ages 45–60 years, shoulder labral tears were present in 72% (determined by one radiologist) and 55% (determined by another) of the subject pool (Schwartzberg et al., 2016). In 39 professional and collegiate hockey players, 77% presented with various pelvic and hip pathologies, with labral tears being of greatest prevalence (Silvis et al., 2011). A follow-up study on the same cohort determined that only 20% of those with hip labral tears eventually reported symptoms within 2 years (Gallo et al., 2013). In 1211 adults ages 20–70 years, MRIs of the cervical spine revealed 87.6% had bulging discs, and of those subjects in their 20s, 73.3% of men and 78.0% of women presented with bulging discs (Nakashima et al., 2015). In a systematic review of 3110 subjects, 96% of those in their 80s presented with spinal disc degeneration, as did 37% of those in their 20s (Brinjikji et al., 2015). *All of the subjects in all of the above studies were asymptomatic.* There are plenty more papers published with even more data, but those I have presented should suffice.

The continuum model of tendon pathology developed out of this poor association between structure and pain and indicates just how widely accepted this notion is among researchers. Yet the sharp departure from conventional thought makes it difficult to swallow for those not immersed in the literature. Once, at a weekend course, I presented

Scientific Literacy

Correlation is not Causation

Correlation is a statistics term that describes a relationship between variables. When the relationship is in a similar direction, this is a positive correlation. For example, height and weight are positively correlated. Shorter people tend to weigh less, but not always. If the association between height and weight were perfect, the coefficient of correlation would be 1.00 (and 0.00 if not at all related). When a relationship exists, but in the opposite direction, this is a negative correlation (where the coefficient ranges between -1.00 and 0.00). For example, if the longer you practice yoga the fewer injuries you have, then yoga and injuries would have a negative correlation. If the longer you practice yoga, the more injuries you have, then yoga and injuries would have a positive correlation.

Probably the most common error in interpreting research is conflating causation with correlation. Just because two variables are correlated, does not mean one causes another. In the above example, if yoga and injuries wear positively correlated, that would not imply that yoga causes injuries, tempting as that conclusion may be. Just because two events occur together, does not mean one causes the other. A popular example can be found on the nutrition blogs. One well known study found that people who drink diet sodas tend to gain more weight than those who drink regular sodas. False causation has bloggers reporting that diet sodas (or the artificial sweeteners they contain) make you gain weight. In order to determine such a causative relationship, the study design would have needed to control for any other variables that might cause weight gain, such as genetics, medications, physical activity, and overall diet. Additionally, correlation studies must be endlessly replicated (as with smoking studies) to establish causal links. Remember, research does not prove causation, it only establishes cause and effect relationships through theory, experiment, and statistics.

all of the above data (and more) to a large group of yoga teachers. My aim was to incite a conversation about yoga and injuries within a group that I had sensed was catastrophizing popular yoga styles and postures. After I listed the staggering percentage of positive imaging findings (i.e. presence of pathologies) in asymptomatic populations, a teacher in the back spoke out and asked, "Is there any good news?" My reply was simply, "This is the good news." So conditioned are we are to conflate tissue "abnormality" with dysfunction, pain, and injury that we cringe and worry at anything other than perfection. Greg Lehman, who created the course "Reconciling Biomechanics with Pain Science," refers to these abnormalities as "wrinkles on the inside." Nobody walks up to an aging person and gasps with horror at her wrinkles asking if her face functions without pain. Personally, at present, I have a grade II rotator cuff tear (tendinopathy). When I announce this during my weekend courses, the teachers in the room visibly recoil and audibly

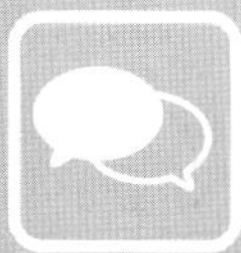

Thought Provoker

Tissue Abnormalities

Spend a moment and take inventory of your relationships with yoga over the years. Consider what you originally believed about yoga and musculoskeletal injury and if this belief is different today. Aside from your own personal experience, consider other influences that helped form those beliefs (i.e. continuing education, social media, teaching experience). With all of this in mind, where do you stand on the prevalence of tissue abnormalities? Does this inspire you to practice yoga with more caution or less caution (within reason, obviously)? For example, what is your position on Headstand – eliminate it to protect or include it to protect?

gasp with worry. When I explain I am absolutely asymptomatic with no loss of function, worry turns to confusion. I must always further explain that I discovered the "injury" after I requested an MRI for some wrist pain. The report also revealed mild scoliosis and bulging discs in my cervical spine and osteoarthritis in my acromioclavicular joint. None of these areas have ever been symptomatic for me and continue not to be years later. Incidentally, my wrist pain went away shortly after, while the diagnoses from the MRI remain unresolved. I realize this is anecdotal, and I'm pushing evidence-based decision making, but sometimes it does help to support data with a personal story when biases are being aggressively challenged.

Returning to the research on tendinopathy, we can learn from recent findings about injury beyond the collagen tearing model to determine that compromises in structure and composition might occur within the ECM and the cellular components. "Pathic" tendons might present with disorganized collagen, greater than normal amounts of type III collagen, increased GAG and proteoglycan (PG) content, hypercellular activity, apoptosis (cell death), abnormal neurovascular growth, and sometimes even calcification of the tendon (Rio et al., 2014). Additional biochemical changes also indicate pathology and will be covered in the next section. The physiological drivers of pain are even more complex and will not be covered here. The burning question now is, "what exactly constitutes an injury if collagen structure is not the only consideration?"

Broadly speaking, load is definitely a factor in musculoskeletal injury – too much or too little is problematic. More specifically, diminished mechanical capacity to bear load might establish presence of, or result in, an injury. Narrowing further and using the continuum model as our guide, diminished capacity could be a sensitivity to load as a result of structure, function, or pain. We could then say, for our purposes, that a musculoskeletal injury is an intolerance to load. In turn, restoring load tolerance (the ability to load asymptomatically) increases capacity and improves structure, function, and/or symptoms. In terms of the role of a yoga teacher in providing a safe class, load tolerance and load capacity are the only appropriate considerations. Any other injury by any other definition, and arguably the prevention thereof, should be referred out to a qualified and properly trained rehabilitation or healthcare professional.

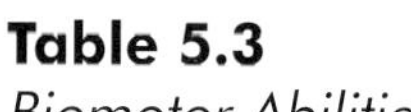

Table 5.3
Biomotor Abilities

Biomotor Ability	Description
Strength	Amount of weight you can move
Power	Speed at which you can move that weight
Speed	Speed at which you can move yourself (or a limb)
Endurance	Length of time you can sustain muscle contractions
Agility	Quality and speed at which you can change direction
Coordination	Ability to integrate complex movements
Balance	Ability to maintain equilibrium
Flexibility	Amount of range of motion you have

In many cases, effectively increasing load tolerance and capacity requires more equipment, and more education/experience in teaching/coaching/training various biomotor availabilities than most yoga education provides. Not all biomotor abilities are well-trained through a conventional yoga practice; only some (Table 5.3). A yoga teacher well-versed in various training modalities will discover she can modify the loading parameters of the postures and vary the pose selection by combining an asana practice with additional body weight drills and the creative use of props/equipment. Skillful and deliberate "exercise selection" with tissue adaptation in the foreground and aesthetics in the background is not presently the standard educational format (quite the opposite, in fact). Why then, is a yoga teacher expected to teach a safe class with confidence and purpose if they are not well versed in these principles?

In the absence of a biomechanics education, yoga teachers are generally advised to keep students safe by avoiding load. It is the ultimate reduction of the complexities of load intolerance. It is not wrong, in that it is not unsafe in the short term, but it does not increase capacity for future safety, and may even decrease capacity. It assumes avoiding loads altogether is the best way to avoid injury, which we now know not to be true. Paradoxically, the same type of stress, or stimulus, that injures also protects. Adding complexity to the paradox, the capacity for the stimulus, or the specifics of the loading parameters are unique to the individual and are nearly impossible to predict. In fact, predicting injury using even well-established screening tests is about as accurate as predicting the outcome of a coin toss (Bahr, 2016). Even teachers with a biomechanics background are left with a 50/50 choice in avoiding injury; exposure to load or load avoidance. There is no other option.

Pause and turn to page 158 for a summary of related research.

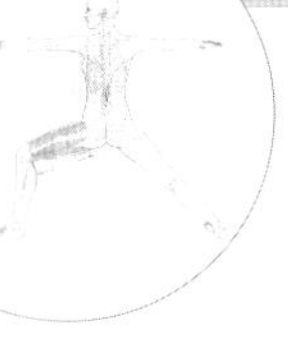

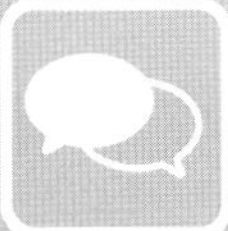

Thought Provoker

Tissues Under Tension

Looking at the shoulder joint during a Side Plank, the soft connective tissues (tendons and ligaments) are under tension and the joint structures (bones and cartilage) are under compression. Remember, the contracting muscles supporting the shoulder are applying the tensile load. A tensile load does not always look like a "stretch." During an isometrically held Side Plank, which shoulder muscles do you think are active? In turn, which soft tissue structures are loaded in tension?

To be clear, nobody is suggesting yoga teachers load without regard to pain. What is being suggested is that a safe yoga practice consider all aspects of capacity. With the current evidence as it stands, tissue pathologies are likely present in the majority of students, many of which are possibly asymptomatic. Moreover, loading those tissues into tension is not likely to cause (further) collagen tearing, as was once thought. Even if they were, the tension on those tissues associated with a yoga practice are relatively low in magnitude and rate when compared with strength and conditioning (S&C) exercises or power exercises (i.e. plyometrics). A yoga student who isometrically loads a slightly uncomfortable rotator cuff in a Side Plank, for example, might find it improves her tolerance for load. If not, the likelihood of tearing collagen because of the pose alone is still slim to none, and she might consider seeking assistance from a qualified and licensed therapist to assist her in restoring load tolerance. The Side Plank, however, is hardly an unsafe pose to teach – barring any other extreme cases (e.g. compound fracture) or non-musculoskeletal conditions (e.g. tumor, neuropathy, etc.), of course. For some populations this pose might be too progressive too quickly, in which case it might exceed capacity and result in greater load intolerance, in which case it should be regressed, and then progressed, appropriately. These are the necessary considerations in a safe and sustainable practice, not in relation to the pose itself.

Tensile Loading

Finally, after several chapters of defining terms and explaining concepts, we arrive in a place where we can deconstruct tensile loading and how it relates to yoga asana. Remember, stretching is an activity which focuses on flexibility and ROM. Loading is an applied force which may result in tension, compression, shear, torque, or bending. Stretching, therefore, is a form of loading.

This is highlighted here, again, because I find it not to be intuitive. Perhaps it's the way we culturally talk about stretching as an act of letting go and loading as an act of building strength. This perception is just as misleading as the long/weak and short/strong dichotomy previously discussed. A stretch, mechanically speaking, is a tensile load, and as with any other load, the parameters can vary.

The proximal hamstring tendon, for example, can be stretched (i.e. loaded) with varying parameters. Just about any forward bend is considered a hamstring stretch, which will, in turn, load the entire muscle tendon unit (MTU) of the hamstrings (tendons included) in tension. A stretch against resistance, or an eccentric contraction, also loads the hamstring MTU in tension, but with a greater magnitude than the former example. Perhaps less obvious is the stretch on the tendon during a concentric contraction. When the hamstring concentrically contracts (e.g. during a hamstring curl), the muscle fibers may shorten, but the tendon is again loaded in tension, also with a greater magnitude than the first example.

One could say the same for the ligaments and joint capsules. A supine squat position (i.e. knees to chest on your back) stretches the connective tissues at the anterior aspect of the knee, as does an unloaded Deep Squat (i.e. Garland Pose), or an overhead squat with a 40 kg barbell. All other factors being equal (e.g. joint position), then mechanically speaking the difference lies in the magnitude of the load.

Soccer players are prone to proximal hamstring strains because of the high demands of the sport. Kicking, running, sprinting, rapid changes of direction, falling/tumbling, and sliding all subject the athlete to high and fast loads. Kicking, in particular, ends in hip flexion combined with knee extension; essentially a high speed hamstring stretch position. If a soccer player were to sustain an overstretch injury, it seems it would be more likely to occur during the demands of the sport than during a comparatively lower load stretch like a yoga pose.

It is well known that high and fast loads are what cause strains and sprains. In terms of tissue capacity, however, because the terms “high” and “fast” are relative, it is more accurate to say that strains and sprains are caused by loads to which the tissue has not yet adapted. Of course, capacity and adaptation are not infinite, and will eventually be limited by the mechanical properties of the tissue. The question is whether these limits are being exceeded, or even being met in a yoga posture. The act of “stretching” as outlined in Chapter 2, generally does not expose tissues to tensile loads of such magnitude and acceleration that one could “overstretch.” These flexibility exercises are relatively low magnitude load, even the resistance stretching when compared with lifting weights, for example. If overstretching were so easily done, we'd have a lot more Olympic lifters overstretching than yoga students.

One could argue that overstretching is the result of time in the pose (e.g. duration and frequency), but with regard to duration, we know that tissue creep during prolonged tension is in part to prevent overstretching from occurring. We also know crimp patterns are modulated by the cells and modified during creep, also thought to prevent overstretching. Moreover, creep recovers, as it's a temporary phenomenon. Frequency relies on the “wear and tear” philosophy, which we are not certain exists. If it did, it would suggest we have a finite number of tensile loads available before the structure cannot sustain another. In the absence of any compelling evidence, I find it difficult to apply “wear and tear” model for an inanimate material, like the suspension bridge, to an adaptable living tissue.

The concept of overstretching further relies on the model of tissue tearing that also has not held up to the research. Normal, healthy collagen is now understood not to tear, it's extremely resilient. Tissues with an underlying cellular or biochemical pathology are those that are prone to tearing and rupture (again, usually at the bone or muscle junctions); and pathological tissues are made more resilient through tensile loading. Optimal loading still applies, of course. With all this in mind, I propose that our concern with overstretching in yoga should be reframed into a concern with underloading. Let me explain.

During a lecture, I was once asked by a prominent and legendary yoga educator what I thought about Standing Forward Bend Pose and how many salutations are too many. With everything you know now, you understand this question has no binary answer. My reply was that there is no way to predict how many will be too many; it would depend on the individual (e.g. age, sex, genetics) and her loading history. I followed up by implying I would have less concern with the frequency of her Standing Forward Bend Pose if she could deadlift her body weight. You see, overstretching is not the driver of my concern; underloading is. And if tolerance to load, be it structural, functional, or symptomatic, is the goal, then we must increase load exposure over time.

Naturally, there are caveats. First, tendons are also subjected to friction (i.e. shear) and compressive loads, which need to be considered. Second, this applies to normal collagen structure, and not collagen structure associated with hypermobility. Let us continue to deconstruct.

Compressive Forces

While the primary focus of this book is tensile loading (i.e. stretching redefined), it does not happen in a vacuum, and tissues are exposed to multiple forces during movement. Friction occurs between the tendons and the peritendinous sheath during movement, and compression occurs at the insertion point at outer ranges (Table 5.4). The latter is sometimes difficult to visualize. The compression is not longitudinal as is the tension, but rather lateral. As the joint approaches end range, the tendon is wrapped over the bone where it inserts and is laterally compressed against it (Fig. 5.3).

Table 5.4
Insertional Compression Sites

Tendon	Compression Site	Joint Position
Proximal hamstring	Ischial tuberosity	Hip flexion
Achilles tendon	Calcaneus	Ankle dorsiflexion
Gluteus medius	Greater trochanter	Hip adduction
Quadriceps	Femoral condyle	Knee flexion
Adductor longus	Pubic ramus	Hip abduction and hip extension
Long head of biceps	Bicipital groove	Shoulder extension
Pectoralis major	Humeral tuberosity	Shoulder external rotation
Supraspinatus	Greater tuberosity	Shoulder adduction

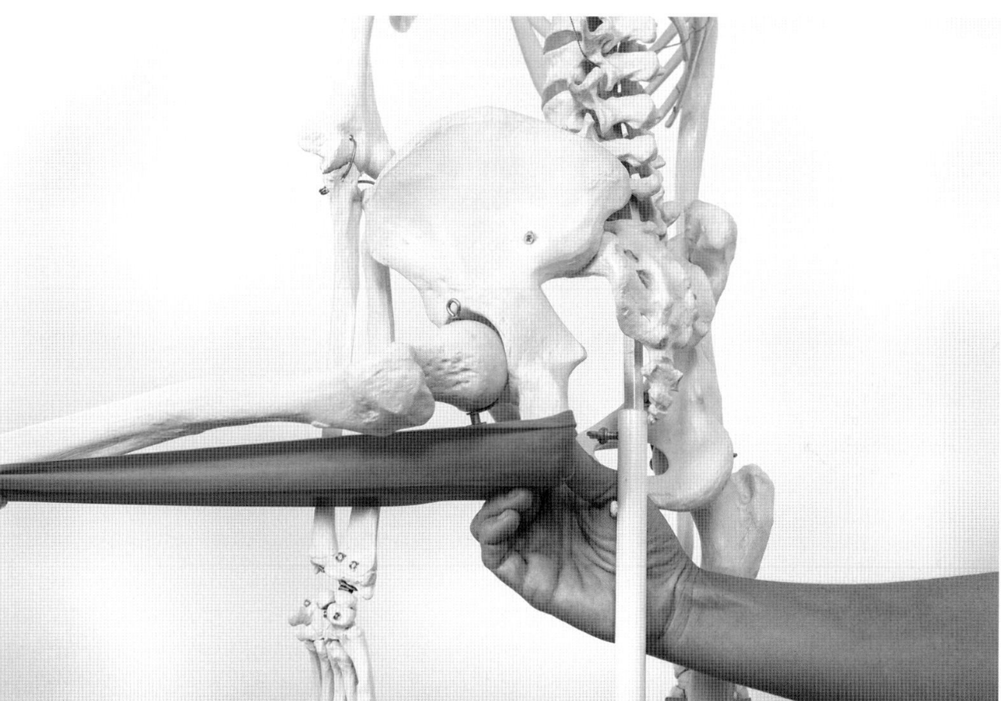

Fig. 5.3
Insertional compression site of the hamstring tendon in outer range.

If form follows function, tendon structure is a design which withstands, stores, and releases large amounts of tension. It has been shown that when tendons are exposed to excessive compressive forces, such as at certain attachments, they begin to develop areas of fibrocartilage. Again, if form follows function because tissue adapts, it is not surprising that tissue structure with a design to withstand compression (i.e. cartilage) develops where compression occurs. What may be problematic in the tendon, however, is the structure and composition of the fibrocartilage areas. Fibrocartilage is indicated by increased PG content, and also by an increase in type II cartilage. Tendinopathy is indicated by increased PG content, and also by a decrease in type I collagen. It is speculated that these compressive matrix changes provoke symptoms but it is still uncertain how, and if, they compromise function in tendons (Docking et al., 2013). After all, healthy tendons must be able to tolerate all types of forces, including compressive forces.

Based on the adaptive response to compressive forces, we can wonder if the prevalence of insertional hamstring tendinopathies in yoga is a compressive issue and not an "overstretching" issue. Over many years of inquiry about hamstring injuries in yoga, this is the first plausible and satisfying answer I have come across. Every educator or teacher I asked had the one single solution to avoid proximal hamstring tendinopathy, but none of them explained a mechanism of action, and many of them contradicted each other. "Standing Forward Bend requires bent knees to prevent microtears of the hamstring tendons." "No, straighten your legs during Standing

Forward Bend so you distribute the stretch to the upper and lower hamstring evenly." "Untuck your tail in Downward Facing Dog Pose to lengthen the belly of the hamstrings." "Don't lift your sitting bones in Downward Facing Dog Pose or you'll overstretch your hamstring tendons." Apologies if you use these statements. I understand, I have used them in the past, too, out of desperation to do my part to minimize the epidemic. In deep hip flexion postures, such as Standing Forward Bend, the proximal hamstring tendon stretches over the insertional tuberosity, causing transverse compression forces on the tendon. Perhaps the frequency of Standing Forward Bend, in addition to all the other forwarding bending types of poses, in conjunction with hamstring underloading that is characteristic of most styles of yoga could pose the greater risk rather than how the pose is done.

As I wrote in the very beginning of the book, "a well-developed vocabulary could lead to richer conversations about how stretching works…the more specific our questions are, the more accurate our answers will be." In the case of insertional hamstring tendinopathies in yoga, I might change the question to ask, "which forces are contributing to the load intolerance?" I might wonder if all the deep forward bending type poses (including poses like Lunges and Warrior Poses that involve hip flexion) in yoga classes are causing diminished capacity?

I'll repeat again, yoga teachers do not treat tendinopathies, but we are tasked with preventing them to the best of our ability, and we do increase the capacity of tissues. I might choose to sequence differently, to reduce the frequency of deep hip flexion and increase the frequency of loading those tendons in tension. I might progressively introduce deeper hip flexion, slowly to allow time for adaptation. For a student who does have an aggravated hamstring tendon, I might suggest she avoid deep hip flexion

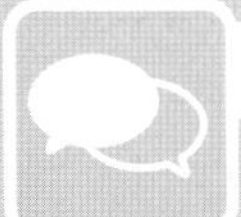

Thought Provoker

Tissues Under Compression

Looking at the ankle joint, dorsiflexion stretches the posterior lower leg structures. As end range approaches, insertional compression at the calcaneus increases. In order to load the Achilles in tension without compression, the ankle would need to be in plantarflexion. Weight bearing (i.e. heel raises) would increase tension over seated plantarflexion, and single leg, heel raises would increase tension even further. To reintroduce compression, stand on a block in plantarflexion and slowly, with control, lower the heel below the block toward the floor (eccentric posterior lower leg contraction).

What would a similar thought process for the quadriceps look like? What stretch position, or pose, compresses the distal quadriceps tendon (i.e. patellar tendon) against the femoral condyle? What position puts tension on the tendon without compression? How can you increase tension? In what position, or pose, can you use eccentrics to reintroduce compression?

for several weeks (as per the biochemistry timeline) and then slowly and progressively load first in extension and, eventually, in flexion. I took this approach to my own aggravated hamstring tendon and several years later I have far more capacity than before and no more sensitivity. I can also deadlift far more than my body weight now and I have not lost any ROM. Again, the outcome is simply anecdotal, but this is an example of how I applied evidence-based decision making to my "exercise selection."

I must point out that there is some debate among researchers and clinicians on whether or not passive stretching introduces compressive loads high enough to provoke load intolerance. For some time, stretching was advised against for people with pathologies (i.e. stretching for plantar heel pain) because of the effects of compression. Now, some suggest that that advice was over cautious and stretching is okay if it improves symptoms. Yoga, however, is not all passive stretching. Many poses, including the Lunges and Warrior Poses, anecdotally aggravate plenty of tendons. Warrior III Pose is probably one of the most provocative, as it combines compression and higher levels of tension. Unfortunately, the research on yoga and tendons is scarce, at best, and we are forced to draw from sports science data. Until we know more, the information provided here is to help you develop a safe and sustainable yoga practice.

Hypermobility

Until now, unless otherwise specifically stated, all the information presented has been for normal tissue, free from genetic variants. I don't mean to use the word "normal" with an implication that hypermobility is "abnormal" or faulty. I use the term normal here to imply "common," or even "typical." Admittedly, that is probably also an inaccurate implication, as I suspect undiagnosed hypermobility is prevalent. Over 1000 types of collagen mutations have been identified (Brodsky and Persikov, 2005), yet the populations exhibiting mutations characteristic of hypermobility are surprisingly underrepresented in the literature.

What we know about hypermobility is relatively new. We understand it is considered a spectrum disorder, where it may present as a debilitating disorder, as a hardly detectable condition in a highly functioning individual, or as anything in between. In addition to capsular laxity induced by an altered collagen structure at the molecular level, symptoms include a variety of non-musculoskeletal conditions including chronic pain (predominantly), anxiety, diminished proprioception, excessive bruising, and gastrointestinal irritability (Cattalini, Khubchandani and Cimaz, 2015; Scheper et al., 2015). It appears hypermobility syndromes are multi-systemic and should, therefore, be discussed with and treated by a qualified healthcare professional. In terms of joint laxity, marked by an overall looseness and sense of instability accompanying these collagen mutations (Wolf, Cameron and Owens, 2011), this also presents on a spectrum. Joint laxity can be localized, systween.

In the context of keeping yoga safe, the considerations for hypermobility are not going to be strikingly different from anything introduced thus far. As with "normal" tissue, load tolerance and capacity should be in the foreground. It may be controversial to say, but an occasional symptom-free hyperextended knee might not be as pathological as yoga teachers make it out to be. Once again, when aesthetics drives

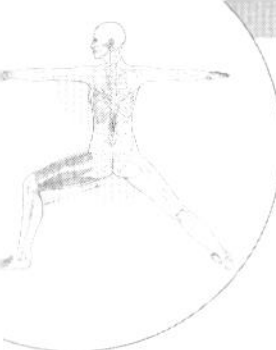

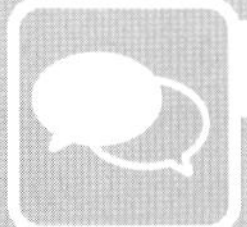

Thought Provoker

Laxity

Laxity has been defined here as either a temporary property which possibly functions to prevent overstretching, or joint looseness as a product of collagen structure variations. Sometimes, laxity is used to infer plastic morphological changes to tissues with normal collagen structure in response to passive stretching, sort of like a creeped and lengthened tissue, but permanent and unable to recover. Do you think this is possible and what is your evidence for your position?

the practice, we lose direction. The common aesthetic instruction for a hyperextended knee is to micro bend the knee to reduce the joint angle. A mechanically driven instruction would focus on the ability to create tension across the joint. If the practitioner has deficiency in mechanical tension (i.e. ratio of resistance stress to strain, or stiffness) due to collagen structure, she must rely on muscle tension to provide it. Offering a position that enables her to find, and sustain, muscle tension would be more effective than a haphazard micro bend, which may do nothing to help her engage the muscles supporting the knee. These positions might include backing off of end ranges (i.e. macro bend in the knee), closed chain options, resistance bands or yoga straps to replace the lack of internal tension, and slow oscillations or rocking motions instead of static poses to "harness" fidgeting (McNeill, Jones and Barton, 2018). Additionally, eccentrics might improve proprioception, possibly through alterations in muscle spindle sensitivity (Hanci et al., 2016). There is no one-size-fits-all joint position for any one person on the hypermobility spectrum, and the best approach to yoga for hypermobile practitioners (and any other practitioner, conveniently) is to increase capacity and tolerance for load.

Safety in Yoga

As with any subject that cannot produce a binary answer, people tend to find it difficult to linger between the two opposites. It is easier to reduce the world to one of two things than to the realm of uncertainty. How many times have you heard someone say, "There are two types of people…, those who…, and those who…"? For example, there are two types of people, those who think yoga is amazing and safe, and those who think yoga is problematic and injurious. Without volumes of research, we cannot claim either position with any definitiveness, and chances are, because we are dealing with biology, it will always depend. A survey in the US (n = 542) tells us that the positive physical changes overwhelmingly outnumber the few adverse events associated with yoga (Park, Riley and Braun, 2016) and one in Australia (n = 9151) that women who do practice yoga report less joint pain than those who do not (Lauche et al., 2017).

Personally, I have been positioned on both extremes of the pendulum swing. During my first decade as a yoga practitioner, yoga was a panacea. Maybe I was younger and more robust, maybe it was an era where yoga had not yet fallen from grace, or maybe my

Scientific Literacy

Surveys

A survey is a type of descriptive research (as opposed to experimental research) that collects information directly from the participants either by a written questionnaire or an oral interview, providing the researcher with insight into how the sample population behaves or what it believes. Open-ended questions (why do you practice yoga?) may give unique insight into behaviors and opinions but require effort from the participants who may feel imposed upon and choose not to complete the survey. Closed questions provide answers for the participants to rank (e.g. in order of preference), scale (e.g. degree of agreement or disagreement), or categorically respond (e.g. yes or no) and are more likely to be completed by the participants. Open-ended questions are sometimes used to develop the answer selections for future closed questions. Surveys seem like an easy method of data collection, but the inexperienced surveyor quickly learns that poorly constructed questions are difficult to extract data from. Focusing on the intent of the research and designing the study questions to reflect the objective are crucial to success. Pilot studies, or practice runs, are especially important for this form of research as they reveal the efficacy of the survey questions. Surveys, because they are inexpensive forms of data collection and allow for a geographically diverse sample pool, comprise one of the most commonly used forms of research.

bias was so strong that I had no room for another narrative. Also, the internet was not what it was today, and personal injury stories were not globally transmitted to a curated audience at lightning speed. In my second decade as a yoga practitioner, yoga was a risk. It was causing injuries, teachers were sequencing and adjusting irresponsibly, and the whole culture needed an overhaul. Coincidentally, or perhaps not, the timing paralleled my own "stretching injuries," left anterior hip, right proximal hamstring, and right anterior shoulder. Maybe I was older, and maybe the internet influenced my bias and I took the opposite position. Today, as I enter my third decade as a yoga practitioner, I am comfortable being uncertain. I allow myself to ride the pendulum as evidence informs me, careful to get off if it swings too far.

This mentality is a practice in itself. It requires me to challenge my own bias, which, as a human, is not in my nature. It would be much easier to write with conviction that students who hyperextend should micro bend to avoid injury, or that stretching is a waste of time and will make you weaker. It would be much easier to write that "research shows" that yoga can result in injuries; therefore, one must worry and be fearful; or to write that "research shows" that yoga is safe, therefore, performing the postures with aesthetic precision will provide one with protection from injury. None of these statements are valid, even if you read them on the internet and especially if it was I who, at one time in the past, wrote them.

Scientific Literacy

Observational Studies

Observational studies are another type of descriptive research where the subject pool is usually analyzed over time in a natural setting. Behaviors and outcomes are recorded, but no intervention is offered. As an undergrad I was an intern for the observational component of the Women's Health Initiative (WHI), which collected data on almost 10,000 post-menopausal women over a 15-year period to determine health issues contributing to morbidity and mortality. It sounds glamorous, but my rather mundane job was to enter the medical records sent to us by the personal physicians of the subjects. We collected these records, in addition to an annual questionnaire concerning health-related behaviors and exposures. At the end of the study the researchers compiled and analyzed the results to reach conclusions about certain risk factors for outcomes such as heart disease, cancer, and diabetes. The WHI did also include several components that were randomized controlled trials, but the key to this observational component was for the women to engage in their normal everyday behaviors. The medical records I entered were not results of any special test ordered by our researchers, but rather the medical care they would have received independent of participation in the study. This ensured the purest data, affected as little as possible by outside influence (considering that simply enrolling in a study has the potential to influence participant behavior).

Research conducted over years or even decades is referred to as a longitudinal study. Longitudinal studies are mostly observational studies but will occasionally be experimental. Cohort studies are those which look forward and are designed to collect future data. Due to the extensive time period, this type of research can be costly and is at risk for a high rate of participant dropouts. To avoid these pitfalls, some longitudinal research is retrospective, which collects data from the past. Unfortunately, when retrospective research relies on the memory of subjects rather than documented medical records, the reliability of data is compromised. All types of research have merits; it is important to consider the strengths and limitations of the study design when interpreting results.

Scientific Literacy

Statistical Significance

The term "statistical significance" sounds very important, as indeed it is; however, it is also helpful to know exactly what it means. The nature of research is that it generally does not set out to prove anything. Research helps us get closer and closer to what

Continued on next page

Continued from previous page

we understand to be the correct solution for the problem or question at hand. We use statistics to mathematically quantify the likelihood that our findings were not arrived at by chance. The unofficially accepted standard for statistically significant findings is a 95% or higher likelihood that findings are no accident, or a 5% likelihood of false findings ($p < .05$). This is the equivalent of saying statistically significant results have a 1/20 chance that the resulting analysis, and consequent interpretations, are false. Remember, it is almost always impossible to control for all variables so, mathematically, there will always be some chance that the experiment could have gone another way (i.e. rejecting or accepting the null hypothesis was in error).

Additionally, the $p < .05$ marker is really just an arbitrary line in the sand. Imagine a research paper found that a certain yoga pose was unlikely to cause an injury. The results were statistically significant ($p = .04$) such that there is a 96% chance that the pose is safe. You would teach the pose confident you were not putting your students at risk. But what if that same study instead found there is only a 94% chance the yoga pose is safe ($p = .06$), failing to reach statistical significance. Would you immediately stop teaching the pose because it is now no longer safe? Would you teach it to begin with, knowing you are putting 4% at risk?

As you can see, statistical significance does not always translate to clinical significance. In yoga, clinical significance means the evidence is so compelling that you change the way you teach – that old instructions have lost their effectiveness and must be replaced by new instructions. In evidence-based teaching methods, this is an important distinction. One paper revealing statistically significant results or the opposite may not be enough evidence for you to change your teaching methods, which may have been effective consistently over time. Statistically significant data comprise just one piece of information to be considered in your decision-making process, which should also include research, experience, and student circumstances.

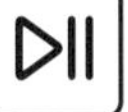

Pause and turn to page 161 for a summary of related research.

By taking the middle road, however, one does not lack conviction. One simply recognizes one's bias and requires evidence to support it. Most of us do not recognize our own bias and require evidence to refute it. Some not only do not recognize their own bias but also deny/reject any evidence that refutes it. It is the difference between an open and a closed mind. With the clarity of this distinction, I lead you into the next and final chapter where we explore perspectives that might challenge the conventional yoga script.

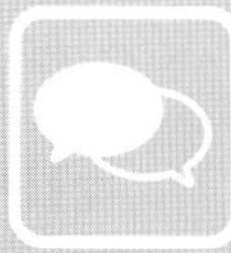

Thought Provoker

Biomechanics of Yoga

The very first thought provoker in the book asked, "If I were to ask you 'What are the biomechanics of Downward Facing Dog Pose?', what would your answer be?"

How has your answer changed between Chapter 1 and Chapter 5?

Research Summary

Symptoms with Exercise

Should Exercises Be Painful in the Management of Chronic Musculoskeletal Pain? A Systematic Review and Meta-analysis (Smith et al., 2017)

Background

Chronic pain associated with musculoskeletal conditions (e.g. back pain) is a leading cause for missed work days. Interventions generally include physical, pharmacological and psychological programs. Physical programs include either exercise or manual therapy, or both. Because tissue damage and symptoms are known to be poorly correlated, recent experimental exercise interventions emphasize load management, as well as reduction in fear and catastrophizing. In such studies, it is conveyed that negative sensations are not necessarily synonymous with increased harm. Previous systematic reviews have not specifically looked at how the acceptance versus avoidance of symptoms during exercises affects overall outcomes.

Purpose

The purpose of this paper was to determine the effectiveness of exercises where some level of pain was either allowed or encouraged versus avoided on symptoms, function, and disability in individuals with chronic pain.

Methods

Relevant databases were searched for randomized controlled trials (RCTs) on various exercise interventions. Interventions had to be targeted toward musculoskeletal symptoms persistent longer than 3 months (i.e. the accepted time frame used to determine chronic pain) where the intervention specifically allowed symptom replication or exacerbation compared with a control where symptoms were to be avoided. Interventions in response to a source of pain from anything other than musculoskeletal conditions were excluded, as were papers with a risk for bias.

Continued on next page

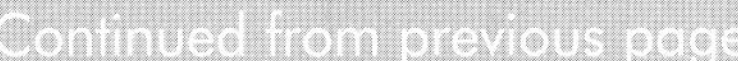
Continued from previous page

Results

Nine papers were accepted for the review, inclusive of 385 subjects suffering from various conditions including or associated with low back pain (with or without leg pain), subacromial impingement syndrome, various types of shoulder pain, Achilles and/or posterior heel pain, and plantar fasciitis. In the long term, there were no significant differences between groups. In the short term, however, there was a significant difference between groups in the reduction of reported pain in favor of the group for whom reproducing symptoms was encouraged or allowed.

Discussion

This paper is noteworthy because it highlights the changing views about musculoskeletal conditions. The narrative of the past, where reproduction of symptoms was to be avoided at all costs or risk further damage, is not holding up well against the evidence. This should not and does not permit a yoga teacher to throw caution to the wind. It does, however, influence the expectation of what a safe yoga practice looks like and reinforces the educated choice to either load or avoid load. More importantly, these evolving perspectives can influence how teachers cue, perhaps choosing language to emphasize robustness over fragility.

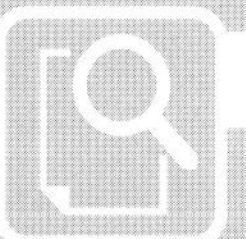

Research Summary

Injuries in Yoga

Musculoskeletal Injuries Related to Yoga: Imaging Observations (Le Corroller et al., 2012)

Background

The authors discuss the popularity of yoga in the West as a relatively low cost and easily accessible form of exercise and stress management. They state yoga can be practiced in classes or at home with video or instruction from a book with little risk. At the time of publication, there was limited information available about yoga injuries in the general population.

Purpose

The aim of this article was to retrospectively report radiology findings on musculoskeletal injury related to yoga over a 9-year period.

Continued on next page

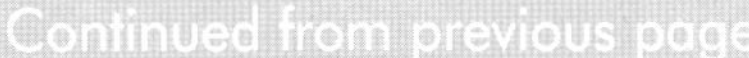
Continued from previous page

Methods

The database of over 2 million radiology reports from a single facility between the start of 2002 and the end of 2011 was searched for the term "yoga." Repeated reports for an individual case were excluded as well as those cases using the term "yoga" in a manner irrelevant to the required imaging.

Results

Thirty-eight reports satisfied the inclusion criteria and were divided into positive imaging and negative imaging groups. Twenty patients, average age 45, presented 23 positive results in the ankle/foot, knee, hip, shoulder, spine, and abdomen. Sixteen lesions/tears were found in the tendons or fibrocartilage (i.e. vertebral disc, labrum, meniscus). The remaining seven injuries included a fractured toe, an inguinal hernia, a hip replacement complication, two swollen joints, and two dislocated patellae. Eighteen patients presented with negative imaging results in the head, spine, wrist, foot/ankle, elbow, hip, leg, and abdomen. The most common of all 38 reports was headache, which returned with negative imaging in all seven cases.

Discussion

The National Institute of Health (NIH) classifies yoga as complementary and alternative medicine (CAM), therefore, the risks and benefits of yoga are an important area of research. At the time of publication, few papers focusing on yoga injuries were available. While this paper presents data from a single care center, the retrospective format of data collection made it impossible to determine which type of yoga was practiced and for how long. Additionally, any preexisting tissue pathologies that may have been related to the incident are unknown. Details of the symptom-inducing occurrence are limited, and do not offer insight into the potential mechanism of injury. It is, therefore, not possible to determine with any certainty that yoga was the direct cause of the positive imaging results. Yoga may have been the adverse event that caused an intolerance to load, but as far as structure goes, there is no way to be certain without prior imaging. On the other hand, the constraints imposed by study design made the methods of data collection vulnerable to oversight due to errors or absence of information in the original medical report. It is possible that many other patients who might have sustained diminished capacity due to years of practice did not mention the word yoga, or the provider simply did not feel it necessary to add this information to the report. While the paper may be insufficient to make sweeping conclusions about yoga and the rates of injury, I do believe the data shed light on the tissues most prone to injury in yoga (i.e. tendons and fibrocartilage).

Research Summary

Safety of Yoga

The Safety of Yoga: A Systematic Review and Meta-analysis of Randomized Controlled Trials (Cramer et al., 2015)

Background

Yoga has a long-standing reputation of having therapeutic effects with little or no risk. In recent years, the mainstream media has challenged this notion as evidenced by the growing number of blogs, news articles, and even books covering the topic of yoga-related injury. Blogs tend to provide mostly anecdotal evidence and many of the consumer oriented publications that do cite research, do so selectively (known as "cherry-picking"). Research published on the adverse effects of yoga is mostly of a descriptive type which collects data by way of observation, case study, or survey.

Purpose

The aim of this article was to run a systematic-review and meta-analysis of injurious incidents associated with yoga during participation in randomized controlled trials.

Methods

Four well-established online databases were searched for randomized controlled trials comparing a yoga intervention to either standard treatment, no treatment, exercise, psychological care, and health education. Interventions that utilized yoga in conjunction with an additional component were excluded, yoga was the sole intervention compared to the control. Interventions comparing one style of yoga to another style of yoga were also excluded and the control had to be something other than yoga. No papers were excluded based on type of yoga, dosage of the yoga intervention, or demographics. Inclusion required reporting of any adverse experience, but those determined to be caused by yoga had to be reported as such in the original research. Subject non-compliance due to extraneous conditions was not deemed yoga related.

Results

Ninety-four studies consisting of 8340 subjects remained after exclusions. Thirty-two studies did not specify the type of yoga, 58 studies did specify, and four studies only pranayama. Iyengar was the most frequently studied style, appearing in 19 studies. Yoga dosages were as little as 1 day and as long as 1 1/2 years. The incidence of intervention-related adverse experiences was 2.2%; 10.9% were deemed non-serious and 0.6% were deemed serious. When compared with exercise, intervention-related adverse experiences were similar in frequency ($p = .92$), suggesting a yoga intervention is no more or less safe than those controls.

Continued on next page

Continued from previous page

Discussion

As with all studies, this one has its limitations. First and foremost, fewer than one-third of RCTs on yoga published any data regarding adverse events and had to be excluded from this analysis. Moreover, the papers that did report potential injuries, both serious and non-serious, evaluated a yoga intervention in a highly controlled setting. These data should not be extrapolated to the incidence of injury in a studio or home practice setting where yoga dosage, technique, instruction, adjustments, and other physical activities are not controlled for and can be highly variable. Such factors make assessing yoga safety for the general public a difficult endeavor. Based on the current paper's results, however, it may be concluded that yoga is a generally safe intervention provided the practice conditions replicate those in studies with high efficacy.

EMERGING PERSPECTIVES

6

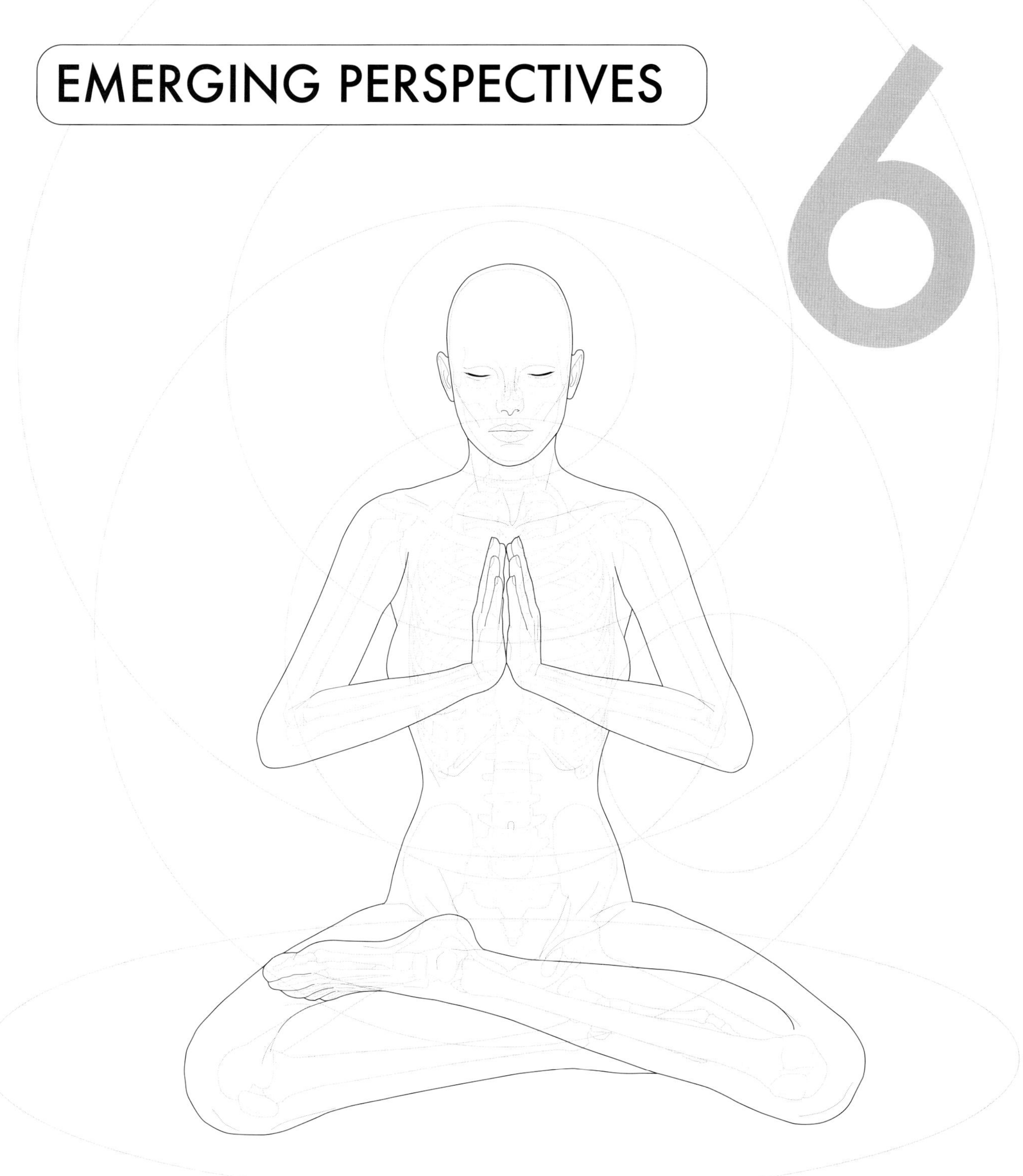

With stretching reevaluated in the framework of tension, and overstretching reframed in the context of underloading, we will explore these concepts, and more, as they relate to yoga asana. The present chapter will build upon concepts of tension and, in many cases, challenge your beliefs and intuition. Interestingly, some of the ideas are not new. I once took a course with Serge Gracovetsky, Ph.D., author of "The Spinal Engine," who said something along the lines of there being no original ideas anymore, and if you look back a hundred years or so you'll see that someone has already proposed your idea, but at a time when it was simply not widely accepted. With critical thinking and the appreciation of uncertainty as a subplot of this book, it seems natural to question certain popularly accepted "truths" as they relate to the conventional yoga script.

Simultaneous to the notion that many modern ideas are not so modern is the recognition that research and conventional thought are separated by a wide time gap. In fact, the average delay between research conclusions and their implementation into clinical practice is thought to be about 17 years (Morris, Wooding and Grant, 2011)! It would take even longer to make its way into the collective awareness of the general public, including yoga teacher training programs, since those groups are neither compelled nor empowered to stay up to date on current research as clinicians and other licensed healthcare professionals are. Furthermore, once a movement system is established, it makes not accepting or accepting contradictory research primarily a business decision instead of a process of scientific exploration. There may be vested interests in refuting conjectures which undermine the entire system.

Conversely, conjecture alone is not a reason to blindly accept or deny new or unconventional ideas. The scientific process never allows us to conclude the absolute truth anyway. If there is an absolute truth, we can be led to it, but we will never know with 100% confidence; the process doesn't allow us to conclude an absolute truth. The best we can do is continue to question, propose, and refute arguments for, and against, these ideas until evidence is consistent and compelling for the theory to be accepted as the most likely to be valid, or not. Bogduk, Aprill and Derby (2013) do an excellent job evaluating the literature on spinal discs as a potential source of pain by testing the refuting position. They conclude that not only can disc pain occur, but it can be diagnosed; therefore, they refute the null hypothesis that it cannot.

Much can be learned about the scientific method by simply reading their process and line of thinking. In this chapter we will explore the ubiquity of tissues under tension and consider positions opposing conventional ideas about stretching. I've titled it "Emerging Perspectives," but it could just as easily have been titled "Uncertainties," or "Unknown Truths."

Biotensegrity

A tensegrity system is one that expresses an equilibrium of forces by balancing the robustness of compression with the durability of tension, and is appropriately named by combing the words tensional and integrity. The 20th-century architect R. Buckminster Fuller garnered fame with a tensegrity structure, the geodesic dome; a structure that brilliantly utilized the inherent stability of geometric shapes. Independent from gravity, these struts under constant compression are combined with non-biologic "tendons" under constant tension, are arranged in geometrical configurations that withstand considerable forces, and

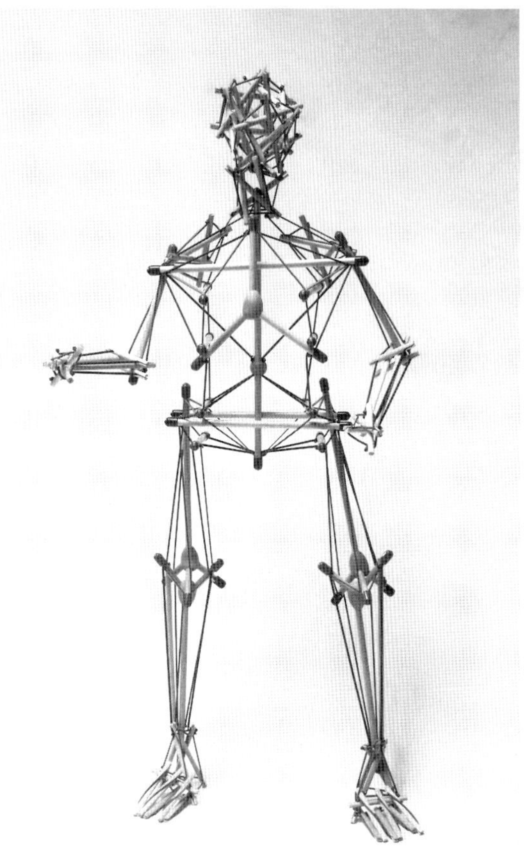

Fig. 6.1
The biotensegrity model. Reprinted with permission. Copyright T Flemons 2006 www.intensiondesigns.ca.

have the capacity to accept loads in any direction, even when tilted on any axis. The interaction and transmission of forces through interrupted, or segmented, compressive components and uninterrupted, or continuously connected, tensile components establish and maintain a stable balance of forces where an increase in compression causes an increase in tension (Pugh, 1976). This continuity of tensional components, actually called tendons, and discontinuity of compressive components, called struts, is the defining aspect of a tensegrity structure and expresses the structure of the human body quite elegantly, and accurately.

From the macro to the micro, the human body can be related to a tensegrity structure, referred to as biotensegrity (Fig. 6.1). Our bones are discontinuous segments separated by fluid or fibrocartilage but connected through the continuous tensional network of our fascia, tendons, ligaments, and joint capsules. Synovial joints can be considered tensegrity structures where the bones are held apart via the tension of the joint capsules (Scarr, 2012). The spine, with its segmented vertebrae bound together by the continuity of the periosteum, intervertebral discs, and ligamentous structures can be likened to a tensegrity system. Our cells even demonstrate properties of tensegrity (Wang et al., 2001), as was suggested earlier in the discussion on cell-matrix adhesions. Finally, tensegrity exists all the way down to the molecular level, including our DNA structure. Biotensegirty is the basis for mechanotransduction (Ingber, Wang and Stamenović, 2014).

Static posture, or how one arranges and aligns one's body parts in an upright position is, or was, mostly assessed from a compression structure perspective. Just like a building with load-bearing walls, the bones of the human body bear the weight of the bones above them, continuously and vertically stacking. By this design, those segments with the greatest load-bearing capacity would be inferiorly located, and those with lesser loads to bear would be superiorly located. The spine, for example, is a structure that satisfies the compression structure narrative where larger bones are found at the base (i.e. lumbar region), and generally decrease in size as you ascend (i.e. thoracic, then cervical regions). This design depends greatly on gravity, as there is a clear bottom, or base, to the structure. If you turned your house made of load-bearing walls on its side, no longer supported by its base, it might not hold up under gravity. Yet the spine maintains its structure independent of gravity as evidenced by any posture or position that requires anything other than a perfectly vertical spine.

It is no surprise early anatomists compared the body to compression structures; it is how we understood architecture design. Historically, humans engineered and assembled such continuous compression structures, in part because of the available construction materials that could best withstand compressive forces. The massive Gothic churches and Egyptian pyramids are a testament to the structural solidity and permanence of compression structures. Logically, our bodies' design was considered similar to these continuous compression structures, where the spinal "column" gives the impression of stacked bones that might provide us with our ability to stand up to gravity. Modern technological advances in materials exhibiting extreme tensile durability, however, have made tension structures like suspension bridges possible where historically they were not (Pugh, 1976). The availability of new materials has spurred a growth of tensional architecture, changing how we understand mechanical design, both man-made and in nature. The tensional capacity of our collagen-based tissues lends itself well to the design of a tension structure, and prompts a renewed reinterpretation of our own bodies.

The entirety of our form exists in a pre-stressed tensional state. This global tension that exists between tissues is present in every element, from hydrogen bonds to cell membranes, from collagen fibers to muscle tone. Even our most superficial epidermal layer is in a state of tension, evidenced by how the skin pulls away from an incision (Guimberteau, 2005). Beneath the skin, contractile muscle proteins regulate the state of pre-stress by increasing tension on the neighboring collagen tissues, as is apparent by the muscular insertions directly into them. Obvious, and well-known, examples include the gluteus maximus inserting primarily (entirely in some individuals) into the iliotibial band (ITB) of the fascia lata, and the transversus abdominis inserting into the lumbodorsal fascia. Less obvious, but logical in the context of biotensegrity, is the revelation that muscle force (i.e. tension) is transmitted not only longitudinally but also laterally and in three dimensions to surrounding structures, including antagonistic and synergistic muscles previously distinguished as separate (Huijing, 2009). In other words, force distribution is global and constant, and our tissues are always under varying degrees of tension.

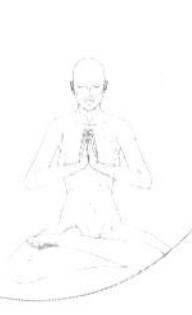

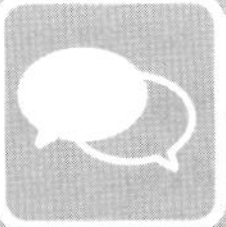

Thought Provoker

Structural Variations

Does the departure from the classic compression model of anatomy change your view of the perfect plumb-line posture, and if so how? What do you think the impact of yoga can be on students who present postural variations such as scoliosis, or "flattened" spinal curves?

In a seminal paper, anatomist Jaap van der Wal (2009) described his observations revealing the interaction between muscle fascicles and otherwise "passive" collagenous structures. His departure from the classical anatomy model, where tendons are in-series with contractile tissues, but ligaments are not (i.e. "tendons connect muscle to bone, ligaments connect bone to bone"), shed new light onto joint structure and dynamics (Fig. 6.2). By adding certain ligamentous structures (which he named "dynaments") to the in-series arrangement, his alternate model could account for the global tension around a joint, where no part is ever slack in any joint position. Tension could now be continuously present, aiding not only in force transmission, but also in mechanoreception (i.e. proprioception). Van der Wal's work is said to have originated as his doctoral thesis in the 1980s, which supposedly garnered very little interest at the time, and only when fascia research gained momentum was he invited to publish it in a scientific journal.

The depth and intricacies of van der Wal's work are beyond our focus here. His revelations, however, support the narrative on the importance of global and perpetual tension, and on how muscle force is captured, stored, and released by these pre-stressed tissues. The muscle force you generate is communicated through connective tissue in all three dimensions, conserving energy by modulating the appropriate stiffness needed to efficiently satisfy the demands of any movement task (Scarr, 2012). Through the deepest

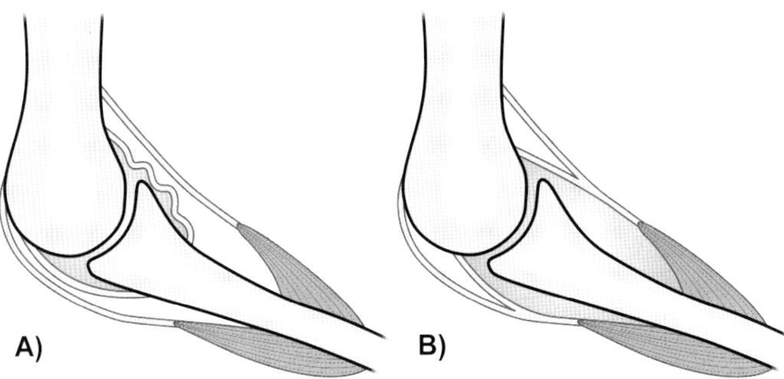

Fig. 6.2

Jaap van der Wal's joints demonstrating (A) the classic bone-to-bone ligament versus (B) an in-series "dynament" configuration. Illustration modified after van der Wal (2009).

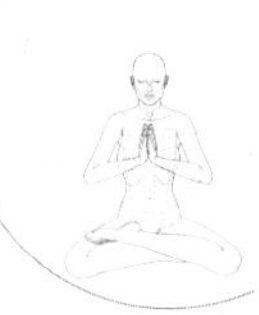

layers of connective tissue, force is distributed and transmitted radially along the fascial network to any and all structures, none of which operate in isolation (Vora et al., 2010).

Although one might find this macro view of the body to be overwhelming, I suggest it simplifies how we practice asana. Rather than worry about which muscle or which structure is affected in a certain pose, we can assume all the muscles around the structure are loaded. Downward Facing Dog Pose becomes a pose that loads the shoulder complex, just as the Warrior II Pose loads the hip and all surrounding structures. If we understand that tension, although it always exists, can be modified through adjusting joint position or muscle recruitment, we can modify the pose as needed to progressively increase capacity. There may be some exceptions to this global perspective where structures are located in relative isolation (e.g. cruciate ligaments inside the knee) from muscle force transmission, but the pre-stressed condition does still apply.

Regarding stretch, if our connective tissues are always under tension, and if overstretching were defined by plastic changes resulting from high levels of tension, then one might conclude that simply existing could have the potential to overstretch our tissues. Skin tends to sag as we age, however we are not generally concerned that the skin over the hamstrings will overstretch and sag while stretching this area in yoga class. Most accept that the loss of elastic recoil might be associated with biochemical factors associated with aging, diet, genetics, etc. In the case of our musculoskeletal connective tissues to which muscles transmit tension, if high magnitudes, frequencies, or durations of tension were to cause plastic changes to resting length, then athletes with strong glutes would be at risk for overstretched ITB and the cue to engage your core would loosen, rather than tighten, your lumbodorsal fascia in the long term. Tissues under tension are a normal condition, one which is not likely to cause plastic changes in response to frequent activities or postures.

Spinal Flexion

Perhaps a carry-over from the compression model is our vilification of spinal flexion in asana. If the spine is a column, and columns do not bend well, then the logical assumption is that the spine should also not bend. Forward bends are then taught with a hip hinge and a "flat" back, in order to protect the spine. But what if the spine is not a column? What if it is designed to be an incredibly stiff, but pliable rod which balances in equilibrium between compression and tension?

In yoga, the typical concern with flexion, particularly lumbar flexion, is the compressive and shear forces to which the intervertebral discs (IVDs) might be exposed (Fig. 6.3). In fear of squishing the nucleus pulposus (loose fibrous inner core of the IVD) out through the annulus fibrosis (fibrocartilage outer layer of the IVD) under these combined forces, safety is promoted by unequivocally hip hinging between and within poses. Transitions such as "rolling up" to standing from a forward bend, or round back forward bends are, in some styles, forbidden. Stylistic preferences aside, whether or not these instructions provide safety is not known. Pilates and Gyrotonic® are two other mind-body practices in which spinal flexion, sometimes even combined with rotation, are commonplace. Tai chi encourages a stance marked by a posteriorly tucked pelvis and lumbar flexion, a position which I found difficult to maintain during my training as I would constantly revert to my

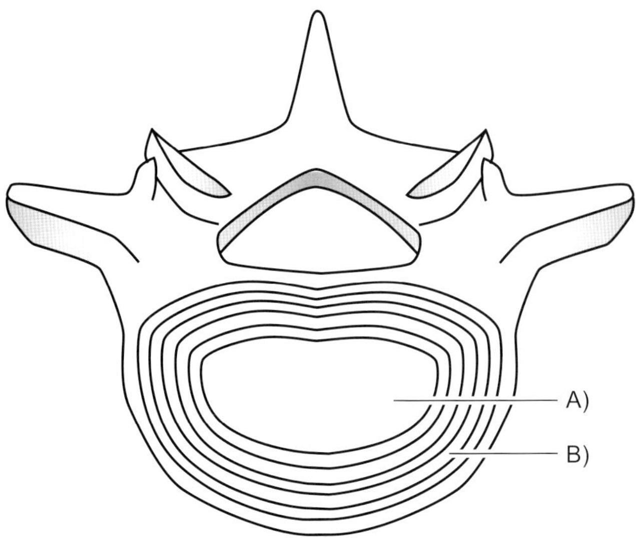

Fig. 6.3
Intervertebral disc. (A) Nucleus pulposus. (B) Annulus fibrosis.

yoga ways. Many recreational sports (e.g. rowing) and daily activities (e.g. playing on the floor with a child) require some degree of flexion, as well. Avoiding spinal flexion in a yoga class is not only physically impractical, and somewhat unavoidable, it also might be a bit counterproductive. Of course, the intent is well-meaning, and protecting students from unnecessary risk is essential to teaching a safe class, but we must wonder if the protective effect actually lies in an avoidance of load, or exposure to load.

While we cannot say with any certainty the impact a yoga class might have on lumbar discs, we can look briefly at the research on disc properties. In the context of tissue adaptation, IVDs have classically been thought to be mostly inert. Much like articular cartilage, the fibrocartilage discs possess an ECM structure that impedes turnover and regeneration. Research today might be suggesting otherwise. First, herniated discs are now known to have the ability to spontaneously regress without surgical interventions (Chiu et al., 2015; Zhong et al., 2017). This raises questions about the finality of disc herniations, and when combined with the asymptomatic cases, everything becomes even more uncertain. Second, the famous Twin Spine Study found genetic factors to be

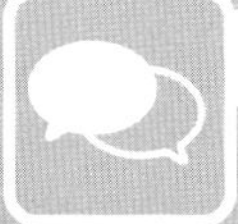

Thought Provoker

Spinal Flexion

What is your position on different types of roll-ups and roll-downs standing, flexed, supine, and seated? Do they increase tolerance for loaded flexion, do they do nothing at all, or do they put the spine at risk?

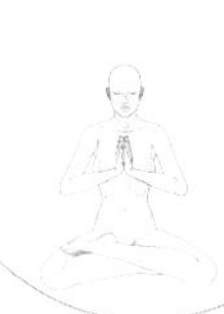

Scientific Literacy

Generalization

Over-generalization is a logical fallacy that leads people to induce broad, sweeping conclusions based on narrow, specific evidence. For example, saying that "people" have greater range of motion (ROM) in a straight leg raise if they inhale during the stretch rather than exhale when the study was conducted with only female subjects generalizes to the entire population. Saying that "all women" have a greater ROM during this experimental condition when the women in the study were runners, of the ages 20–25, or n=3, generalizes to the entire female population. Claiming that some women have greater "overall" ROM if they inhale during the stretch rather than exhale when only one joint in one position was measured, generalizes to all joints. In yoga, because the biomechanical research is scarce, it might be tempting to over-generalize in our search for answers. Running, although it may also axially load the spine, is not the same as Headstand.

a determinant for disc degeneration but loading associated with daily physical activities did not appear to cause wear (Battié et al., 2009). Third, we understand that certain loading conditions promote a structure and composition which might promote disc health (Steele et al., 2015). Two such loading conditions found to increase disc hydration include running (Belavý et al., 2017) and, unexpectedly, slouched sitting (Pape et al., 2018). None of these perspectives are intended to promote spinal flexion with reckless abandon; they are insightful inquiries to the larger question of how we can increase capacity while maintaining safety with the practice of yoga.

Pause and turn to page 189 for a summary of related research.

The topic of spinal flexion leads us back to Newtonian physics and the biomechanical model based on the lever system. A lever is a simple machine whereby one force acts across a fulcrum to move another, overcoming the resisting force. There are three classes of levers with different configurations, providing varying degrees of mechanical advantages (Figs. 6.4, 6.5, 6.6). In the human body, the 2nd class lever is less common, and the 3rd class lever is the most common. The spine is classified as a 1st class lever. Knowing what we know today about tensegrity systems and 3-dimensional force transmission these simple machines seem too…simplistic…to be complete biomechanical models.

Some scholars have adopted a healthy skepticism of the lever system model and reevaluated the dynamics of the spine and surrounding tissues. One such revised model highlights the mathematical impossibilities of the Newtonian physics model and reconciles them with the inclusion of the lumbodorsal fascia. The premise rests on the geometry of the

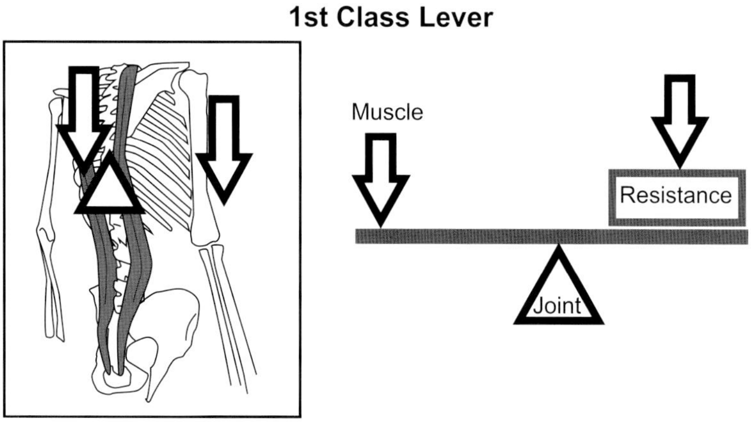

1st Class Lever

Muscle

Resistance

Joint

Fig. 6.4
1st class lever. The generated force (muscle force) and the resistance force (body/object) are on either side of the fulcrum (joint).

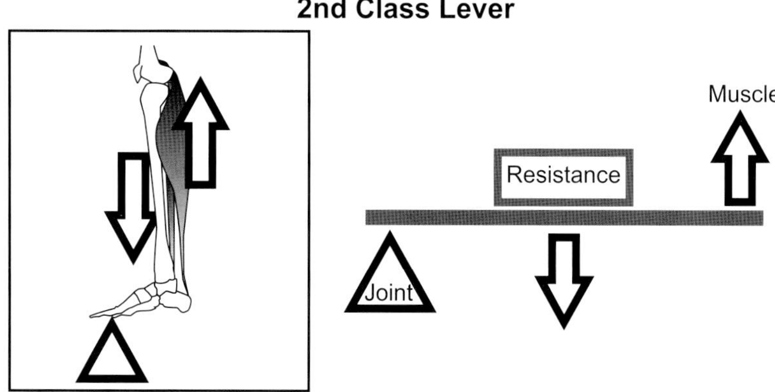

Fig. 6.5
2nd class lever. The generated force (muscle force) and the fulcrum (joint) are on either side of the resistance force (body/object).

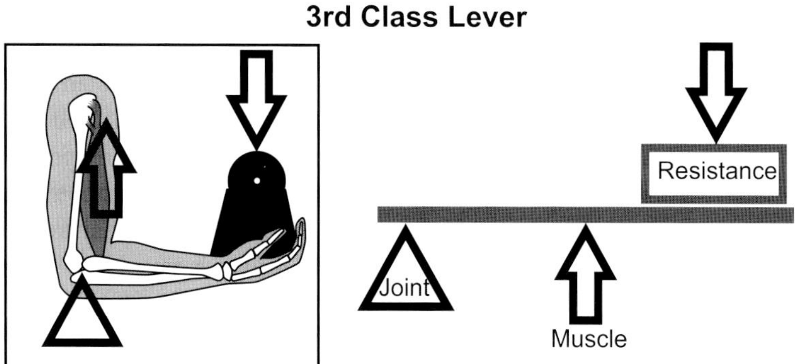

Fig. 6.6
3rd class lever. The fulcrum (joint) and the resistance force (body/object) are on either side of the generated force (muscle force).

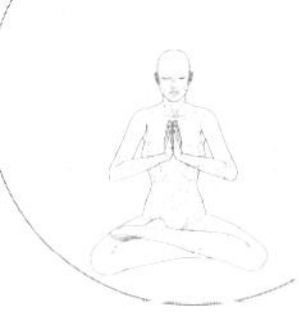

1st class lever. In order to generate enough force to move a substantial resistance force (e.g. picking up a heavy box) the spinal muscles would need to either be much, much larger than they are, or much more dorsally distal from the fulcrum (i.e. facet joints). Indeed, our spinal muscles are quite small, and very close to the fulcrum, thus the model can be refuted. By adding the tensional network of the connective tissue, mainly the deep lumbodorsal fascia, the burden of the load can be shared (Gracovetsky, 2008). A flexed spine narrows and lengthens the thoracolumbar fascia, in turn storing energy to maximize the efficiency of the spinal erectors when extending the spine (Willard et al., 2012). Admittedly, this perspective fits nicely into the narrative of stretch and tissues under tension, so I am prone to entertain it. Those trained by other, well-known and highly respected scholars who stand behind uncompromising intolerance of spinal flexion at any load might vehemently disagree. And, of course, a student who does suffer from flexion intolerance should be referred to a licensed healthcare professional for treatment and management. In regard to healthy backs in active individuals, what constitutes a safe spine during a yoga practice employing body weight postures is not determinable by our current knowledge.

Another consideration in the spinal flexion debate is a response referred to as the flexion-relaxation phenomenon. In normal, healthy backs, when the lumbar spine flexes at its end range, the lumbodorsal fascia is pulled taut and takes on the majority of the load. This allows the spinal muscles to minimize activity, measured by electromyogram (EMG). Upon return from flexion, the stretched lumbodorsal fascia slackens enough for the spinal muscles to increase activity and contribute to the movement. Some subjects with chronic low back pain (CLBP) are known to have an altered, or sometimes absent, load sharing mechanism typical of the normal flexion-relaxation response. The resulting overuse of spinal muscles is thought to cause muscle fatigue and potentially contribute to low back abnormalities (i.e. diminished capacity) (Zwambag and Brown, 2015).

Finally, viscoelasticity should always be taken into account. Prolonged spinal flexion (even as little as 5–10 minutes) creeps the lumbodorsal fascia, temporarily impairing the load sharing mechanism. Upon returning from prolonged flexion, the spinal muscles will require increased activity, potentially contributing to fatigue (Shin, D'Souza and Liu, 2009). As would be expected, the lumbar flexion induced by prolonged desk sitting (i.e. 1 hour) is also enough to interfere with normal flexion-relaxation patterns (Howarth et al., 2013). Regular periods of recovery may mitigate creep and reestablish the flexion-relaxation response. If you aren't doing warm-ups in your classes before introducing standing forward bends (i.e. Sun Salutations), here might be a good reason for you to start (even if it goes against tradition).

Of course, in the yoga setting, there is no access to EMG, so how well one load shares cannot be determined. It is also not necessary. Instead, teaching global as well as segmental spinal movement in a progressive way should be the focus. The hip hinge is still a valuable practice to teach because it is an additional requirement needed to achieve the end range of standing forward flexion (Figs. 6.7, 6.8, 6.9). There is not one superior movement; the process will always be task dependent and individually driven. Yoga, as a mindful practice, provides an opportunity to evaluate one's movement deficits and deliberately select yoga poses (and sometimes non-traditional drills or exercises) to help restore range of motion (ROM) while simultaneously, and gradually increasing capacity.

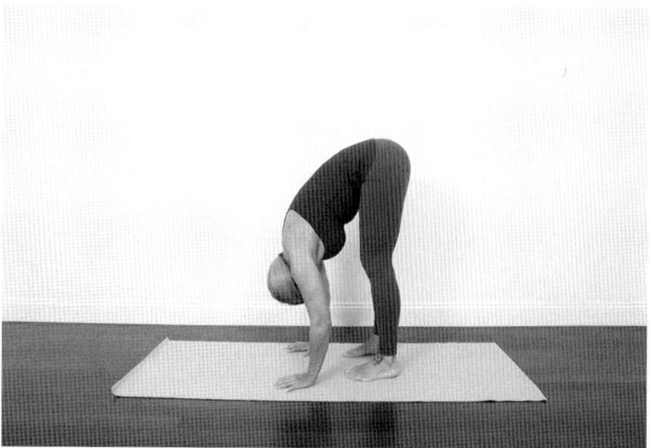

Fig. 6.7
Full range lumbar flexion with hip hinge.

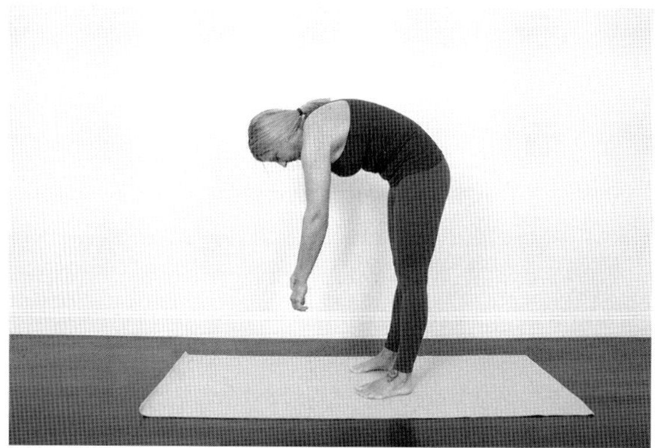

Fig. 6.8
Lumbar flexion with no hip hinge.

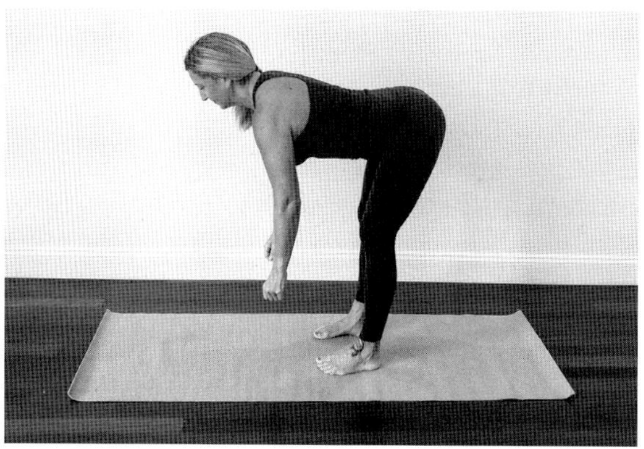

Fig. 6.9
Hip hinge with no lumbar flexion.

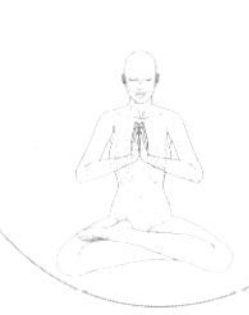

If "Asanas keep the body healthy and strong and in harmony with nature" (Iyengar, 1979), then applying science, instead of tradition, can help us satisfy these goals with greater accuracy and success.

Squatting vs Stooping

Following on from the analysis of spinal flexion during forward bending, comes the debate on whether squat lifting or stoop lifting is the superior method for picking up objects from the floor (Figs. 6.10, 6.11). So ingrained is it in our collective belief system, that most people, without hesitation, will say that squat lifting is the safer option. Entire workplace training programs hinge on this position and costly education programs have been implemented resulting in the loss of hours of productivity. Are these ideas based on conjecture or supported by the evidence?

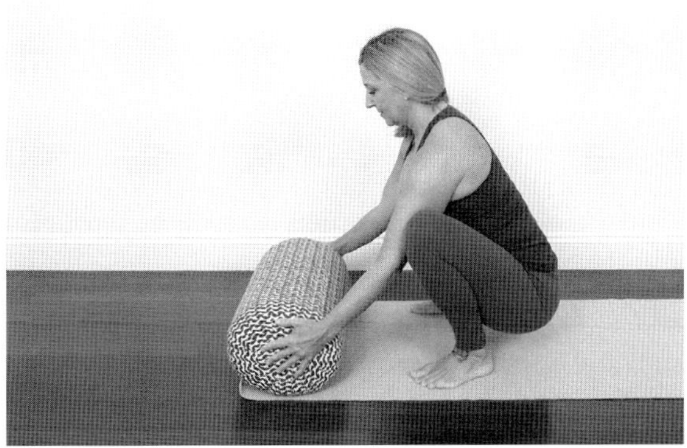

Fig. 6.10
Squat lift.

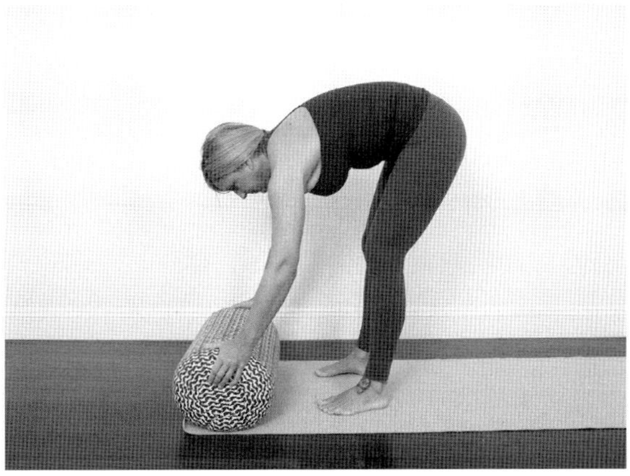

Fig. 6.11
Stoop lift.

As mentioned previously, most new ideas are not in fact new at all. It is just a matter of how well they were received, initially. To highlight this I'm citing a literature review from almost 20 years ago that evaluated the available evidence from 1980s and 1990s. It was determined that neither the squat nor the stoop lifting technique stands out as superior. In terms of efficiency, stoop lifting is marked by a lower heart rate and lower oxygen consumption. Biomechanical studies revealed that compression forces vary and conflict across studies, possibly due to modeling assumptions and task requirements (e.g. size of the object, proximity to body, etc.). Overall, the compression data between squatting and stooping were determined to be similar enough to deem the results inclusive. Shear forces also vary but do tend to be greater overall in stoop lifting (Straker, 2002). It seems that both squatting and stooping are viable options and might be selected based on task, preference, and capacity.

In more recent systematic reviews the superiority of one method over the other is still be determined. Technique training appears to be ineffective at reducing work-related musculoskeletal injuries (Clemes, Haslam and Haslam, 2009), and, in fact, has no effect on changing people's preferred technique (Hogan, Greiner and O'Sullivan, 2014). Even if one could confidently say squatting improves safety outcomes, which one cannot, these workplace training programs are not even successful at changing behavior. Yet, society still holds on. Another paper also determined technique training in the workplace to be ineffective in reducing injury and back pain, but strength and flexibility showed promise (Smith, Littlewood and May, 2014). Once again, increased capacity holds on firmly.

Again, none of these perspectives are intended to promote stooping or squatting with reckless abandon. It should be remembered that the typical yoga practice does not involve lifting objects from the floor. A Deep Squat (Garland Pose) or a Standing Forward Bend only involves moving one's own body weight. Presumably, the compressive and shear forces acting on the spine during a yoga class are even less than those reviewed in the above studies where the subjects were lifting loaded objects.

Alternatively, stress on the spine is known to increase when loads increase, such as when lifting a heavily loaded barbell. In this case, technique does matter. In essence, the greater the load, the less options we have. Since there are typically no barbells in yoga, our options are greater than those of a personal trainer. With the inquiries of

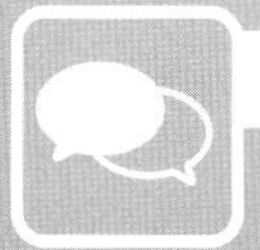

Thought Provoker

Picking up a Yoga Mat

At the end of your next yoga class, try to observe all the different ways the students roll-up their mats and pick up their props to put away. Is anybody in a perfect Squat Pose or a perfect Stoop Pose, or is a hybrid more common? Consider messages you have received in yoga about safety versus how people move when they are not instructed how to move.

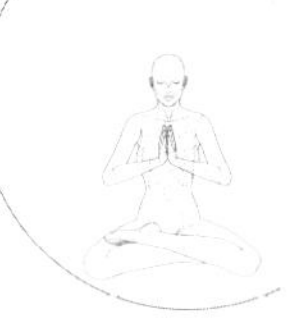

optimal loading as our guide, we can assert that poses imparting loads to which we have not adapted are those that carry the most risk. In order to increase options, desirable adaptation must occur, and in order for desirable adaption to occur, gradually increasing, optimal loading must eventually be introduced.

Core Stability

Still on the topic of the robust human spine, and in succession to the earlier statement regarding increasing loads and the resulting decreasing options, a deconstruction of spinal stability is finally due. Stability is a term that lacks, well, a stable meaning. It can imply a variety of things (e.g. joint stiffness, joint stillness, joint strength, structural integrity, and so on), thus the term may lead to confusion and contradiction when used without specific clarification. In regard to the spine and other single- or multi-joint segments of the body, because they are inherently dynamic structures, the term stability must account for movement (Reeves, Narendra and Cholewicki, 2007).

In a dynamic context, stability is not the opposite of mobility. A stable structure is one that can return to its center following a perturbation. I grew up near a fault line in southern California and my father was an earthquake engineer. I learned at a very young age that the most stable structures were the ones that could bend, twist, and sway with the force of the earth's moving surface. One could say a stable structure is one that has full ownership of all potential mobility; one that can return to a center point, a neutral point, or a state of rest (Fig. 6.12). The viscoelasticity of connective tissue is highly stable. It can be stressed to great degrees, for long periods of time and yet return to its resting tension.

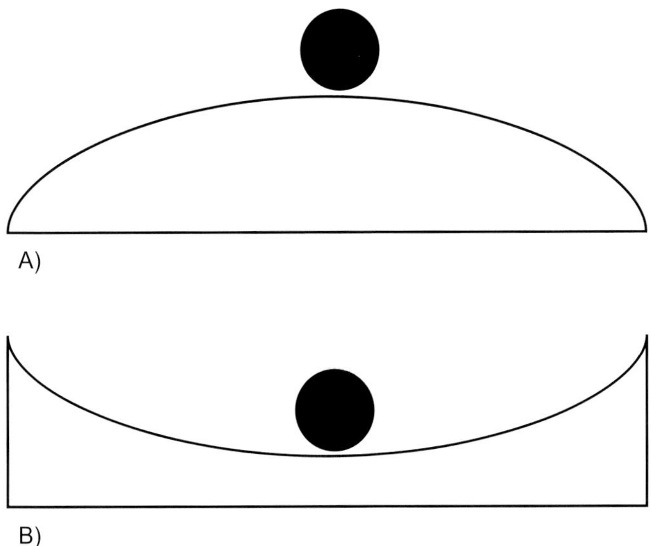

Fig. 6.12
Stability of a ball. (A) Unstable and unable to return to center. (B) Stable and will return to center. Illustration modified after Reeves, Narendra and Cholewicki (2007).

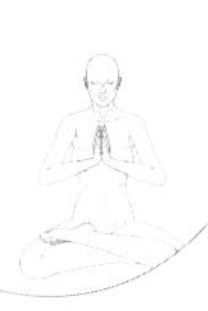

Where a joint, or the spine, lacks mobility, it is limited in its opportunity to maintain stability. In subjects whose lumbar spine movement was restricted with a rigid corset-like devise, their ability to maintain an upright posture was compromised. The title of the paper, "Movement of the lumbar spine is critical for maintenance of postural recovery following support surface perturbation," could not be clearer (Mok and Hodges, 2013). Stabilizing the spine, therefore, becomes a factor of having a well-moving spine, not one of stillness. During certain supine core drills where solely the limbs are moving, the instruction "stabilize the spine" implies keeping the spine statically still (also a good skill to have, just different). If you walked into the room and lay down on your mat with ease, your spine is a dynamically stable structure.

Let's consider breathing for a moment. In yoga, expansive breathing is often encouraged. During an inhalation, the concentrically contracting diaphragm descends, and the ribs stretch and rotate open. The decrease in intrathoracic pressure relative to atmospheric pressure draws air into the lungs. During an exhalation, the eccentrically contracting diaphragm ascends, condensing and rotating the ribs closed. The increase in intrathoracic pressure relative to atmospheric pressure forces air out of the lungs. In upright standing poses, with each breath individual ribs are moving, the spine is moving (as the vertebrae articulate with the ribs), and the entire rib cage is moving relative to the pelvis. A stable spine, and all of its viscoelastic tissues, is always responding to the oscillating levels of tension associated with breathing, even when it appears to be still. Holding a yoga pose is anything but static. Rather, it is an equilibrium of the fluctuating forces within living, breathing bodies and tissues whose mechanical properties adjust over time, and with repetition.

Any student of anatomy has learned that the core muscles are those responsible for the stability of the spine. Core stability has become synonymous with spine stability, spine safety, and back protection. Often the abdominal muscles get more credit than the muscles of the entire core cylinder, and more often than that, the transversus abdominis (TvA) gets all the credit. In an ab-obsessed society, this is to be expected. In actual practice, the muscles of the trunk coactivate, so an abdominal exercise becomes a core exercise anyway. The question is exactly how much core activation is required to maintain a posture with the spine in a neutral position.

In my weekend courses, when I ask yoga teachers what percentage of maximum voluntary contraction (MVC) is needed to maintain a stable spine, the numbers are usually pretty high. In all fairness, we already covered MVC in relation to tendons, where it is of a high value, so my question is somewhat misleading. By now, you should have your own guess. One of the classic papers on spine stability tells us an unloaded upright spine requires about 1.7 +/- 0.8% MVC in a neutral position. The EMG values increase during upright extension and flexion, but in the neutral zone the values are surprisingly low. Those same subjects were loaded with a 32 kg (70.5 lbs) mass strapped to their shoulders and then asked to repeat the movements. Loaded, the MVC in neutral was only 2.9 +/- 1.4% (Cholewicki, Panjabi and Khachatryan, 1997). Try engaging your core maximally and then scaling down to 2.9%. It's hard. Of course, there are valid performance reasons to brace your core, especially as load increases, but spinal stability is not one of them. Spines are inherently stable and robust structures, in tensional and compressive equilibrium.

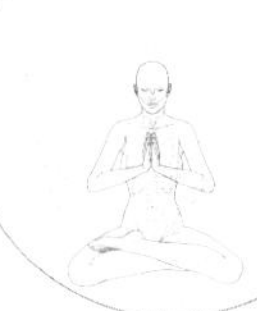

Thought Provoker

Bandhas

The *bandhas* probably did not originate in an era where spine stability was a concern, but in today's modern postural yoga, they can potentially be conflated. As the conversation around safety in yoga grows, we might look to the yoga tradition to guide us. If you teach or practice the *bandhas*, how does the spine stabilization research inform you in terms of intensity?

It is worth pointing out that the take away message is not that core strength is irrelevant. Increasing one's core strength translates to success in a far greater repertoire of movement challenges than simply remaining upright and stable. Most arm balances in yoga, for example, seem to benefit from core strengthening exercise. It all comes back to force and, specifically, direction of force. When one is standing upright the load stacks vertically and the "support cables" to the spine provided by core muscles need not tether very much. When one changes position, as in Plank Pose, for example, the core muscles will increase their tension as the body is now perpendicular to the force vector of gravity. Handstand is vertically stacked and therefore demands less muscle tension than pressing up into it. Developing core strength is highly advisable for increasing skill and adding heavier loads.

Incidentally, the evidence for core stabilization exercises being superior to any other exercise in modifying symptoms in subjects with low back pain is lacking (Smith, Littlewood and May, 2014). The propagation of this belief is likely due to a combination of factors including an underlying assumption that the spine needs stabilizing to avoid pain, followed by a misinterpretation of the literature, generalizations, and inflated conclusions. It goes back to another classic paper which found a timing discrepancy of TvA activation between subjects with and without back pain (Hodges and Richardson, 1999). The delay, measured in milliseconds, in the back pain group has been mistaken for weakness in the great game of research telephone. Somehow the timing became strength and, in some cases, endurance; the distinction between these biomotor variables has collapsed. It is now standard advice to recommend abdominal strengthening to anyone and everyone with a minor back complaint. Even further extrapolated, it is now standard advice to strengthen one's core in the pursuit of protecting one's back from potential future problems. In the many anecdotal cases where abdominal strengthening exercises are effective, it is likely, again, to be a non-specific result of an overall increase in load tolerance rather than the result of the TvA specifically being trained.

Anyone managing back pain should be referred to a licensed healthcare professional, but it is still worth discussing here. "Yoga for healthy backs" is a popular theme in workshops and on the internet. I do believe that yoga can have both positive and preventative effects on low back pain, but not because of TvA activation or any predetermined selection/sequence of poses. Breathing and meditative aspects of yoga are not the topic here, neither is the treatment of back pain. We will, therefore, set the breathing and meditative aspects aside, although still appreciating their value.

For many, yoga postures provide novel mechanical stimuli. If guided well, the practice is variable and progressive. Any positive or preventative effects of yoga could be reduced to simply providing a means by which one can increase load tolerance. Practitioners who enjoy core stabilization exercises can certainly continue to do them. Practitioners who see benefits, for whatever personal or performance objectives they may have, can also continue to do core stabilizing exercises. Selling core stabilization exercises as a magic pill for back pain, however, is not only irresponsible, but also unsubstantiated. Without a foundation in the research, it might be difficult to spot the pseudoscience.

Posture and Alignment

A static posture, whether an upright military stance (such as Mountain Pose) or any yoga posture, is how one arranges the parts of one's body and holds it in a moment in time. Yoga alignment is similar, although the verbiage around it tends to be a bit more inclusive of joint actions and muscle activations due to the complexities of the shapes. In both cases good posture (or good alignment) is praised and poor posture (or poor alignment) is met with concern. The very fact that a binary judgment of posture exists, tells us we value an appropriate norm to which all should strive to achieve.

The history of posture is a fascinating allegory dating back to 1750s when the aristocratic norms of slouch and leisure became unfashionable (Yosifon and Stearns, 1998). The stiff postures of military and dance started a trend which eventually became a sign of good character in the Americas. A sign of good etiquette, stiff and upright postures were supported by fashion (i.e. corsets and stiff vests) and furniture (i.e. rocking chairs were reserved for the feeble). Posture was eventually medicalized as it developed into a diagnostic tool that could be monetized, establishing a vested interest in its use and perpetuity. In the 1920s, good posture was identified as proper etiquette by social conservatives, and as proper function by the medical field. In the early 20th century, a staggering number of conditions, illnesses, assessment tools, and corrective devices emerged, further pathologizing poor posture. In schools children were particularly targeted in the pursuit of slouch prevention. Today, while our posture attitudes are far looser, these influences maintain a firm grip, especially in the therapeutic arena. One could deduce that the present day focus on yoga alignment is an artifact of these western postural beliefs.

Yoga alignment cues tend to fall into a correct/incorrect dichotomy. Some examples include specific foot angles, pelvic tilt, spinal curves, shoulder position, and head placement. There are more, but these sufficiently make a point. Unfortunately, bone morphology varies greatly (e.g. not all feet point forward, some spines are side bent and rotated, and most everyone has differences between the right and left sides). These variations will not only affect an upright standing posture, but also be amplified when the arrangement of parts is more complex. For example, Chair Pose will look different based on limb lengths (Fig. 6.13). Someone with long femurs and a short spine must align her body over her center of gravity differently from someone with short femurs and a long spine.

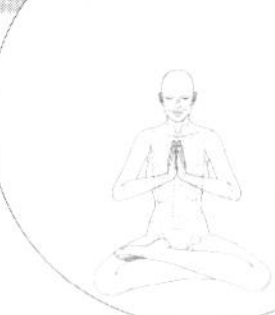

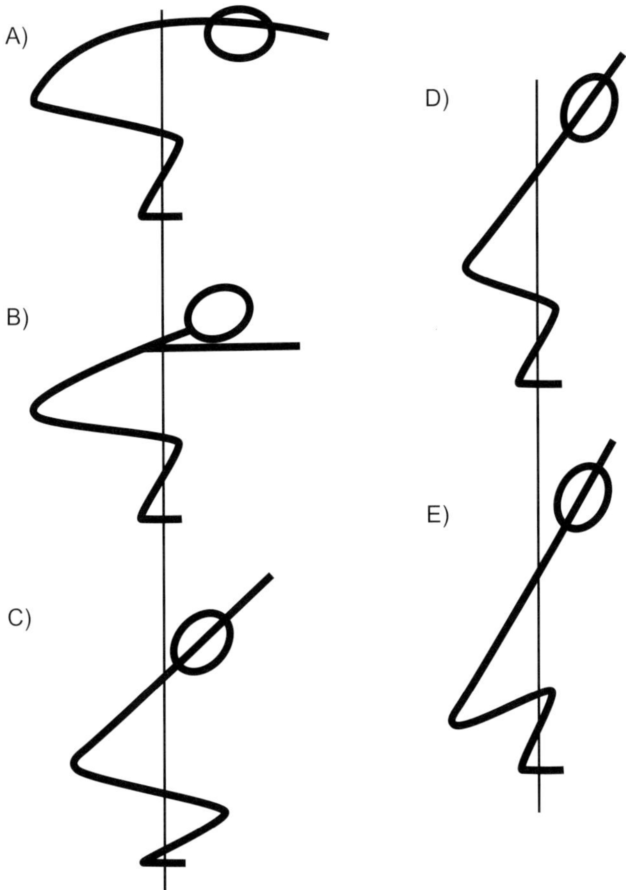

Fig. 6.13
Chair Pose. (A) A practitioner with long femurs and short spine may need to posteriorly tilt and flex her spine to maintain her center of gravity as her pelvis goes back. (B) She may use her arms in front of her as a counter lever. (C) If she has the dorsiflexion (or the permission) to move her knees far forward over her feet, she might find a more neutral spine. (D) A practitioner with short femurs and long spine may easily "lift her chest" while maintaining her center of gravity as her pelvis will not travel backwards much. (E) She will be able to lower her pelvis with ease while keeping her knees behind her toes. Note: These models are for conceptual purposes only and are not geometrically or mathematically accurate.

Neither of the postures is incorrect, and no amount of cueing or teaching will change the laws of physics. Geometry, not pathology, dictates such differences here.

Inherently, imperfect alignment cannot exist without a constructed value system, thus "bad" postural alignment is not faulty. We don't judge a tree by its alignment; it is either stable and stands proud or it has lost stability and fallen. Our constructed value system might lead us to judge an erect and upright tree more beautiful than a mangled, yet

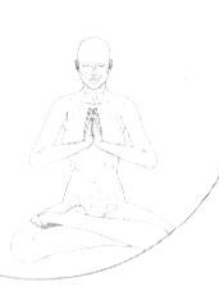

stable tree. Our values are often based on familiarity; standards of beauty tend to revolve around what we recognize. In general, most human bodies have an average morphology, one we typically see. There will always be outliers, however, who still have "normal" morphology, just not common. It is within our constructed value system where we label anything beyond the average, or "normal," as improperly aligned.

To further highlight that "normal" is an arbitrary construction, it must be pointed out that an average can be expressed in three different ways, and a data set could provide three distinct values (Table 6.1). Arithmetic mean is probably the most commonly used in research. In some instances, what society perceives as "normal" contradicts the averages. For example, most people would assume a neutral pelvis is the average, correct alignment, thereby establishing it as normal, proper, and even healthy. A study of 120 asymptomatic adults in the UK (average age 23.8 years), however, showed that most had an anterior pelvic tilt (85% of males, 75% of females). Only 9% of males and 18% of females had a neutrally aligned pelvis, the rest had a posterior tilt (Herrington, 2011). These values tend to vary by race (Endo et al., 2014), too, so it is advisable to avoid overgeneralization by immediately deducing that an anterior pelvic tilt is the new normal. At this point in the book, you know now not to do this. The variation across, gender, race, and culture also brings into question the degree to which we embody the cultural constructs we created around our bodies. It's the classic nature versus nurture inquiry, and the answer most likely lies somewhere in the in-between.

The larger issue at hand, however, is how well the evidence stands up to the postural-structural-biomechanical model of health we have constructed and injected into modern postural yoga. The identification of culturally (and medically) agreed upon malalignments as a cause or source of pathology has come under fierce criticism in light of the last two decades of research findings (Lederman, 2011). Because many have a vested interest in perpetuating this model of health, and even more have anecdotal evidence to support it, I imagine the debate will persist far longer than the expected 17 years referenced earlier in this chapter; understandably so. A yoga teacher who teaches an alignment-based class risks her brand falling apart if she suddenly rejects all her claims of the past. Additionally, she has possibly helped a lot of people feel better using these methods, which feels like good enough evidence to continue. The intent here is not to decide for you, but to refute the prevailing line of thinking when valid arguments against these conclusions exist, so that you may also consider your own position with a larger overview of possible mechanisms.

Inarguably, many have benefited from an alignment-focused yoga practice, and I have no reason to challenge those experiences. I am more interested in getting closer to

Table 6.1
Mathematical Averages

Mean	The sum of the values in a data set, divided by the total number of values
Mode	Most frequent value appearing in a data set
Median	Middle value in a data set, separating values on either side evenly

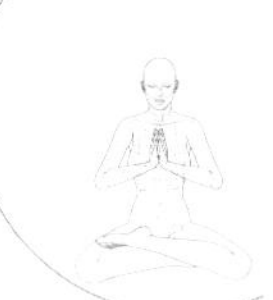

understanding why success is prevalent when proper alignment might be an illusion. One potential mechanism for the perceived improvements in physical health among yoga practitioners (Park, Riley and Braun, 2016) might be as simple as yoga postures imparting varied loads across tissues. Machines made of fixed behavior materials perform best in absolute repetitive loading. Our viscoelastic bodies perform best when loads are inconsistent, and the parameters vary (Gracovetsky, 2005). Therefore, it is entirely possible that an alignment-based practice works because the postures are just different, not necessarily correct, and stimulate adaptation. Once the body has adapted to the different, a new measure of different will be preferred.

I articulate this theory in an effort to reconcile the emerging perspectives within this chapter with my extensive yoga alignment background. So much of the yoga conversation today, at least among long time teachers, is about safety and avoiding injury. I wondered how we shifted so quickly from yoga being great to yoga being harmful. Perhaps we have all been practicing yoga in a certain way for long enough that the postures are no longer beneficial. As Dan Jones, a strength and conditioning coach, has famously said, "the benefits of an exercise decrease as expertise increases." Likewise, the benefits of proper yoga alignment are profound when novel, but they tend to decrease over time. If yoga is the only form of loading we participate in, as it has been for many of us long time teachers, then are we essentially underloading and failing to increase capacity? Through the biomechanical lens it is no surprise that the undesirable musculoskeletal adaptions do not emerge until years of practice are behind us.

Naturally, the implementation of this theory has greatly influenced how I teach and practice. First and foremost, it led me away from alignment-based yoga and more toward variability in the postures. I question some of our sacred cows of alignment, especially those that are intended to protect us from injury. I'll repeat that this is not an invitation to load with reckless abandon. It is an invitation to question, challenge, and refute the status quo when evidence supports it. In no way does this suggest alignment-based yoga is faulty or incorrect. Assuming morphology and anthropometrics are taken into consideration (which would take an entirely separate book to thoroughly unpack), practicing with proper form is an endeavor driven by a postural-structural-biomechanical model of health. It just happens to be one way, and not the only way, to practice yoga.

Additionally, I have expanded my yoga practice beyond the traditional postures. Purists vehemently disagree with me here, but every word I've written until this very point in the book supports my reasoning. Themes such as optimal loading parameters (i.e. specific, variable, progressive), tissue adaption, capacity, and load tolerance, which I have carried through this book, all influence my expanding movement repertoire. Probably the most effective and rewarding addition has been the implementation of basic strength and conditioning principles. I hesitate to share this with yoga enthusiasts because I, like them, will always be more at home in a yoga studio than in a fitness facility. Further, I do not wish to come across as anti-yoga, but nothing seems more anti-yoga than the gym culture (although this is changing). Biomechanics and biology, however, compel me to propose the blasphemous notion that yoga asana is limited in the loading parameters it can satisfy.

Regarding the swinging pendulum of the benefits and risks associated with yoga asana, one might now see the answer will always be "it depends." Depending on the yoga authority, certain poses are fervently declared either critical or hazardous. Depending on

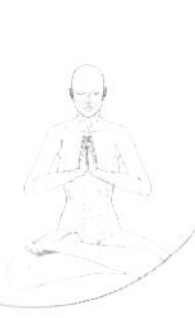

Scientific Literacy

Video Motion Analysis

Video motion analysis is a method of data collection that gathers kinematic and kinetic information about human movement. Reflective markers are placed at prominent bony landmarks and captured by the video equipment during movement. The number and placement of the markers depend on the joint angles and limb displacement data that need to be captured. Video (or still) images are then converted into digital data that can be analyzed. There are many uses for video motion analysis, and it is often found in the biomechanics literature to study gait, evaluate athletic performance, or discover skill deficits. In yoga research it might be used to determine opposing moments of inertia (resistance to angular acceleration) in the poses or the velocity of the limbs when entering a pose, such as Headstand.

the practitioner's loading history, certain poses will either stimulate adaptation or fail to. Depending on morphology, the accepted standard aesthetic cues of any given pose are favorable or problematic. Often this includes poses with extreme ROMs, particularly in the hips and shoulders. The truth is, we cannot say with any certainty who will benefit and who will suffer, and whether structure or symptoms will be affected. Headstand is probably one of the most controversial poses, followed by Shoulderstand. Of my highly esteemed colleagues, some are proponents, others are assailants. Where do I stand? I

Pause and turn to page 191 for a summary of related research.

say with great confidence, "I don't know." I would consider the individual, and all the variables that might play a role, and still, I would not know. Not knowing might feel crippling, but I find it liberating. The best I can do is implement sound evidence-based practices into my yoga and then step back, wait, assess, adjust if necessary, and repeat.

Cueing and Kinematics

I imagine it must be frustrating to arrive at the last section of the book only to be told, "it depends," and "I don't know." I urge you to recognize the power in those words, and to realize the wide-angled lens through which you can now look. After zooming all the way in to appreciate the complexities of the microscopic aspects of our tissues, we now zoom all the way back out to appreciate the complexities of the entire person. Early on I told you there would be no binary answers. As you now can see, biology won't allow them.

This revelation, however, should simplify how one applies biomechanics to asana, not complicate it. Instead of searching endlessly for the safest way to practice or teach a pose, it now clear that the best we can do is manage loads. The ways in which we can do that are: (1) specific to an area of the body, (2) progressive, and (3) variable.

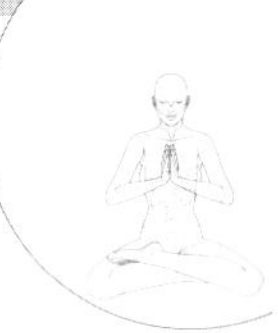

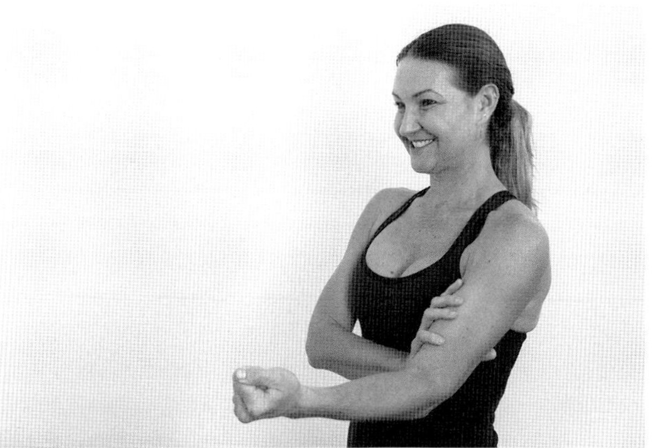

Fig. 6.14
Co-contraction.

Once again, I must remind you that I am not suggesting teachers lead their classes with reckless abandon. We know a few things about yoga and biomechanics now, so we can deconstruct how a yoga teacher might go about managing load. We can also bring ROM back into the conversation, because it is can help guide us in how to manage load.

Since most yoga postures are held for several breaths, they can be categorized as isometrics. During isometrics, muscles co-contract around a joint and hold the joint position static. You can try this by bending one elbow to 90 degrees and using the opposite hand to wrap around the upper arm area. The fingers will cover the biceps area and the thumb will cover the triceps area. Engage your biceps isometrically and the triceps also engage, as do other surrounding muscles (Fig. 6.14). Specific muscle cues, particularly once someone is already in the pose and holding it isometrically, are not necessary and, further, assumes everyone knows their muscles by name.

Instead, co-contraction can be encouraged through creative cueing. Most yoga cues already do this in some way (i.e. "hug the muscles to the bone"). Many styles of yoga encourage cues to provide an action with an opposite action. For example, in Plank Pose, one might say, "push your hands into the floor and lift up out of your wrists." These opposing actions encourage co-contraction in the isometric posture, thereby encouraging greater force transmission across the related joints. As with the spine, co-contraction here is not about "stabilizing the joints," but about stimulating tissue adaptation and increasing capacity.

ROM is of interest in two ways. First, co-contraction might not be achievable in end range positions among the very flexible (including the hypermobile). In that case, the practitioner has gone too far and could benefit from backing off until they can feel muscle tension. Second, co-contraction might not be achievable among practitioners with compromised ROM who circumvent mobility in one joint by borrowing it from another. The classic example is someone who has limited shoulder flexion extending her back so that she appears to have more shoulder flexion. Another circumvention is to adduct the shoulders while simultaneously flexing the elbows, which we often see in Downward Facing Dog Pose. Obviously, as per the principle of specificity, spinal extension will not promote shoulder flexion, and neither will adduction, but co-contracting at her end range of shoulder flexion before she circumvents it might (Figs. 6.15, 6.16, 6.17).

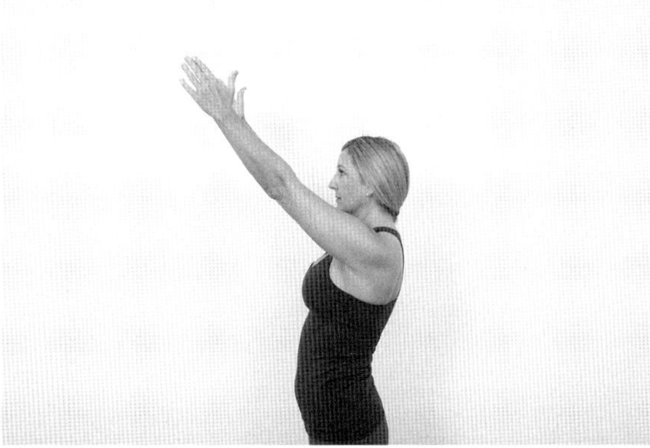

Fig. 6.15
Shoulder flexion.

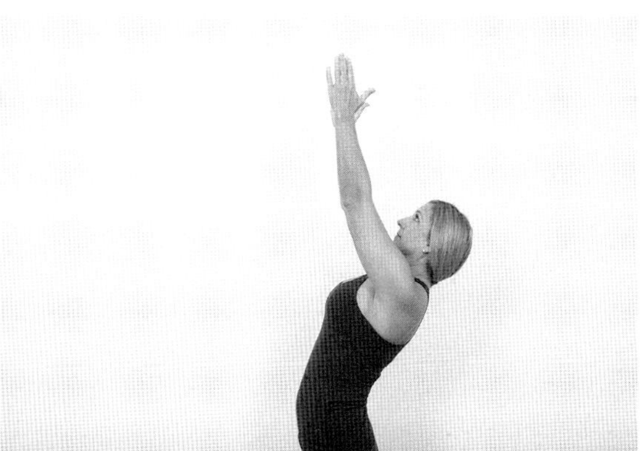

Fig. 6.16
Shoulder flexion with spinal extension.

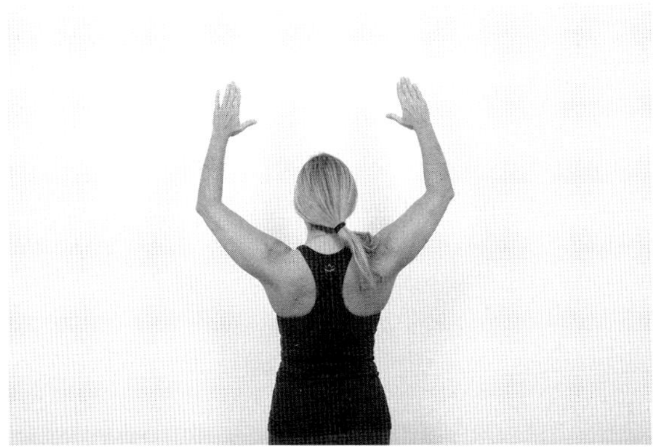

Fig. 6.17
Shoulder adduction with elbow flexion from a flexed shoulder position.

In both cases, either abundant or deficient ROM, using co-contraction as a guide allows for muscle force production to inform the pose.

The resulting appearance of the pose may not be aesthetically pleasing to someone trained to look for the shape, so it might take some getting used to. It may appear as if the practitioner is not "finishing" the pose, even though she is practicing with awareness and intention. If ROM does change over time, then a greater joint angle can be accessed, and co-contraction can be implemented there. If ROM does not change over time, then it is possible that the practitioner has reached her morphological limit and she can continue to increase capacity at that joint position. In either case, the function of the pose is placed before aesthetics.

Another benefit of co-contraction is that it leads teachers away from instruction that is based in diagnosis and rehab. "Faulty" kinematics, muscle "imbalances," and "compensations" are terms used by the rehab industry to determine "dysfunction" and then attempt to "correct" with targeted exercises. Somehow, this language has made its way into the yoga classroom, with well-meaning intent I'm sure. But the rehab industry has its own uncertainties and emerging perspectives that it has not yet sorted out. For example, exercise has been shown to improve strength, ROM, and symptoms, but not to alter kinematics (Ferrer et al., 2018). In fact, kinematic assumptions of the past decades are coming into question as technology advances. A recent study determined that subjects with full supraspinatus tears presented with the opposite arthrokinematic translation than was expected, where the humeral head migrated inferiorly, just as those with a fully intact tendon did (Millett et al., 2016). This means that even if exercises did alter kinematics, the assumptions as to which exercise would alter them, and how, might be incorrect. These types of assessments and corrective treatments can remain in the realm of researchers and clinicians, while the yoga teachers can focus on managing load to improve capacity, ROM, and possibly strength.

Here we arrive once again at how biomechanics can inform a yoga practice. Remember, biomechanics is about force. This book has focused primarily on tension and showed how muscle force increases tension on the surrounding connective tissue. If load parameters are sufficient enough to stimulate adaptation, then hopefully we better promote a safe and sustainable practice. Which specific muscle needs to be trained is not important as muscles don't act in isolation anyway. It has been shown that as the mechanical demand increases in shoulder flexion, the muscle recruitment pattern remains consistent with flexion at lower loads (Wattanaprakornkul et al., 2011). As long as shoulder flexion is being trained, and the manner in which it is being trained carries over to the skills needed to achieve the pose, then kinematic variables are not that important for the yoga teacher.

Yoga teachers are not physical therapists, even though the term "therapy" is often used in conjunction with yoga, implying otherwise at times. Instead, yoga, and specifically the asana component, provides an opportunity for the practitioner to develop a relationship with herself and her body. A yoga teacher who is always correcting and fixing what might be wrong could be interfering with the practitioner's own experience. Of course, instructions need to be given, but to what extent?

In certain poses, where skill must be acquired, instruction is useful. For example, telling a student to press her hands into the floor during a handstand may help her come off the wall. Does a student who is holding a handstand already in the middle of the room, provided that is the end goal and she is not in any pain, need to be told how to do it correctly? If you believe certain scapular positions may eventually cause "wear and tear," you might try to correct her. If you believe there is more than one way to achieve a Handstand Pose, you might choose to leave her to explore her own pose.

In other poses, where skill is generally not required, I advise teachers to say less. For example, in Bridge Pose, it is not necessary to instruct what to do with the glutes, especially once the student is in the pose. The student will use as much glutes as necessary to hold the pose isometrically, and that amount will fluctuate. In my first decade of practice, the instruction to "relax the glutes" in Bridge Pose was ubiquitous. Teachers then swung the pendulum to the other side and started insisting we "engage the glutes" in the pose. As usual, the correct method lies somewhere between the two. The gluteus maximus (Gmax) is a high-load muscle and EMG tends to go up when the demands of the activity go up; sprinting shows greater Gmax EMG than running, and even more than walking (Bartlett et al., 2014). If I wanted to increase the demand on the posterior hip muscles in Bridge Pose, I might choose to walk feet further way from the pelvis to bias the hamstrings, or turn the feet out (externally rotating and abducting the hip) to bias the Gmax. Neither of these is an incorrect or unsafe modification of the pose.

If any version of Bridge Pose, or any pose for that matter, caused adverse symptoms in a student, I would suggest trying another way. Again, as the load increases, options decrease, but yoga poses are generally lower load activities, especially when compared to lifting heavy weights where technique might matter more. Almost every weekend in a course, I offer the option of elevating the scapula somewhat when raising the arms over the head, or internally rotating (instead of externally rotating) the humerus somewhat in Downward Facing Dog Pose for students who complain about shoulder discomfort when doing the poses. In most cases, they immediately feel better and have not lost the ability to achieve the shape of the pose. If their symptoms persist, this signals to me they are good candidates for being referred out to a healthcare professional. Since scapular depression and humeral external rotation seem to be the standard protocol in any pose requiring the arms to be overhead (although not exclusively, I've taught at many studios where this rule has been abandoned), I sometimes must give permission several times before the students are willing to try it; they need to be convinced it is not wrong.

I am an advocate for open-ended questions and saying less because I believe sometimes yoga cues are too specific and interfere with the student's self-inquiry. Students will have unique strategies for raising their arms overhead. Learning to identify those strategies is a skill that can be honed but requires the teacher to be more curious than authoritative. I like to remind teachers that they are, in fact, also students and the pupils that attend their classes are giving the "teachers" the gift of learning yoga from them. Yoga is not about instructing, but about learning and, sometimes, instruction can be a form of obstruction.

I have offered you a fresh perspective on yoga that, I hope, disrupts the way we teach and practice yoga. It is not that I object to how we currently teach and practice yoga, but I do worry that we have become polarized in the pursuit of the right way over the wrong way. If biomechanics informs your approach in any way, it is my wish that you experience the joy in yoga and movement, that you inject creativity and variability into the practice, and that you build trust in your body and in your students' bodies.

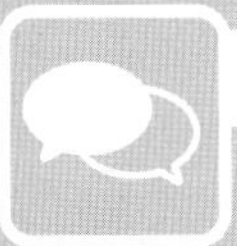

Thought Provoker

Instruct Less, Teach More

Modern postural yoga, with its external aesthetics rooted in alignment, has become somewhat of an externally driven practice where the shape is valued more than the experience. The next time you either teach or do your own home practice, I invite you to replace one common instruction (i.e. "stand with your feet parallel") with an open-ended question that incorporates force. You can reference an external load such as ground reaction force (i.e. "what happens further up the leg when you press your heel into the floor?"), or an internally generated muscle force (i.e. "reach out with the arms with as much effort as you can as you attempt to draw them in and observe how the pose changes"). If you watch your students or observe the subtle changes in your own body, you may discover that the body becomes better at identifying its own unique alignment when given the opportunity.

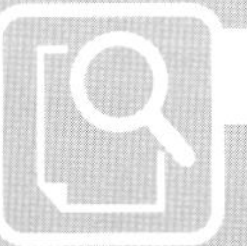

Research Summary

Adaptive Potential of Spinal Discs

Running Exercise Strengthens the Intervertebral Disc (Belavý et al., 2017)

Background

To date, it is believed that intervertebral discs (IVDs), which are made of fibrocartilage, do not have the capacity to positively adapt within one's lifespan. In spite of the general acceptance that tissues adapt to load, the current evidence on IVDs instead focuses on damage and degeneration caused by overloading in compression, torsion, and shear. We have evidence in animal models that IVDs might have a loading "window" in which conditions for an anabolic state can occur. Based on the methods of those studies, it might be possible that walking or running activities in humans could replicate those loading parameters.

Continued on next page

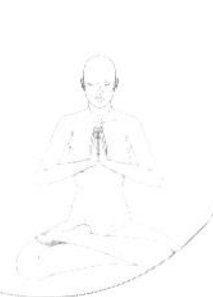

Continued from previous page

Purpose

Researchers hypothesized that in participants with no previous spinal condition, those who jogged or ran regularly would show greater IVD volumes than in individuals who were otherwise sedentary.

Methods

Seventy-nine non-smoking subjects with no history of spinal trauma or irregularity were recruited into three groups. Each group consisted of only subjects ages 25–35, to best control for degenerative changes natural to the aging process, who were required to have been consistent with their physical routine for at least 5 years minimum. The first group, the non-exercise group, did not perform more than 150 hours per week of moderate activity and did not walk more than 15 minutes to/from work. The second group, the joggers, ran 20–40 km weekly, but did not participate in any other sport or workouts. The third group, the runners, ran more than 50 km weekly and did not participate in any other sport or workouts, with resistance training as the exception (because many distance runners benefit from resistance training). On test day, MRI scans were performed later than noon, after 20 minutes in a seated position, and subjects had not exercised yet that day.

Results

Runners and joggers had significantly elevated proteoglycan (PG)/glycosaminoglycan (GAG) content (the negative charge of which binds with water), thereby greater lumbar disc hydration ($p < .01$) and lumbar IVD height, thereby disc hypertrophy ($p < .05$) than the non-exercisers.

Discussion

This paper showed that in this particular age group, people who were exposed to upright/vertical loading in compression and decompression cycles associated with running, had increased disc hydration. It is important to note that running dosage was specific and that generalizing to say one should run more is not yet warranted. While the results do suggest that running might have positive adaptive potential on the fibrocartilage of the IVDs, it is unclear if the increased hydration is purely a factor of mechanical loading. Running is an aerobic activity which increases oxygen uptake and leads to increased mitochondria (the organelle in which the biochemical metabolism of the cell is regulated), increased capillarization, and much more. Perhaps the stimulus is mechanical or chemical in nature, or possibly both or even neither.

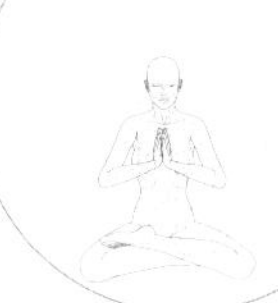

Research Summary

Headstand Safety

Sirsasana (Headstand) Technique Alters Head/Neck Loading: Considerations for Safety (Hector and Jensen, 2015)

Background

Headstand, often referred to as the "king of poses," has some evidence behind its effect on decreasing both heart rate and blood pressure and increasing respiratory capacity. In regard to the loading effects of Headstand, no previous research is known. Prior research cited by the researchers, based upon which they made their background conclusions on cervical spine loading, is varied in nature. Some were cadaver studies in which cadaver necks were either loaded in compression-flexion, or the cadavers were dropped on their heads. Some referenced African populations where head-loading was indigenous to their culture. Others applied large sustained or repeated loads, respectively, to segments of mouse tails in vivo or bovine tails in vitro. None were on axial or flexed compressive loading on inverted humans in vivo. They concluded that safe cervical loading limits lie between 300 and 17,000 N (roughly between 30 and 1730 kg, or 65 and 3820 lb), with an increased capacity of 600 N (roughly 60 kg, or 130 lb) in men versus women; also that age and exposure to load contribute to disc degeneration.

Purpose

Force data were collected on three different modes of entry/exit into/out of Headstand) to determine if techniques varied. No hypothesis was stated.

Methods

Forty-five individuals over 18 years of age who could hold Headstand without assistance for at least five full breaths were divided into three groups of 15 (only two of which in each group were men). The first group, average age 32.3 (+/- 9.2) years, kicked up/down one leg before the other with bent knees (angles varied). The second group, average age 37.9 (+/- 11.1) curled up/down with both legs together and bent knees. The third group, average age 36.9 (+/- 8.8) piked up/down with both legs together and straight knees. After a 10-minute personal practice warm-up, they stood upright on the force plate to determine baseline ground-reaction force (GRF) and were then affixed with reflective markers. Each participant performed three consecutive Headstands with a 2-minute rest between trials on a specially constructed platform consisting of a yoga mat with a force plate under the area where the crown of the head was placed. Kinematic data (velocity of distal lower extremity) were used to determine the entry, hold, and exit phases; GRFs (both average and maximum) were calculated; cervical angle as measured around C3 was collected; and center of pressure was estimated.

Continued on next page

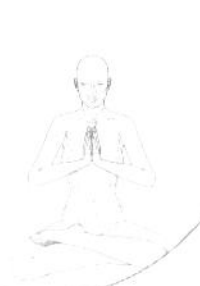

Continued from previous page

Results

Overall, maximum force on the crown of the head was measured between 40% and 48% of participant body weight, with the remainder distributed to the forearms. Just over half of the participants (51%) reached forces upwards of 300 N. Across all techniques, the hold phase of the pose resulted in the greatest maximum force and the exit phase the least. When separated by technique, the first group (split leg kick up/down) had the greatest force on entry and hold, but the least on exit; the second group (curl up/down) was in the middle for entry and hold, but the greatest on exit; and the third group (pike up/down) was the lowest on entry and hold, but in the middle on exit. Differences were significant across phases, but not across technique of each group overall. Neck angle was mostly in extension during entry and neutral or flexed during holding and exit, but not significant across technique. Center of pressure data showed that frontal plane variations occurred more during the entry and exit phases than holding phase.

Discussion

Piking up resulted in lower force and less cervical flexion during entry and holding than the other two techniques. Piking up, however, is generally the harder technique, as the straight legs create a longer lever against which the upper body muscles must produce force and might not be achievable by beginners (a group not represented in this study). Important anthropometric data such as limb lengths (e.g. neck and head, humerus, upper and lower leg) which could potentially affect results was neither collected, nor reported. Additionally, how one interprets this research depends greatly on how one interprets capacity and load tolerance. Most force data were reported as absolute or relative and compared against the cadaver and animal studies to evaluate risk. Comparing rat tails to human necks is probably not the best way to judge whether or not Headstand is safe. Adaptive potential was not discussed, and since cadavers have no adaptive capacity, they are probably not the best source of data either. Finally, the asymptomatic disc degeneration associated with 60% of US population currently practicing yoga was framed as a risk factor with no mention of genetic factors.

Appendix

The series of postures contained in the appendix are intended to provide a framework by which a yoga teacher might utilize yoga asana to increase capacity. The goal of increasing capacity, however, does not automatically imply that capacity is in some way diminished and must be reinstated. It also does not imply that yoga alone can provide the load parameters necessary to sufficiently promote positive tissue adaptation. Exposure to load is dose dependent and its effect will depend greatly on the practitioner, her biology, and her loading history. In the absence of research on tissue mechanics specific to yoga, all we can do is apply the available evidence to the way we teach. I have compiled for you here some of my own approaches to instructing asana with the goal of increasing one's tolerance to load.

The series of poses to follow are categorized by specific anatomical regions. They serve as models for you to develop your own series of poses for the same regions or different regions altogether. The first series is a bit more comprehensive than the two series which follow it, and deliberately so. It is my intention for you to come up with even better pose progressions and variations than I have provided, particularly as you navigate through the appendix. If you have read the book, and embraced its message, I challenge you to draw on your previous knowledge of yoga poses and combine it with your new-found knowledge of tissue mechanics to develop your own series. If you have not yet read the book, or perhaps want to review it a few more times before embracing the message, you may reference the series in the interim. I find that when given the educational foundation provided here, most yoga teachers quickly discover how to adapt the cues they already use and the poses they already teach. This improves their teaching skills and student loyalty base through the ability to make a profound difference in how their students experience yoga.

Modifying Loads for the Proximal Hamstring Tendon

The following series is suggested for yoga practitioners wishing to increase proximal hamstring tendon capacity. As outlined in the text, the specific, variable, and progressive loading parameters are intended to optimally load as best we can using only our body weight. In cases where a student's hamstrings might be underloaded, we wish for the series to provide a protective effect against future possible hamstring aggravation.

In other cases, the series may serve students who have returned to yoga after rehabbing a proximal hamstring tendinopathy but might still be in the time window where an emphasis on increasing capacity is essential.

The suggested isometric hold time for each pose is 30–45 seconds. If you are working toward substantially increasing capacity, then 5 isometric repetitions (reps) are recommended, allowing for 2 minutes rest in between reps. One should progress only when ready, when the suggested 30–45 second holds are sustainable, meaning it might take months for some of the later progressions to become appropriate. If considering the injury recovery timeline as a model for tissue adaptation, remember it could even take 1–3 years for capacity to substantially increase. Patience and adherence (i.e. no large gaps in loading periods) are crucial. If increasing loads are introduced too quickly and symptoms present, resting for a few days is suggested before resuming with a regression. If symptoms persist, a referral to a qualified healthcare professional is recommended.

When trying to incorporate elements of the series into a yoga group class setting, creative sequencing might utilize the rest period by loading a different muscle group in a different type of pose. For example, certain standing poses or poses bearing weight on the arms might give the hamstrings a rest between reps. "Stretching" between reps is not necessary, nor is it encouraged. If the series is followed sequentially, loading will, eventually, occur closer to the end range positions, introducing tension at a lengthened hamstring.

The Hamstring Bridge

Because Bridge Pose is often practiced as a replacement for Upward Facing Bow Pose, the emphasis tends to be on spinal extension. In this variation, the emphasis is on the posterior hip muscles and less on the paraspinal muscles.

Action/skill to bias the posterior hip

From the back of the knee, reach from the top of the calves toward the heel and into the floor. Maintain that action and also reach from the bottom of the hamstring up to the sitting bone. Cultivating a *sense* of pushing and pulling with your muscles, you should feel the posterior leg and hip deliberately engage. Maintain during transition into and out of the pose, while holding the pose, and during all variations and progressions (Figs. A1-A4). Relax during rest.

Vary the series by externally rotating and abducting the hip to bias lateral hamstring (biceps femoris) and gluteus maximus (Figs. A5-A8).

Vary the series by internally rotating and adducting the hip to bias the medial hamstrings (semitendinosus and semimembranosus) and adductor muscle group (Figs. A9-A12).

In some instances, students may struggle to access tension across the posterior leg, particularly the hamstrings. This is commonly the case in students with hypermobility. Applying a constraint may help them access the action/skill. The first option is to change the contact point of the feet to the heels (Fig. A13). The second option is to

The Hamstring Bridge

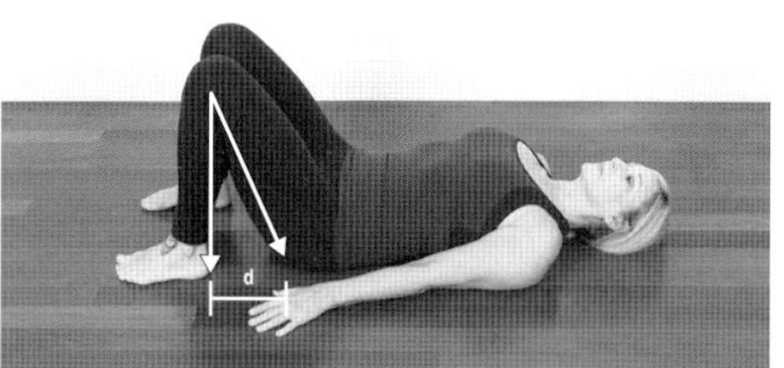

A1 Starting position for the Hamstring Bridge.

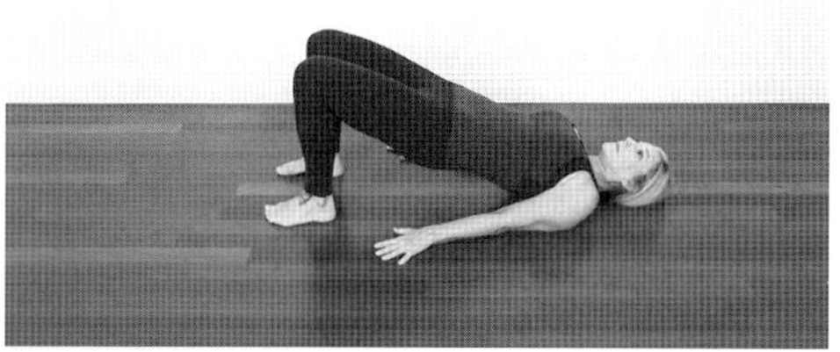

A2 Hamstring Bridge with neutral spine and hips.

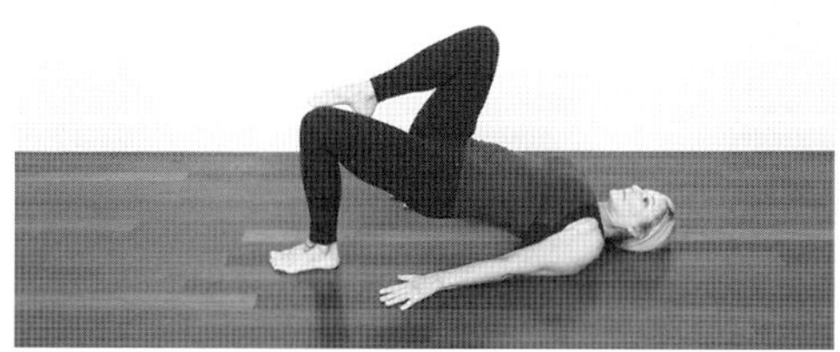

A3 Single leg progression for the Hamstring Bridge.

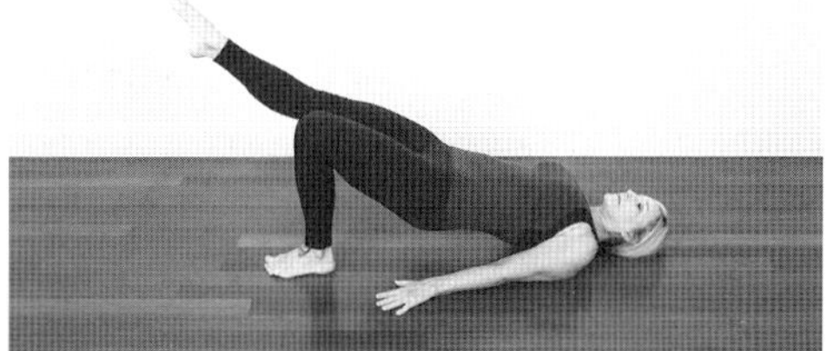

A4 Single leg progression for the Hamstring Bridge with longer lever.

Externally Rotated Variation

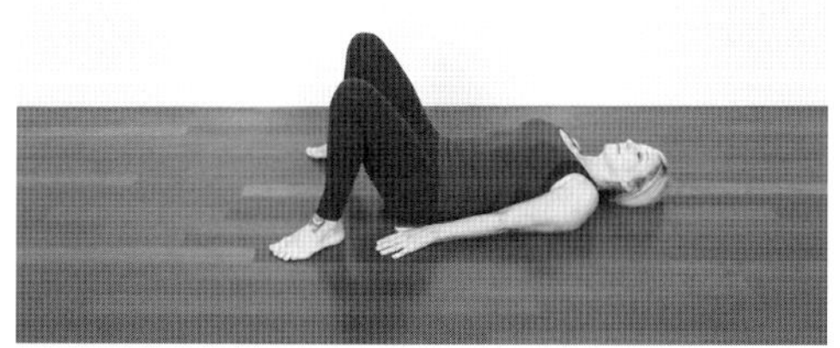

A5 Starting position for the Hamstring Bridge, externally rotated variation.

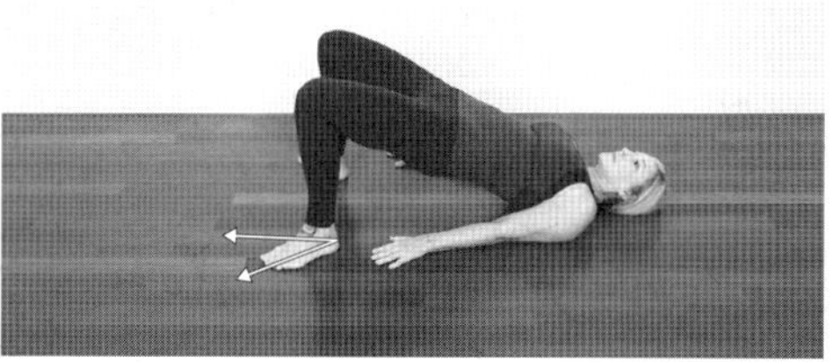

A6 Externally rotated Hamstring Bridge.

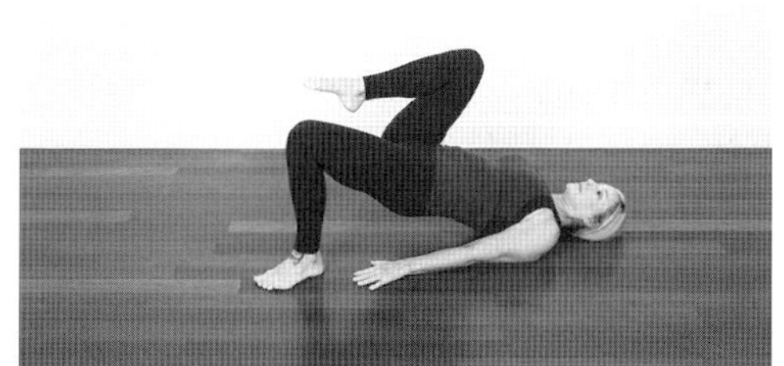

A7 Externally rotated, single-leg progression for the Hamstring Bridge.

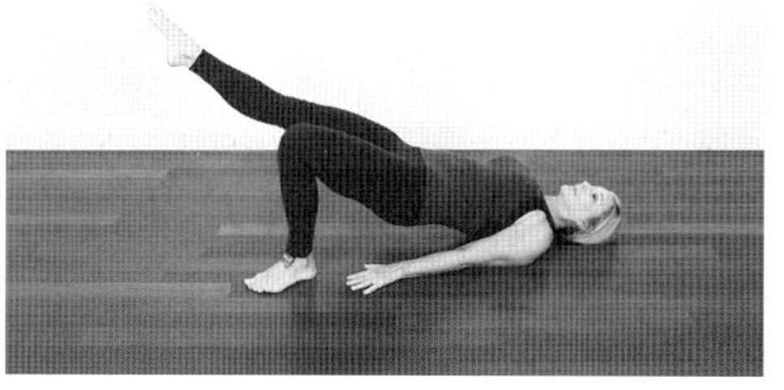

A8 Externally rotated, single-leg progression of the Hamstring Bridge with longer lever.

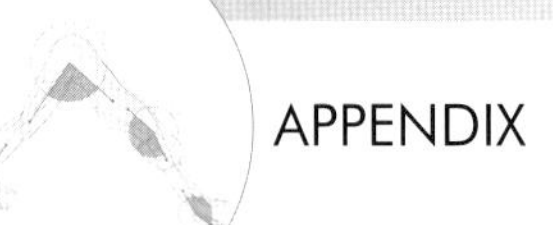

Internally Rotated Variation

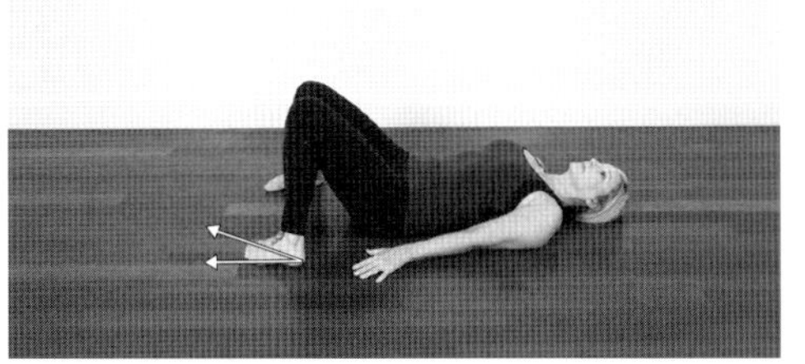

A9 Starting position for the Hamstring Bridge, internally rotated variation.

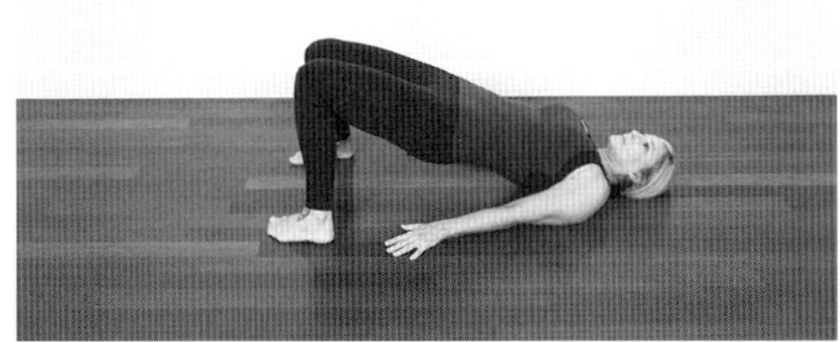

A10 Internally rotated Hamstring Bridge.

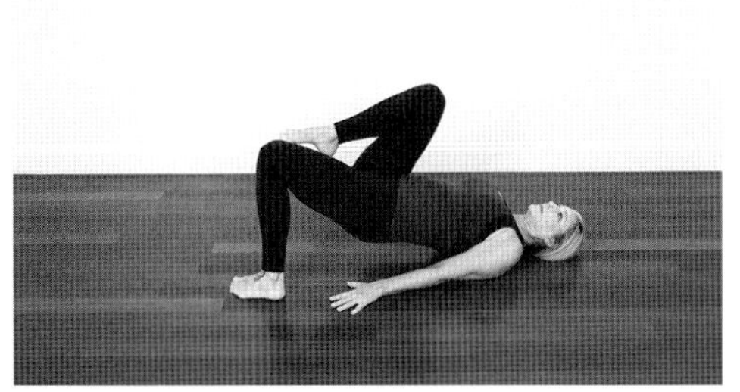

A11 Internally rotated, single-leg progression for the Hamstring Bridge.

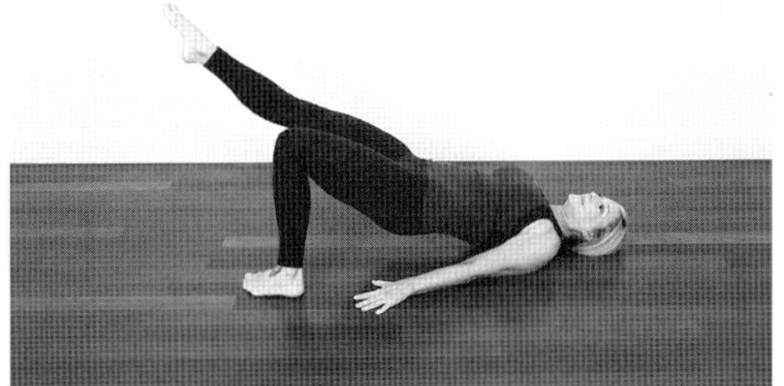

A12 Internally rotated, single-leg progression for the Hamstring Bridge with longer lever.

Options to Assist in Finding the Skill/Action

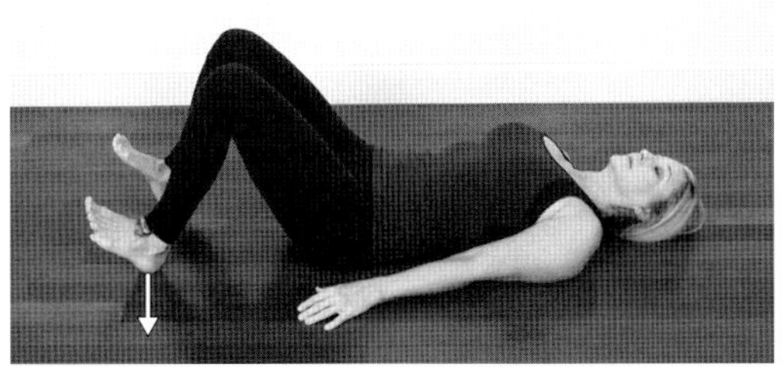

A13 Starting position for Bridge Series with heels dug in and forefeet lifted.

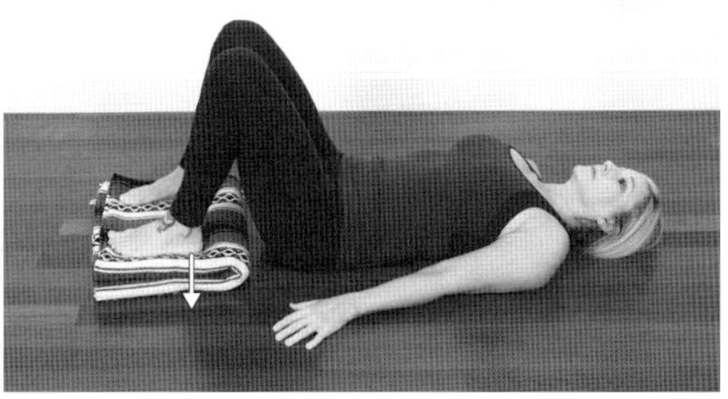

A14 Starting position for Bridge Series with feet on blanket on slippery surface.

provide a sliding surface and instruct the student to avoid letting the feet slide away where a slight action of pulling the feet toward the pelvis will be needed (Fig. A14). Either of these two constraints can be applied throughout the previous series, as well as the series ahead.

Progress the series by moving the feet further away from the hips to change the lever length, and to further bias the hamstrings (Figs. A15-A18, A19-A22, A23-A26).

Hamstring Bridge Progression v.1

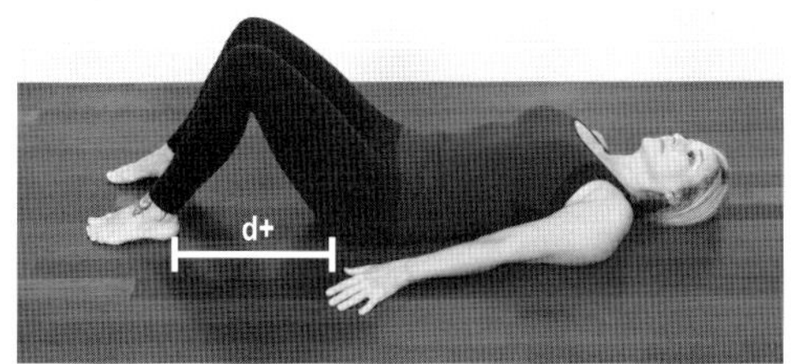

A15 Starting position for the partially Extended Bridge.

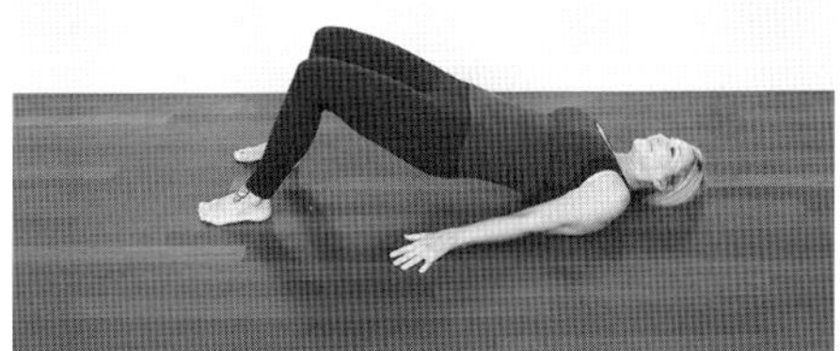

A16 Partially Extended Bridge.

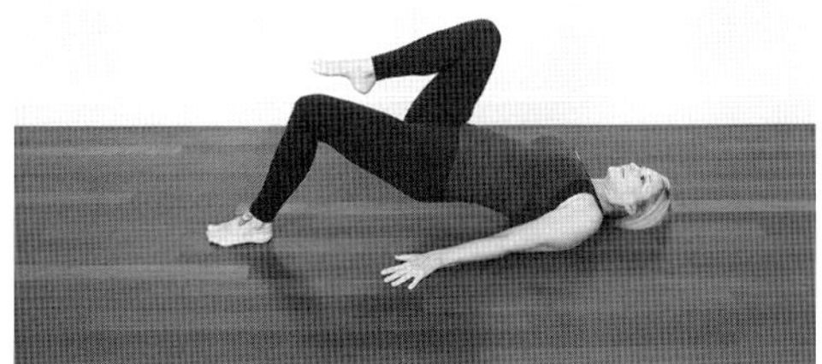

A17 Single-leg progression for the partially Extended Bridge.

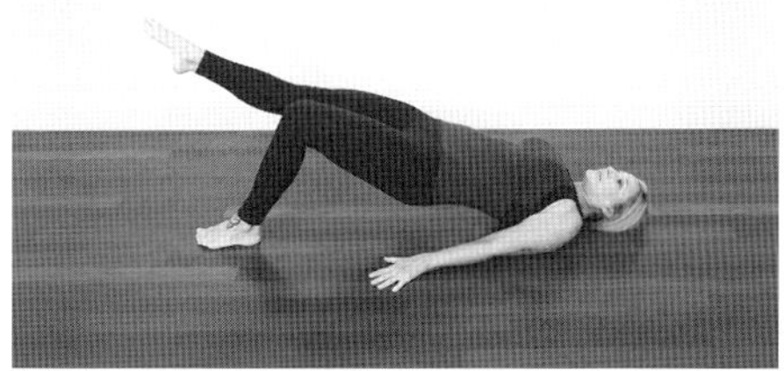

A18 Single-leg progression for the partially Extended Bridge with longer lever.

Hamstring Bridge Progression v.1, Externally Rotated Variation

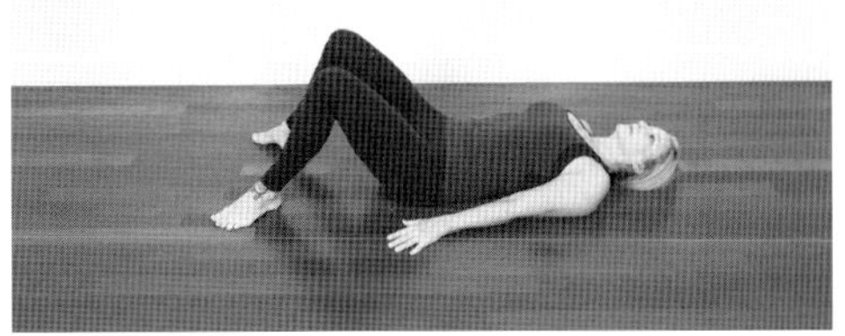

A19 Starting position for the partially Extended Bridge, externally rotated variation.

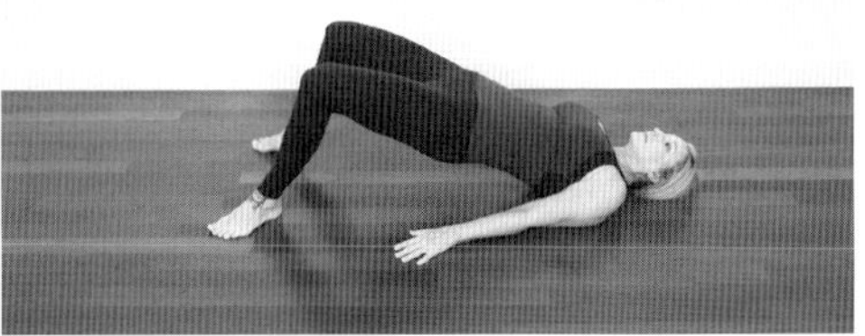

A20 Externally rotated, partially Extended Bridge.

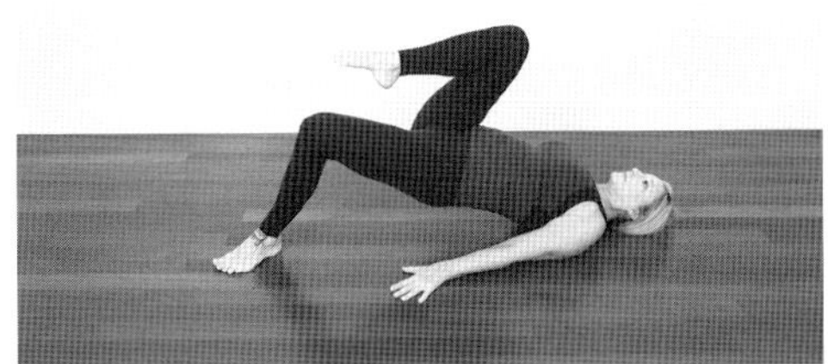

A21 Externally rotated, single-leg progression for the partially Extended Bridge.

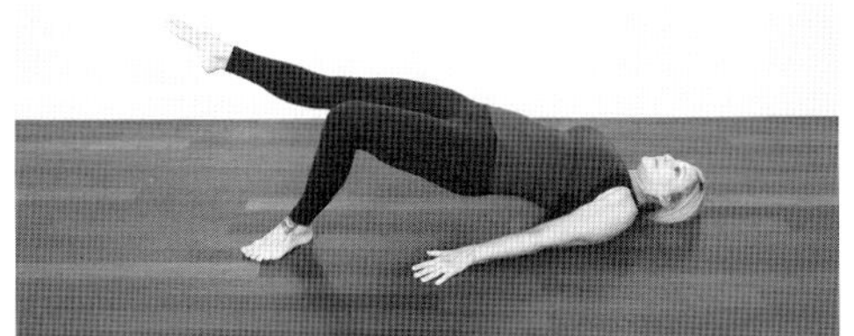

A22 Externally rotated, single-leg progression for the partially Extended Bridge with longer lever.

Hamstring Bridge Progression v.1, Internally Rotated Variation

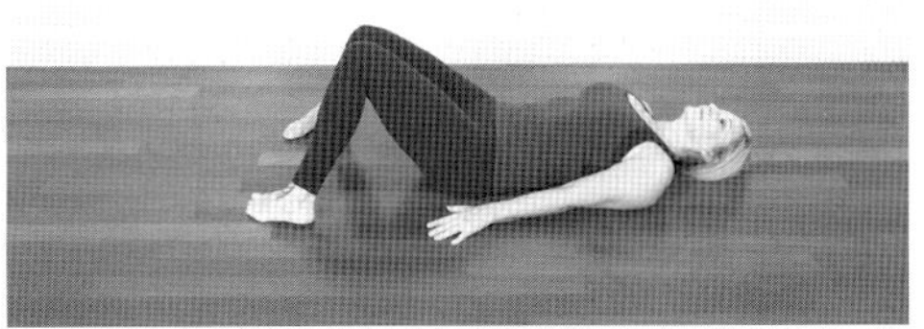

A23 Starting position for the Extended Bridge, internally rotated variation.

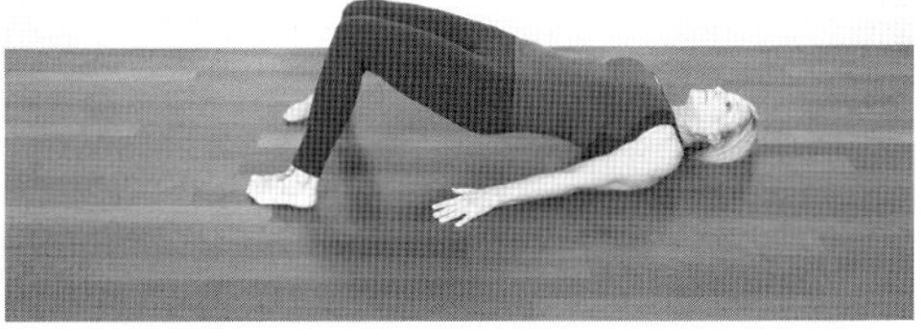

A24 Internally rotated partially Extended Bridge.

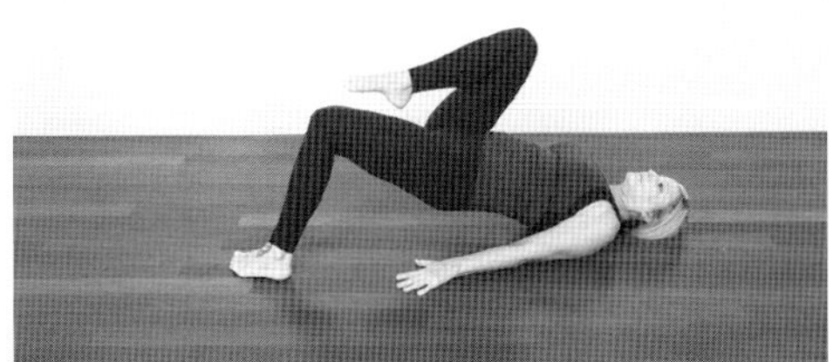

A25 Internally rotated, single-leg progression for the partially Extended Bridge.

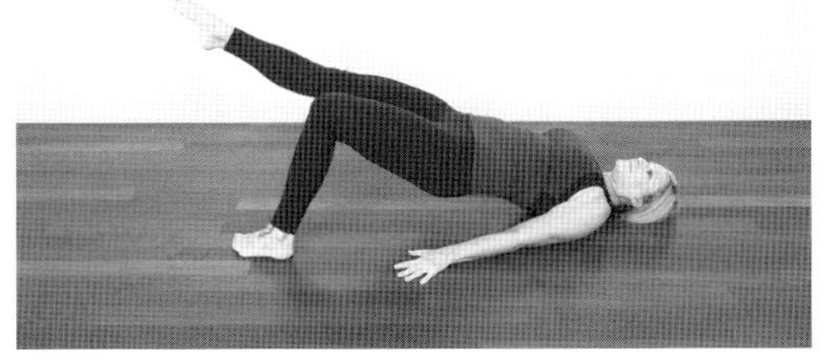

A26 Internally rotated, single-leg progression for the partially Extended Bridge with longer lever.

The distance between the feet and the pelvis can be increased incrementally by about 10–15 cm (4–6 inches) over time. At a certain distance, the forefoot will lift and the heels will be the main point of contact with the floor.

As the distance between the feet and the pelvis increases, the series eventually progresses to a straight leg (or almost straight leg) variation. Elevating feet on blocks will provide space for the pelvis to lift into Extended Bridge Pose (Figs. A27-A30, A31-A34, A35-A38).

Eccentric Hamstring Slides

After isometric Hamstring Bridges, eccentric Hamstring Slides can be introduced. You will need a sliding surface, such as a hardwood floor or linoleum, and a yoga blanket or small towel. Fitness sliders or furniture sliders also work, and even paper plates will do if practicing on carpet.

Suggested reps are 15 with relative competency. If working toward substantially increasing capacity, 3 to 5 sets are recommended, allowing for 2 minutes rest in between sets. Creative sequencing for a group class setting might utilize the rest period by loading a different muscle group in a different type of pose.

Hamstring Bridge Progression v.2

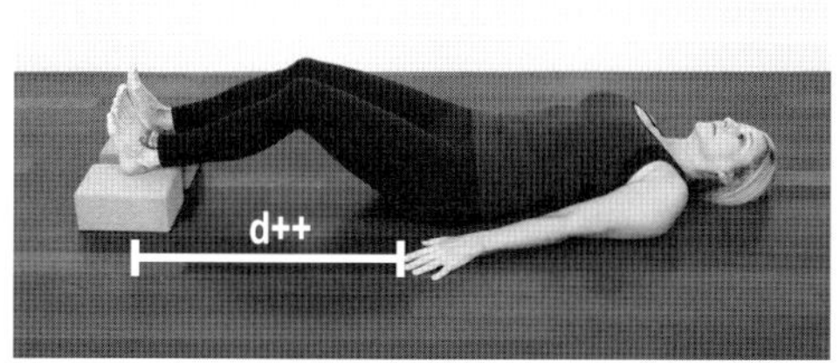

A27 Starting position for Extended Bridge.

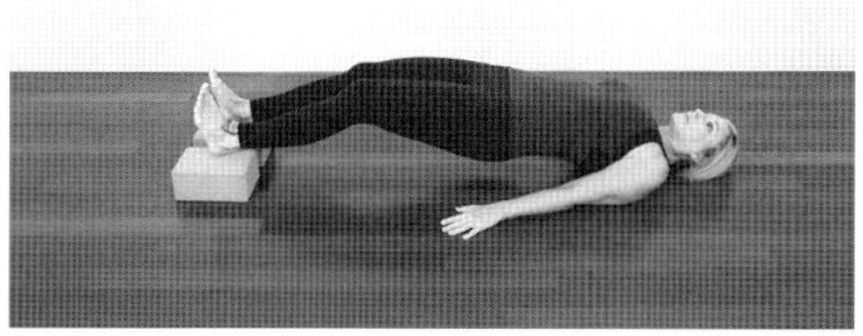

A28 Extended Bridge.

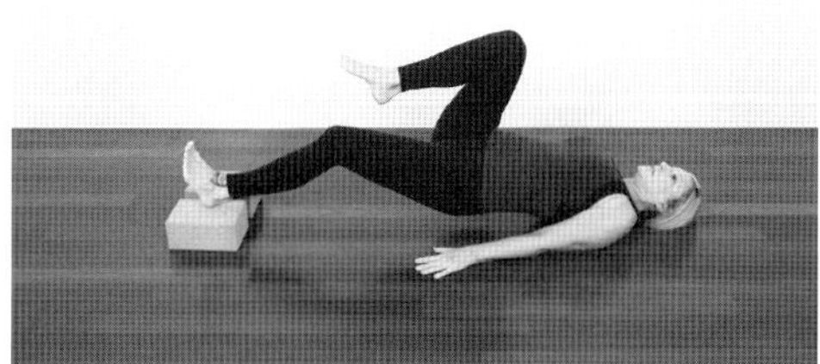

A29 Single-leg progression for Extended Bridge.

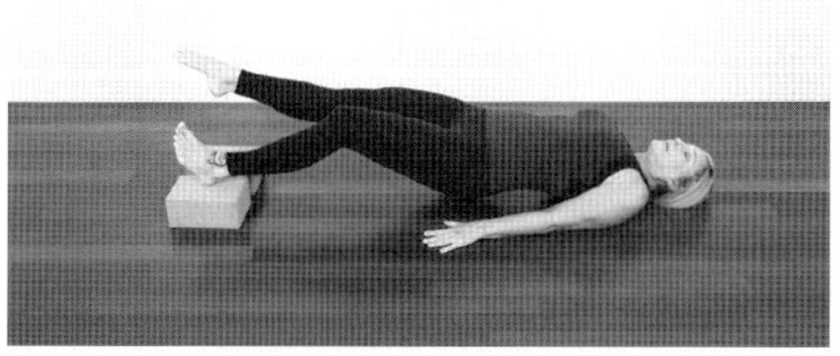

A30 Single-leg progression for Extended Bridge with longer lever.

Hamstring Bridge Progression v.2, Externally Rotated Variation

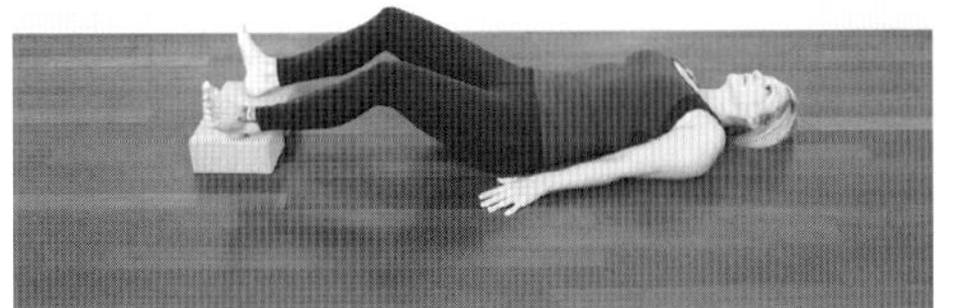

A31 Starting position for Extended Bridge, externally rotated variation.

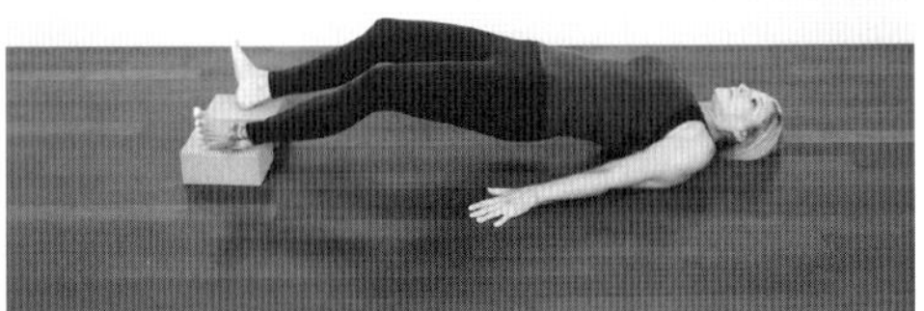

A32 Externally rotated Extended Bridge.

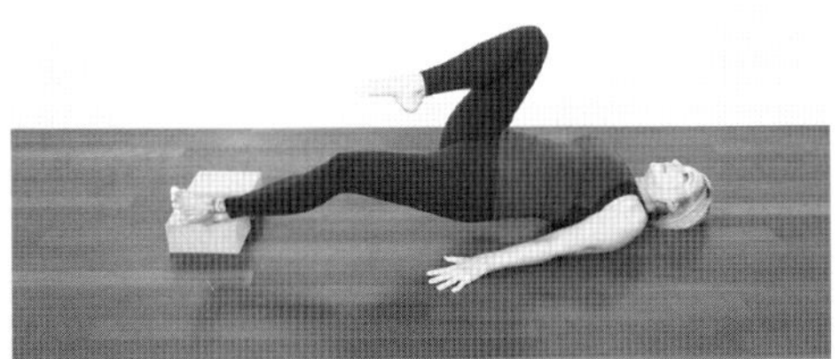

A33 Externally rotated, single-leg progression for Extended Bridge.

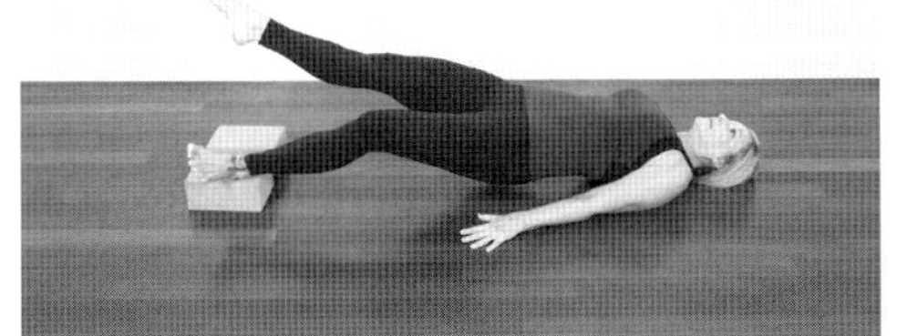

A34 Externally rotated, single-leg progression for Extended Bridge with longer lever.

Hamstring Bridge Progression v.2, Internally Rotated Variation

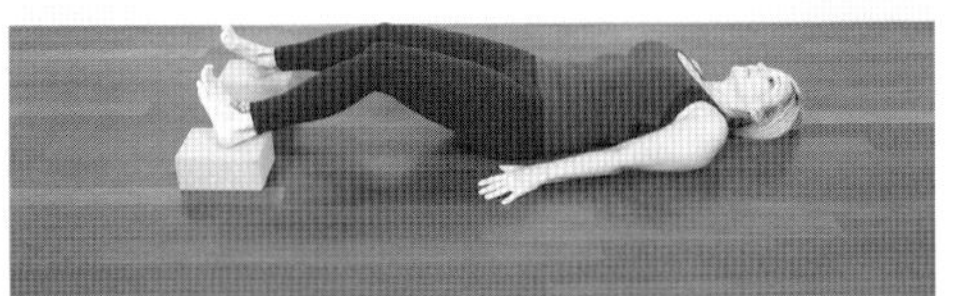

A35 Starting position for Extended Bridge, internally rotated variation.

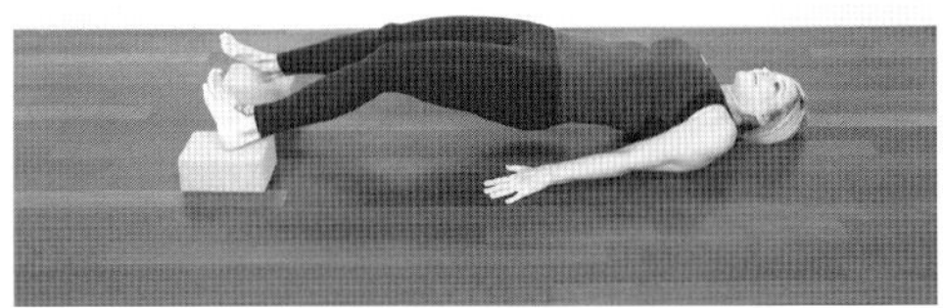

A36 Internally rotated Extended Bridge.

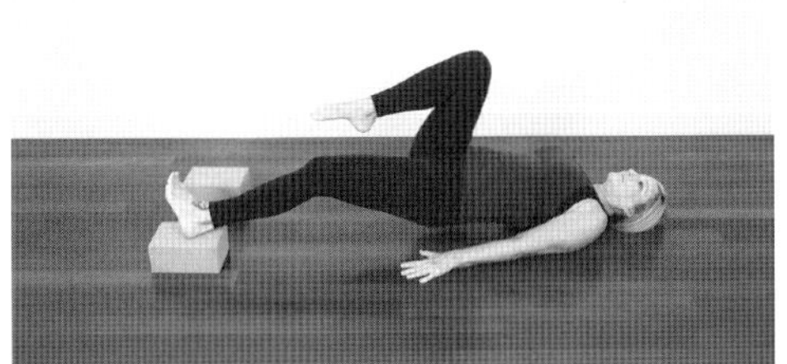

A37 Internally rotated, single-leg progression for Extended Bridge.

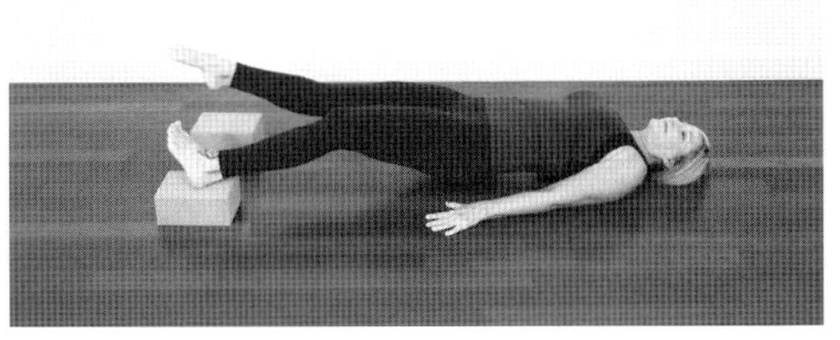

A38 Internally rotated, single-leg progression for Extended Bridge with longer lever.

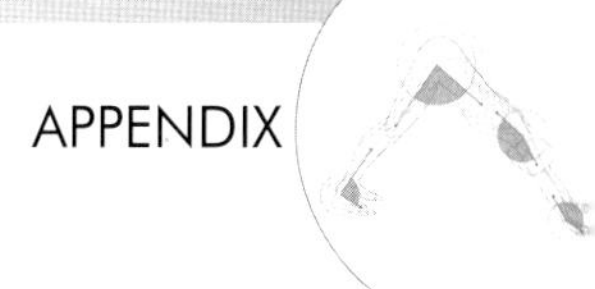

Action/skill

To start, lift pelvis without letting the blanket slide away from you. Then slowly, while keeping the pelvis lifted, slide the blanket away from you, not quite straightening the knees. Go slow, taking about 3–5 seconds to get to end range from the starting position. At the end, lower your pelvis and slide the blanket back to the starting position, then lift the pelvis and repeat (Figs. A39-A45). Vary the sequence by adding external rotation or internal rotation at the hip (Figs. A46-A47). Progress sequence by adding single-leg options (Figs. A48-A50).

Concentric Hamstring Slides

After eccentric Hamstring Slides, the concentric component can be introduced. Repeat the entire eccentric series, but keep the pelvis lifted during the return to the starting position. Suggested reps are 10–15 (or to fatigue, whichever comes first) with relative competency. If working toward substantially increasing capacity, 3 to 5 sets are recommended, allowing for at least 2 minutes rest in between sets. Creative sequencing for a group class setting might utilize the rest period by loading a different muscle group in a different type of pose.

Action/skill

To start, lift pelvis without letting the blanket slide away from you. While keeping the pelvis lifted, slide the blanket away from you, almost straightening the knees. Keep your pelvis lifted and slide the blanket back to starting position in a smooth, controlled manner (Figs. A51-A57). Vary the sequence by adding external rotation or internal rotation at the hip joint. Progress sequence by adding single-leg options.

Lunges

Lunges introduce hip flexion to the front leg (i.e. greater stretch) in the hamstring series. Depending on the student's sensation, deep Lunges (i.e. deep hip flexion) may be postponed until capacity increases. Ideally, Lunges should eventually be weighted to encourage greater muscular recruitment, but Lunges using only one's body weight are a good place to start developing capacity.

Action/skill to bias the posterior hip

In the front leg, reach from the top of the calf toward the heel. Maintain that action and also reach from the bottom of the hamstring up to the sitting bone. Cultivating a *sense* of pushing and pulling with your muscles, you should feel the posterior leg and hip of the front leg deliberately engage (Fig. A58). Maintain during transition into and out of the pose, while holding the pose, and during all variations and progressions. Relax during rest.

These are just some suggestions for Lunge variations and progressions (Figs. A59-A64). With a little creativity, you'll find the options endless. Considerations might include joint angle and limb placement, percent of maximum voluntary isometric contraction, duration, and frequency.

Eccentric Hamstring Slides

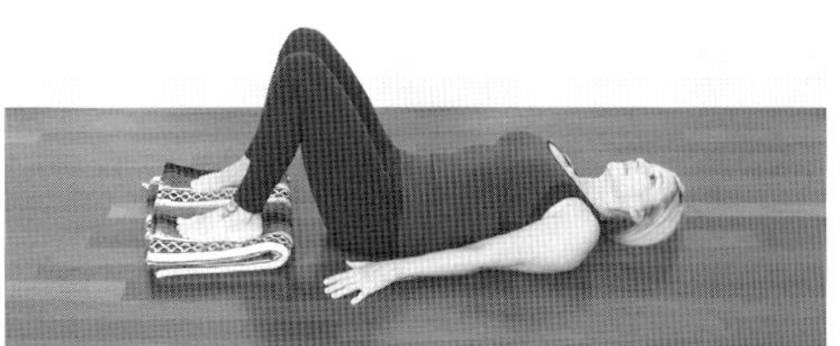

A39 Starting position for Eccentric Hamstring Slides.

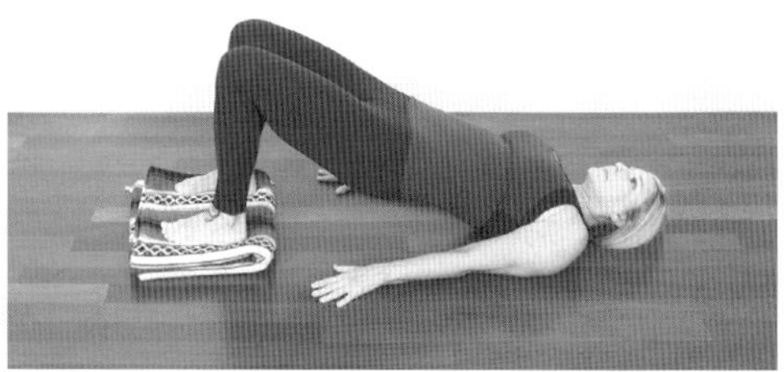

A40 Eccentric Hamstring Slides, pelvis lifts keeping blanket stationary.

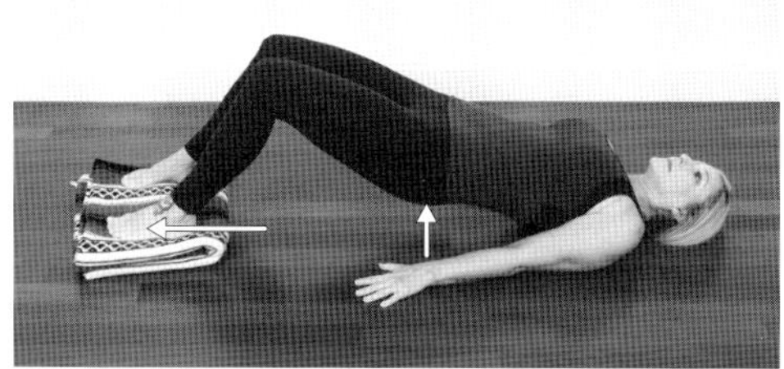

A41 Eccentric Hamstring Slides, blanket slides away from pelvis.

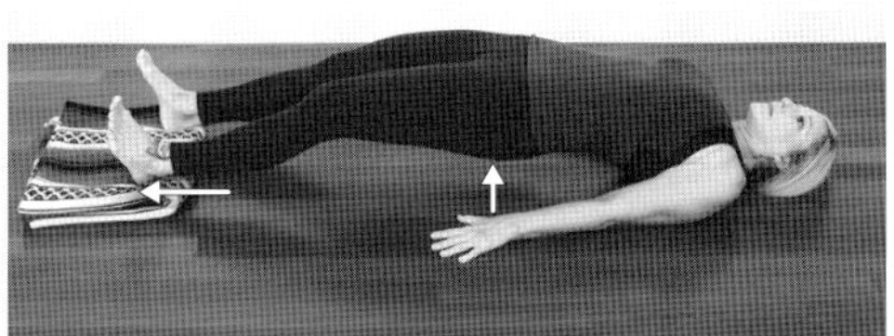

A42 Eccentric Hamstring Slides, blanket continues to slide until knees almost straight.

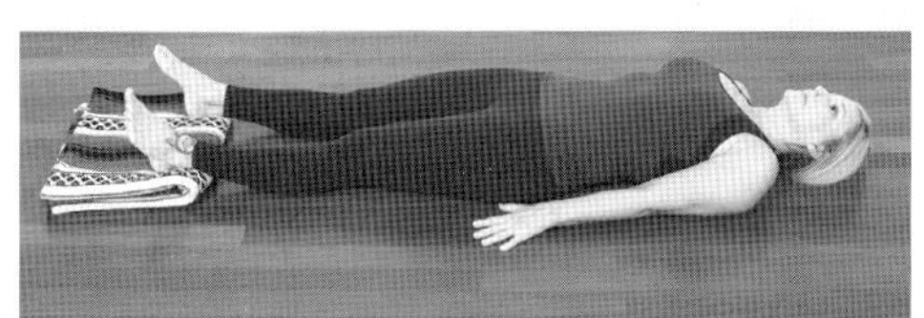

A43 End range, Eccentric Hamstring Slides, pelvis lowers to floor.

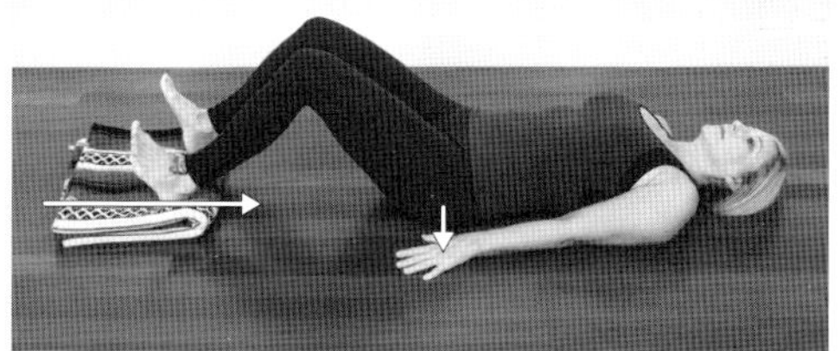

A44 With the pelvis on the floor, blanket returns to starting position.

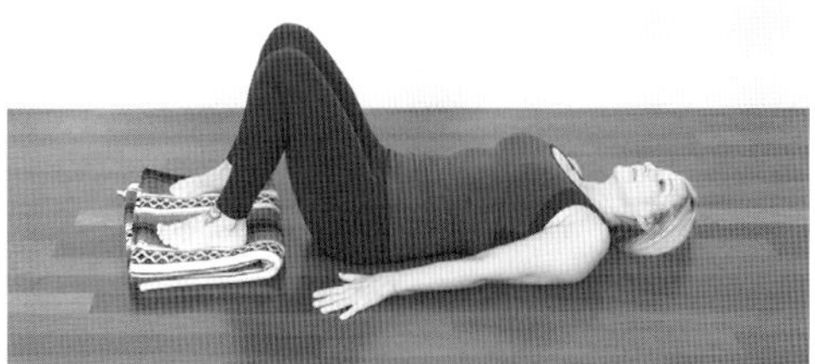

A45 Starting position for Eccentric Hamstring Slides. Repeat.

Variations and Progressions

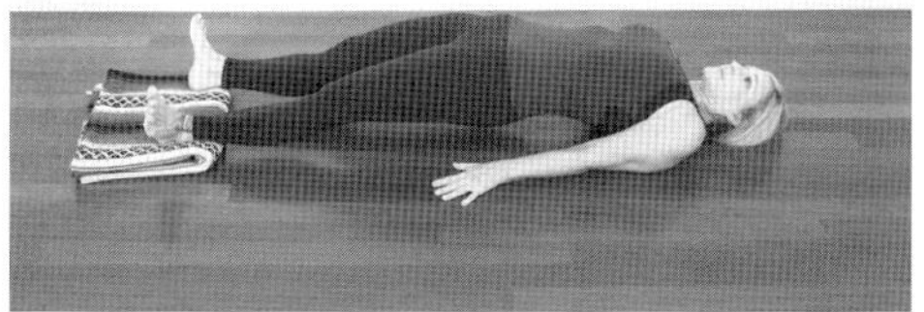

A46 End range, Eccentric Hamstring Slides, externally rotated.

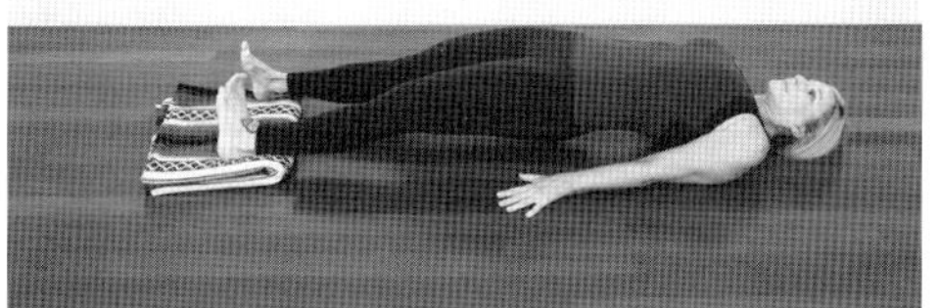

A47 End range, Eccentric Hamstring Slides, internally rotated.

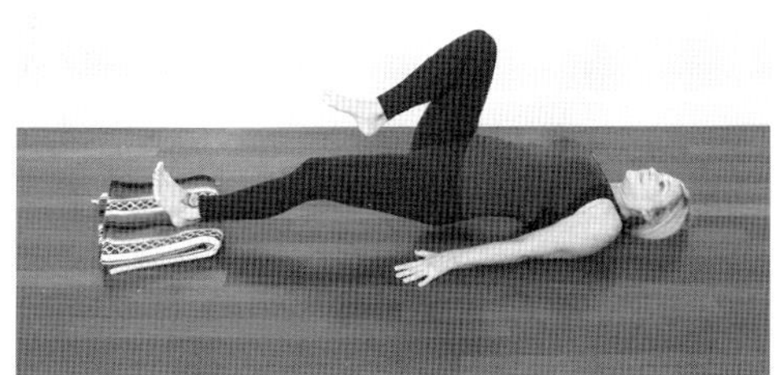

A48 End range, Eccentric Hamstring Slides, single-leg progression.

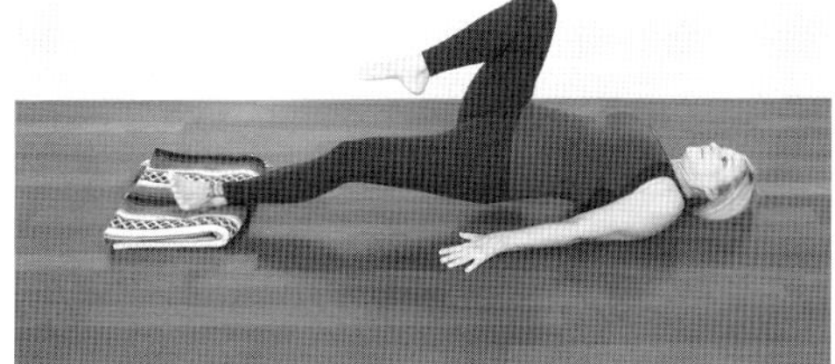

A49 End range, Eccentric Hamstring Slides, externally rotated, single-leg progression.

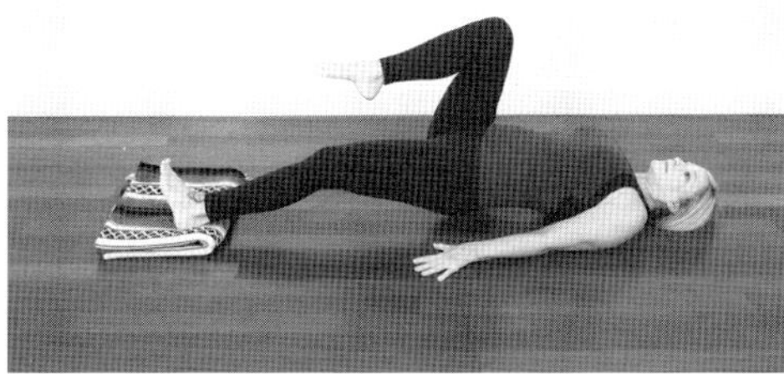

A50 End range, Eccentric Hamstring Slides, internally rotated, single-leg progression.

Concentric Hamstring Slides

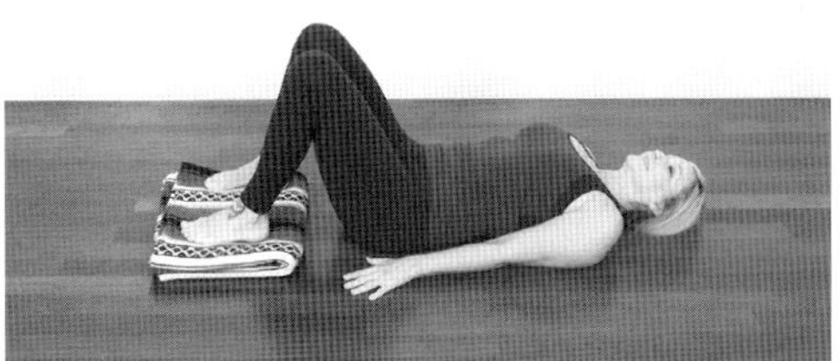

A51 Starting position for Concentric Hamstring Slides.

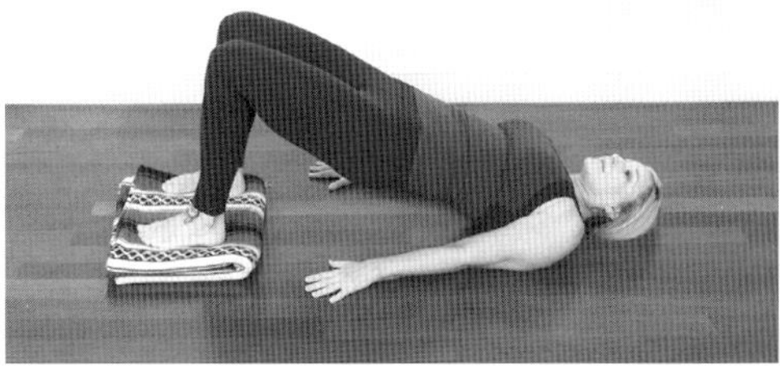

A52 Eccentric phase, pelvis lifts keeping blanket stationary.

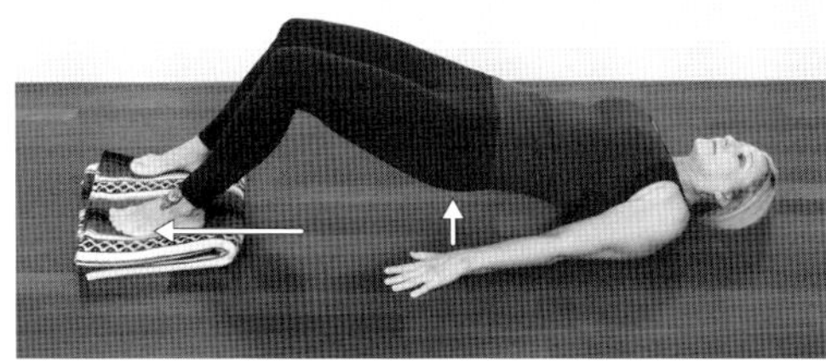

A53 Eccentric phase, blanket slides away from pelvis.

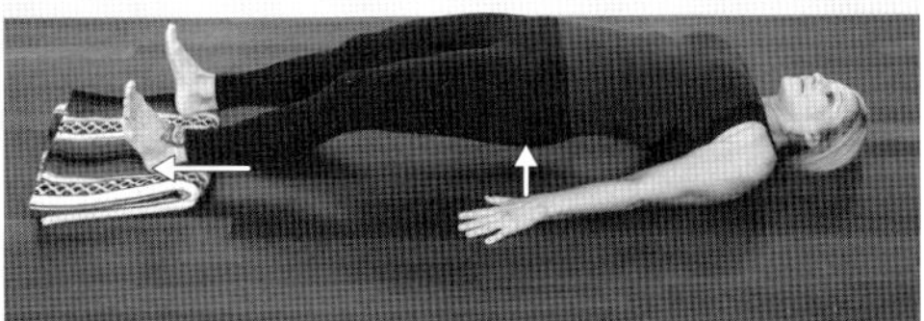

A54 Eccentric phase, blanket continues to slide until knees almost straight.

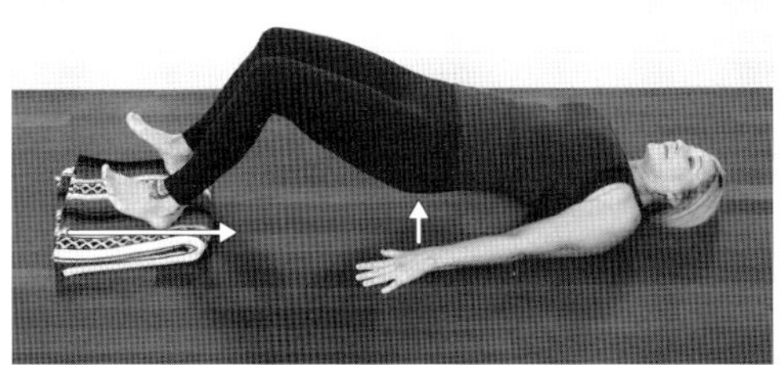

A55 Pelvis lifted, blanket returns to starting position.

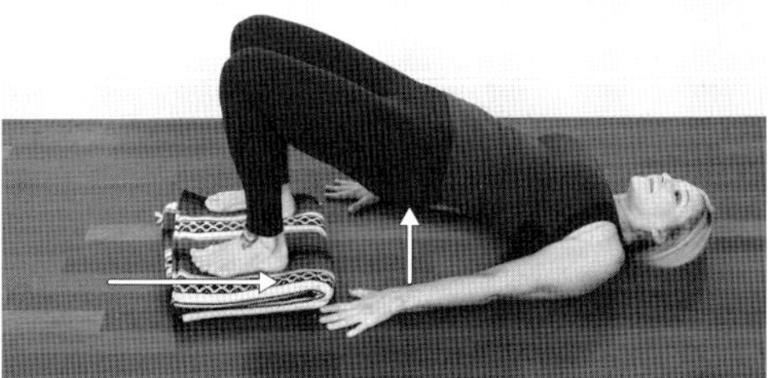

A56 Concentric phase, maintaining lifted pelvis, blanket returns to starting position.

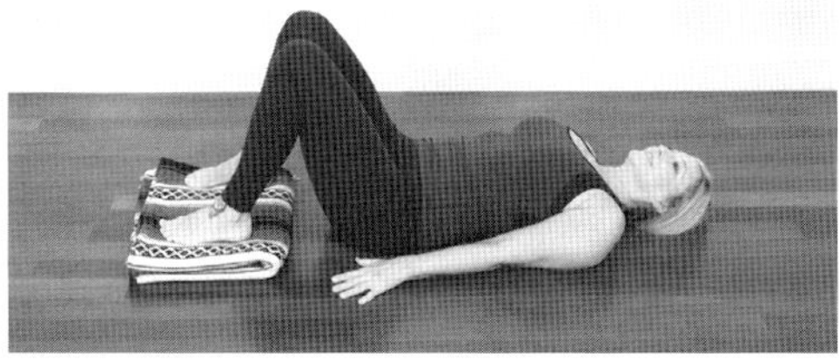

A57 Starting position for Concentric Hamstring Slides. Repeat.

Lunges

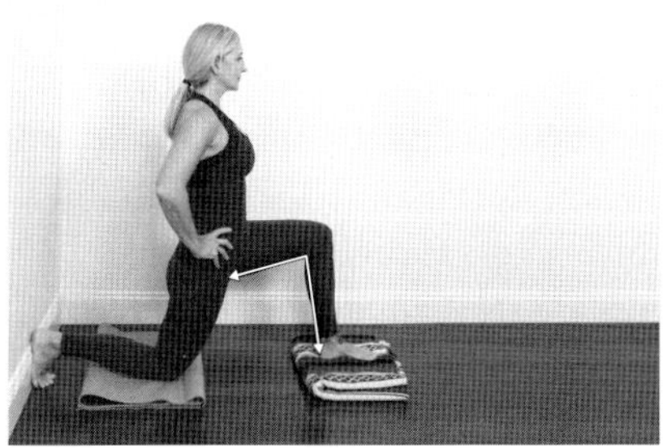

A58 Kneeling Lunge. Isometric, eccentric, and concentric variations.

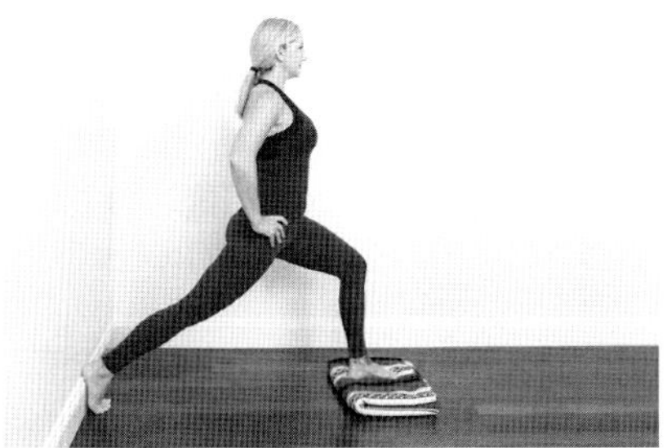

A59 Crescent Lunge. Isometric, eccentric, and concentric variations.

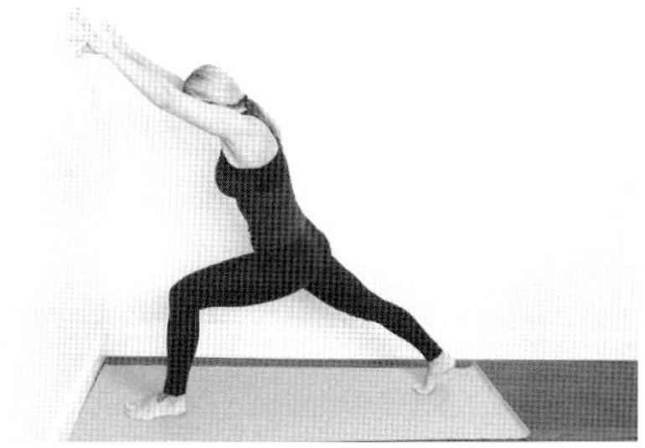

A60 Supported Lunge, hands on wall, resulting in least hip flexion.

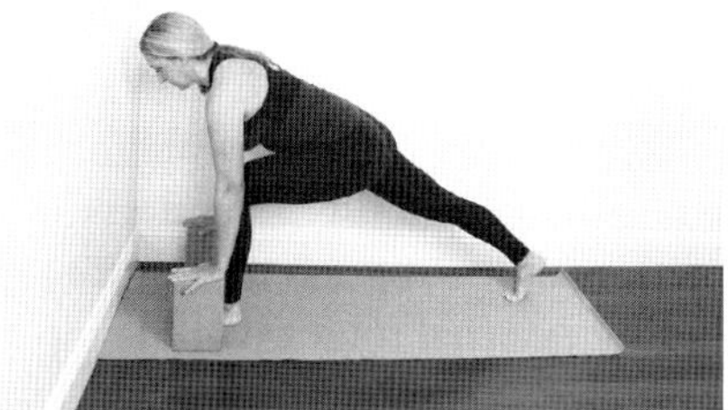

A61 Supported Lunge, hands on tall blocks, resulting in moderate hip flexion.

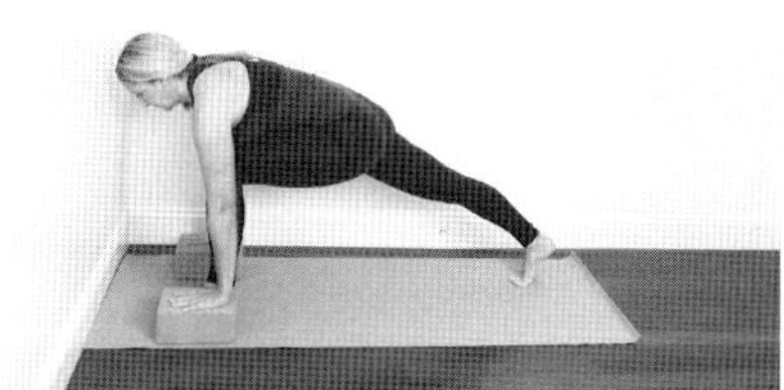

A62 Supported Lunge, hands on low blocks, resulting in greater hip flexion.

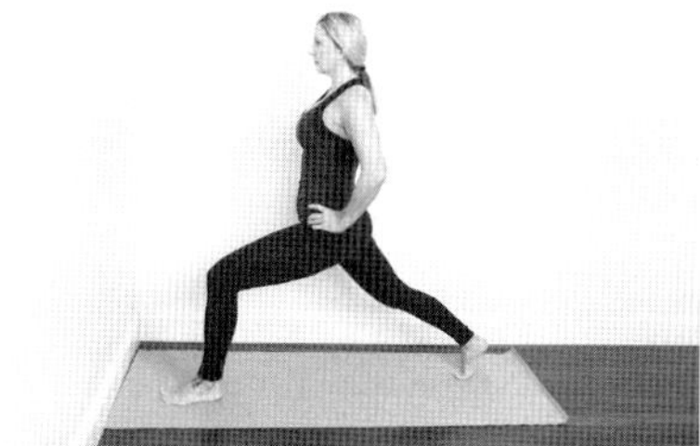

A63 Crescent Lunge, unsupported.

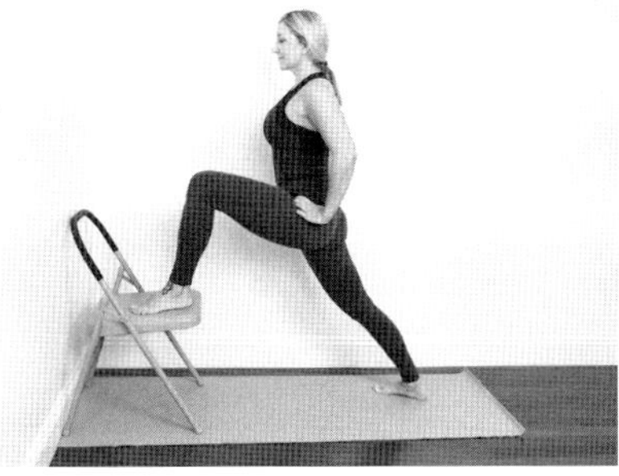

A64 Warrior I Pose with chair, greater hip flexion, shorter moment arm relative to hip.

Forward Bends

Deep Forward Bends tend to be the most aggravating poses for underloaded hamstring tendons. It is not that Forward Bends should be avoided altogether, but I do find that many popular styles of yoga tend to emphasize Forward Bends in the absence of hamstring loading. As per the length–tension curve, muscles tend to produce less force at lengthened positions than at mid-range, therefore backing off end range is recommended at first. As the hamstrings are trained, deliberate tension should become incrementally achievable at longer muscle lengths. Students who are post-rehab after a tendinopathy may choose to progress the depth of their Forward Bends at a more conservative rate than other students. Finally, students with hypermobility may find it useful to oscillate between a bent knee and straighter knee position to help maintain tension in the hamstring.

Action/skill to bias the posterior hip

Reach the tops of the calves to the heel and the bottom of the hamstrings to the sitting bone until you feel the posterior leg and hip deliberately engage (Fig. A65). Only stretch as deep as you can while maintaining hamstring tension (Figs. A66-A72). You may need to keep a slight bend in the knees and/or minimize hip flexion to access the action/skill. Progress to standing single-leg variations (Figs. A73-A77). Vary by including external rotation at the hip (Figs. A78-A81).

Forward Bends

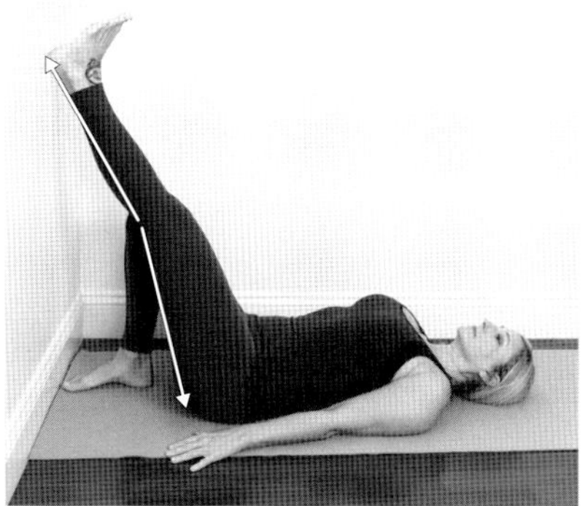

A65 Supine Hand-to-Big-Toe Pose, supported against the wall, less than 90° of hip flexion.

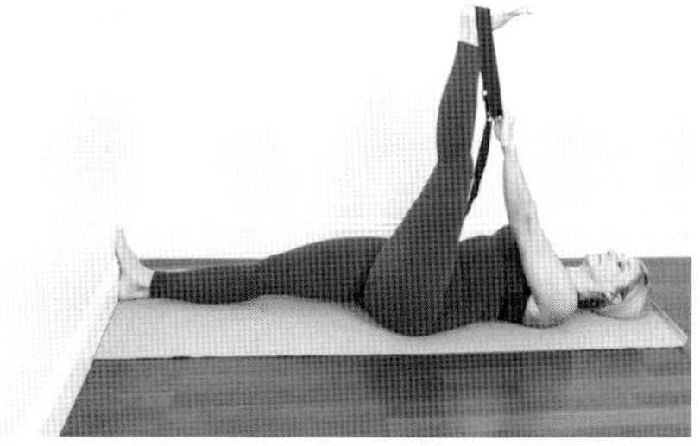

A66 Supine Hand-to-Big-Toe Pose, increasing toward and upwards of 90° of hip flexion.

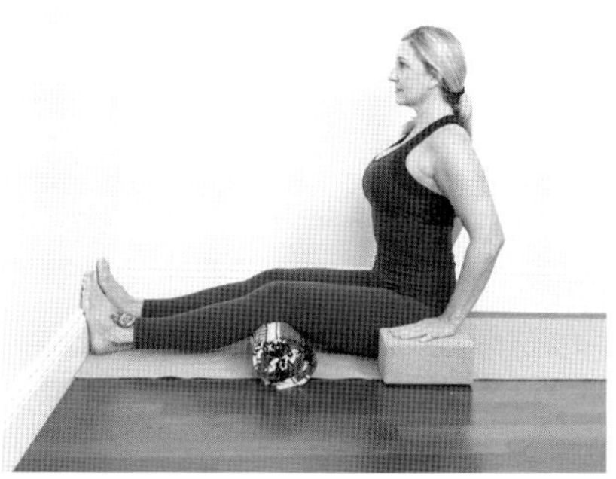

A67 Staff Pose, rolled-up blanket under knees to help access action/skill.

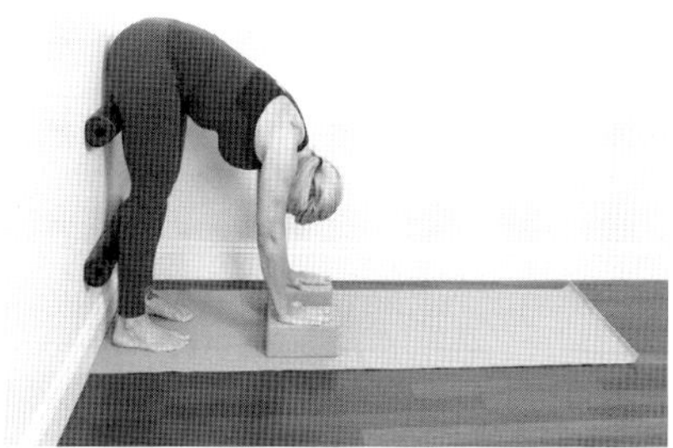

A70 Standing Forward Bend, hands on blocks, pressing into rolled-up mat behind calves and hamstrings to help access action/skill.

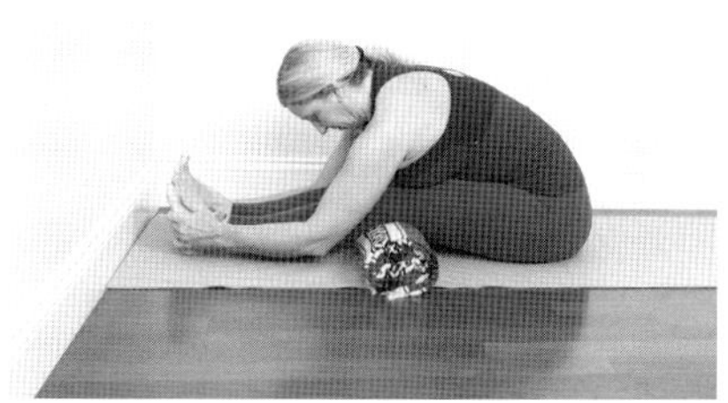

A68 Seated Forward Bend, rolled-up blanket under knees to help access action/skill.

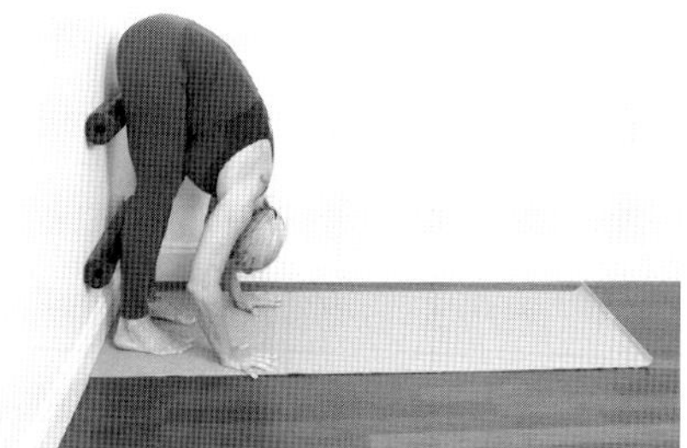

A71 Standing Forward Bend, pressing into rolled-up mat behind calves and hamstrings to help access action/skill.

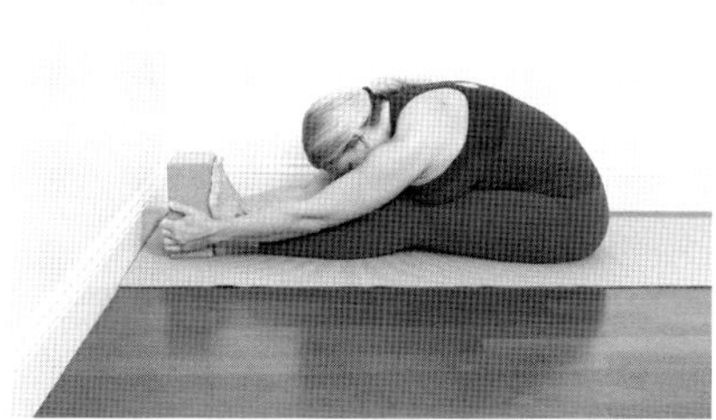

A69 Seated Forward Bend, maximum hamstring length while action/skill still accessible.

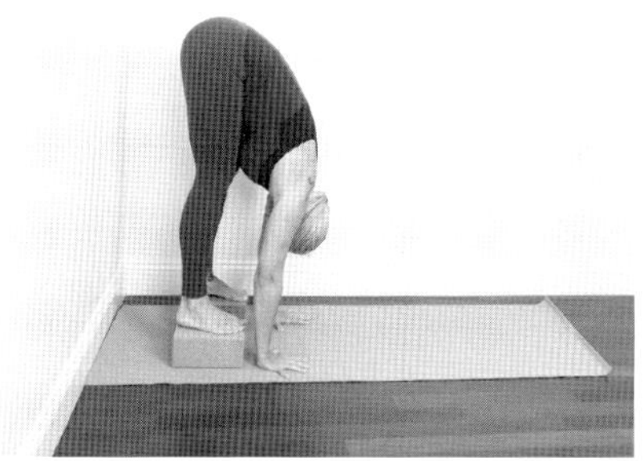

A72 Standing Forward Bend progression with feet on blocks if action/skill can be maintained.

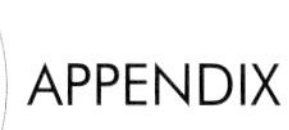

Single-Leg Progressions

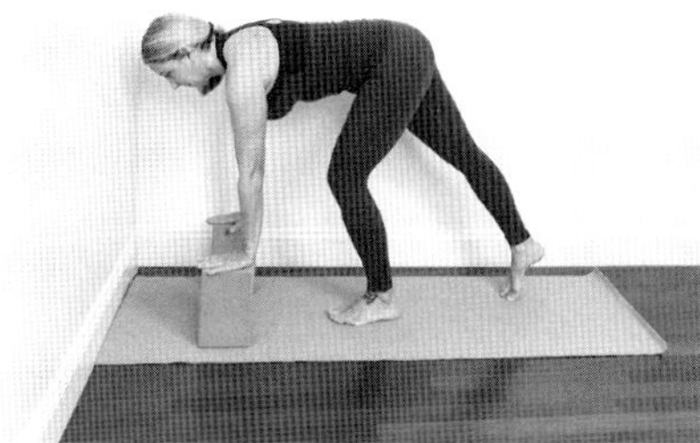

A73 Warrior III Pose variation with hands on blocks, back foot on the floor. Knee might stay bent to access action/skill.

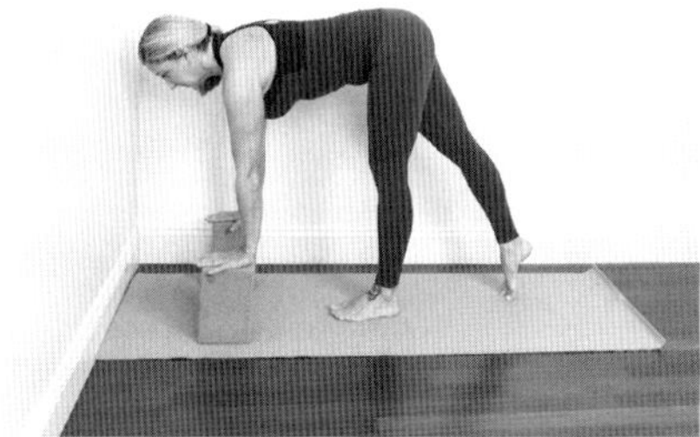

A74 Warrior III Pose variation with hands on blocks, back foot on the floor. Knee straightens if tension can be maintained.

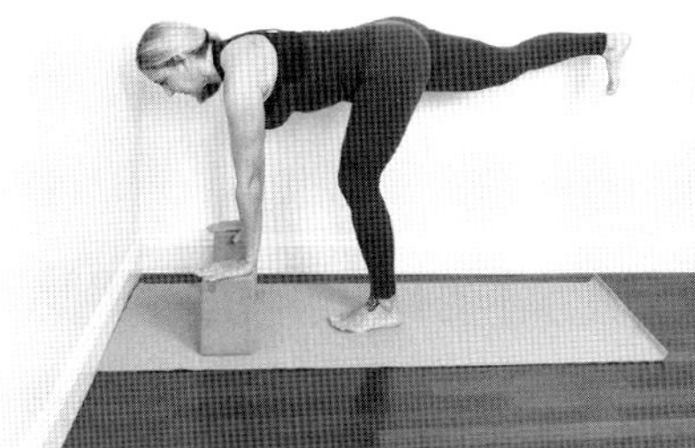

A75 Warrior III Pose variation, hands on blocks. Knee might stay bent to access action/skill.

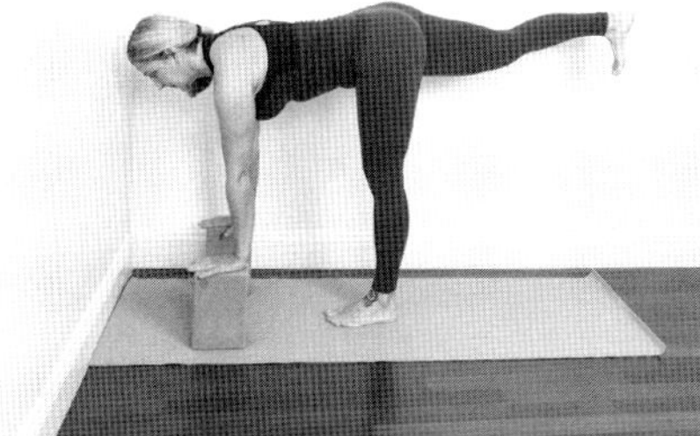

A76 Warrior III Pose variation, hands on blocks. Knee straightens if tension can be maintained.

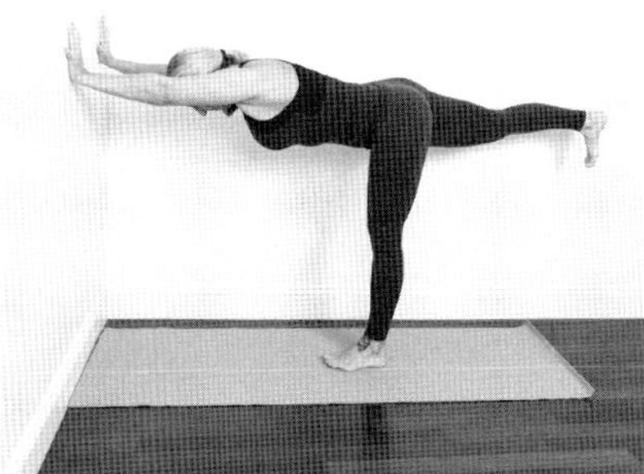

A77 Warrior III Pose variation, hands on the wall. Progress to coming away from wall when tension in hamstring can be maintained.

Externally Rotated Variations

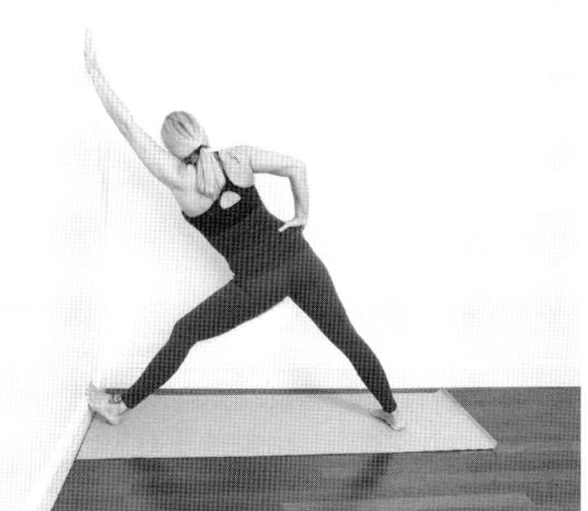

A78 Triangle Pose variation with foot at the wall to help access action/skill. Bottom hand reaches up the wall to minimize hip flexion angle.

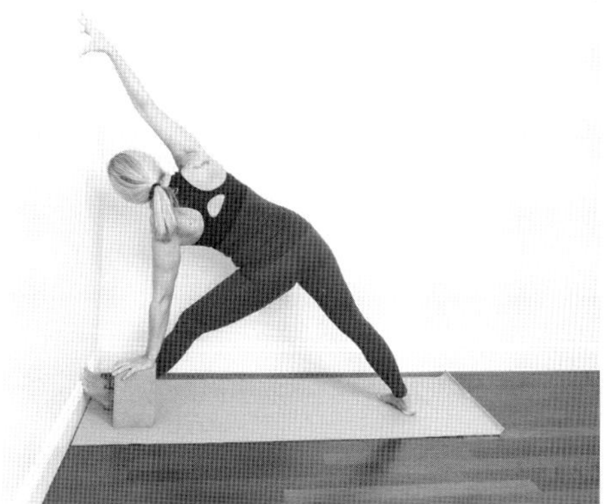

A79 Triangle Pose variation with foot at the wall to help access action/skill.

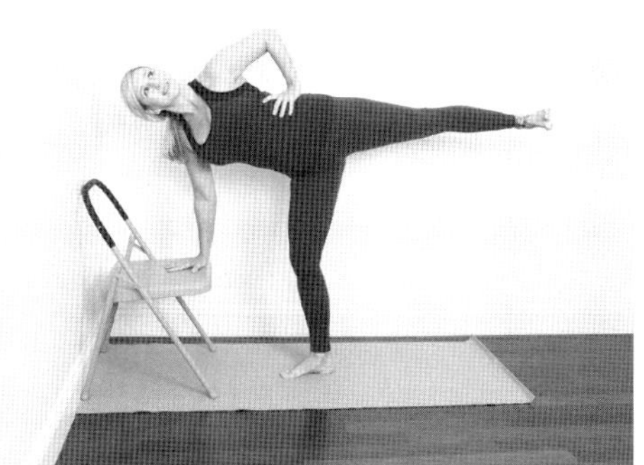

A80 Half Moon Pose variation with hand on a chair. Knee might stay bent to access action/skill.

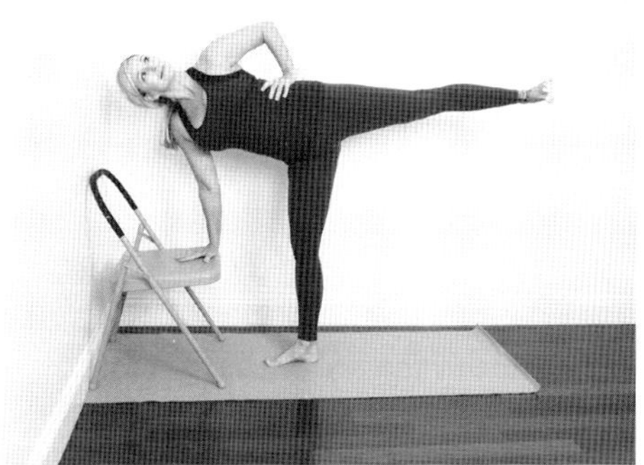

A81 Half Moon Pose variation with hand on a chair. Progress by coming away from the wall when tension in hamstring can be maintained.

Modifying Loads for the Anterior Hip

It is my experience that whenever there is a disturbance in the anterior hip, whether it feels tight, pinches, pops, or aches, the common response is to stretch it out. The assumption is that passive stretching will resolve the minor issue and funtionality will resume with ease. In my teaching experience, I have found that loading the anterior hip generally has the best results.

Hip flexors tend to be underloaded in sedentary people (i.e. sitting at a desk all day does not actively load the hip flexors, the hip is passively postitioned in flexion). Using yoga poses to introduce loads to the anterior hip is generally sufficient as a starting point for increasing capacity in untrained individuals. As always, if symptoms present or persist, a referral to a qualified healthcare professional is recommended. If symptoms are not present or diminish quickly, loads specific to the anterior hip can be varied and progressed.

As with the posterior hip, examples will begin in the shortened range and progress to the lengthened range. The poses listed here are by no means an exhaustive list, they are a few ideas to get you thinking creatively. Ultimately, your student(s) will guide your pose selection.

With the anterior hip in particular, I like to test and retest before and after the practice. Choose any one of the following poses (Figs. A82-A84) to test how your hips feel in deep flexion (maybe compare the right to the left as a reference). Then load the anterior hip at an appropriate progression, or creatively incorporate elements of the series into a group class. Afterward, retest the anterior hip in the same pose and observe the difference in sensation, ease of movement, or ROM. Even if there was no aggravation present in the original test, a greater sense of ease in hip flexion is often experienced.

Supine Resistance Work

Providing resistance in hip flexion is a surprisingly easy and effective way to bring attention to the underloaded anterior hip. It can be done with a partner, or alone. From a supine position, provide an external force in the opposite direction of hip flexion. This opposing load can be applied to achieve concentric, isometric, or eccentric contraction of the hip flexors (Figs. A85-A87), which is a practice that, with further study, can be expanded into isometric or resistance stretching techniques. Loads can be relatively low (20–40% MVC) and resistance should remain relatively constant throughout the arc of movement.

Short Range Postures

Anecdotally, hips flexors are often referred to as short and tight, thus the resolution tends to emphasize passive stretching. Knowing what we know now about muscle length and tightness, we might choose to expand our considerations. If chronic sitting were to have a maladaptive effect on hip flexors, it is likely that the hip flexors are underused, thereby underloaded. Sitting does passively position the hip flexors in a short range, yet it does nothing to strengthen this muscle group. Moreover, if one were to strengthen a muscle at its short range, it would not automatically preclude it from lengthening under tension. Fortunately, short range hip flexor training can be easily incorporated into some common yoga poses.

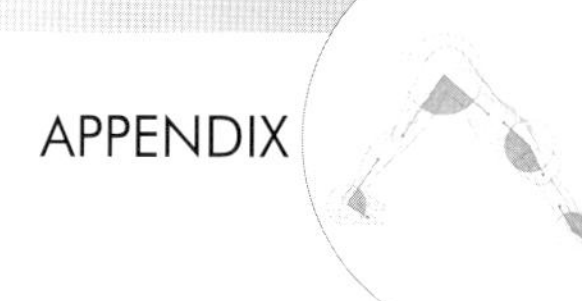

Test Positions

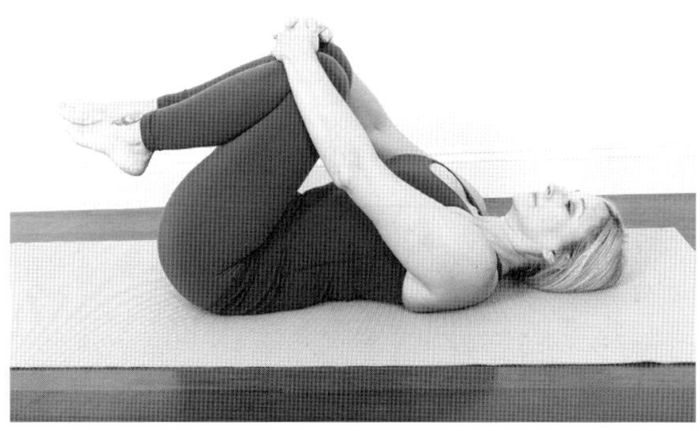

A82 Supine Knees-to-Chest, test position A.

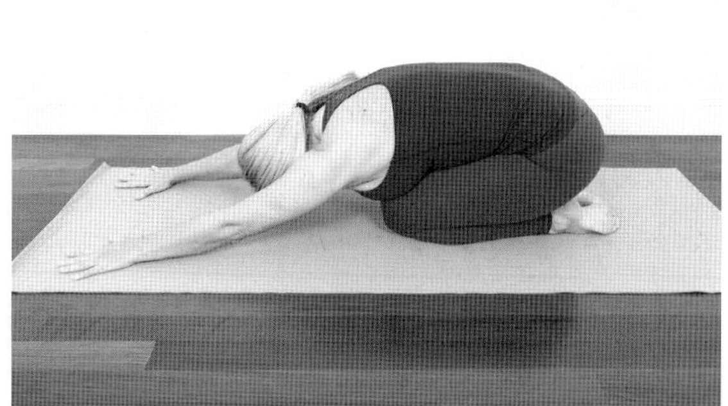

A83 Child's Pose, test position B.

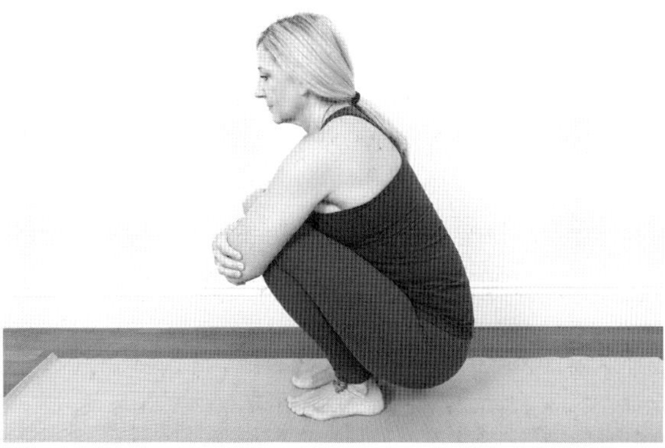

A84 Garland Pose (Deep Squat), test position C.

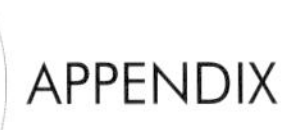

Supine Resistance Work

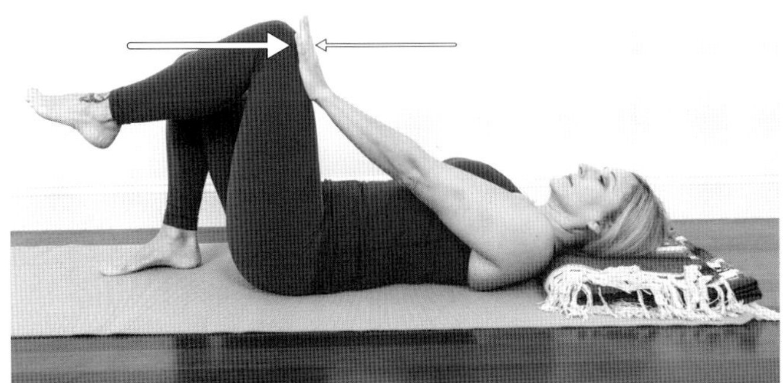

A85 Supine resisted hip flexion, concentric.

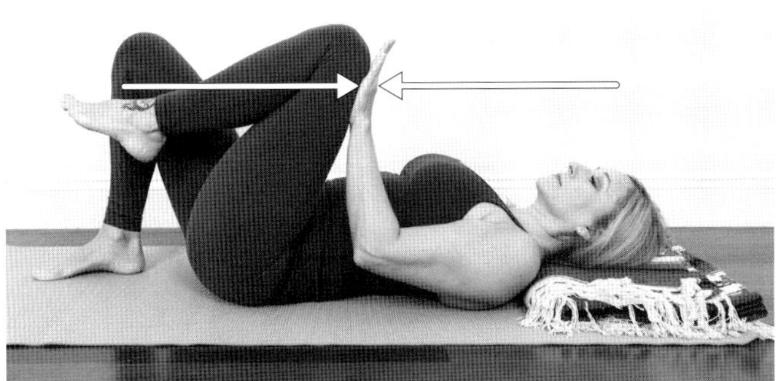

A86 Supine resisted hip flexion, isometric.

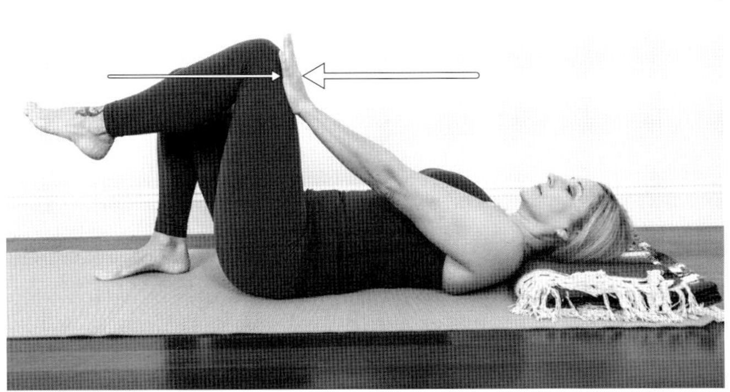

A87 Supine resisted hip flexion, eccentric.

Action/skill to bias the anterior hip

Lengthen from the hip crease toward the knee while simultaneously lengthening the hip crease up toward the shoulder, cultivating a *sense* of lifting both of the thigh and of the chest (Fig. A88). Establish the action in a starting position and maintain during transition into and out of the pose, while holding the pose, and during any variations and progressions you may come up with. Relax during rest.

Marichi's Pose can be adapted to challenge the anterior hip of the extended leg (Fig. A89). Be sure to utilize the action/skill to keep the spine from noticeably flexing, or the pelvis from tilting significantly in a posterior direction.

Boat Pose with straight legs is a challenge for many, particularly when introducing the action/skill. A single, straight-leg version is, therefore, a suitable regression (Figs. A91-A92). To prevent the spine from flexing, one might want to support the

Short Range Postures

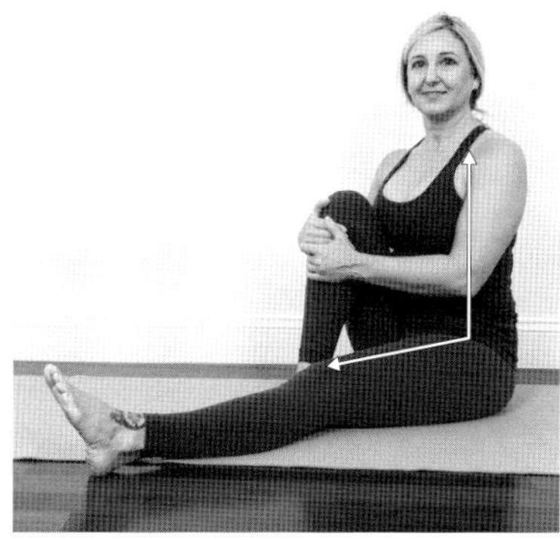

A88 Marichi's Pose variation, start position.

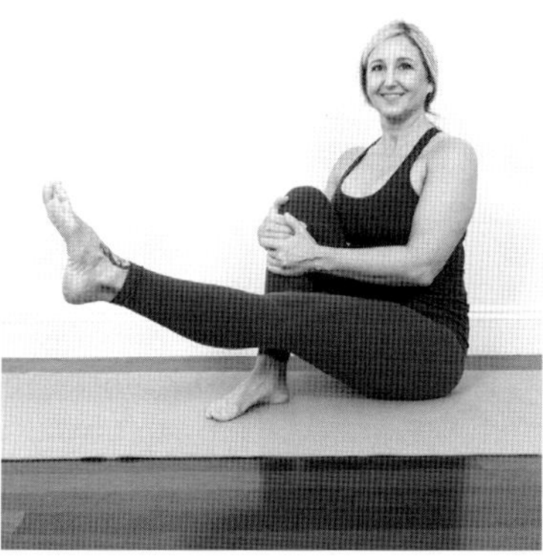

A89 Marichi's Pose variation, increased hip flexion.

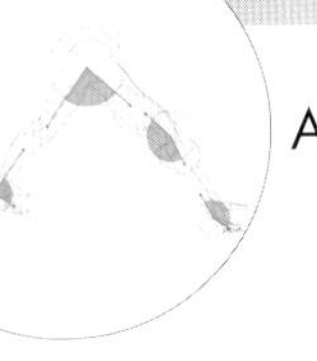

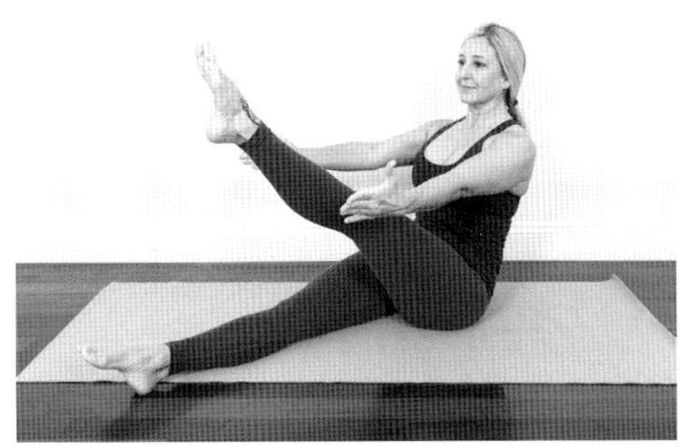

A90 Boat Pose, single leg.

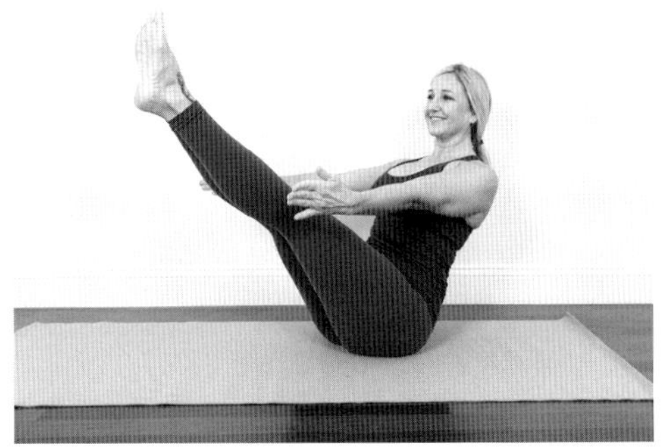

A91 Boat Pose, double leg.

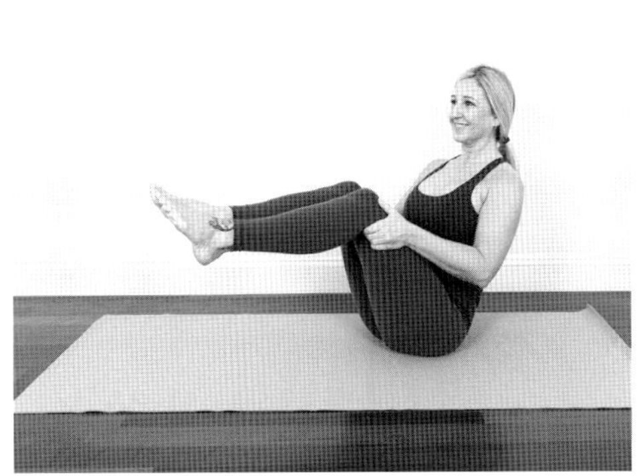

A92 Boat Pose, bent knee. Not recommended.

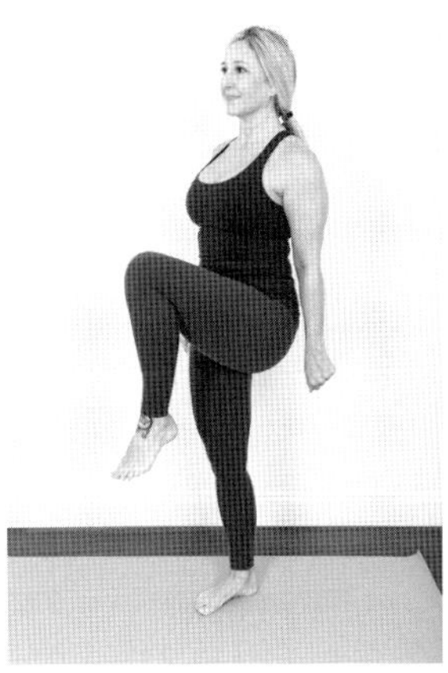

A93 Standing Marichi's Pose.

back against the wall until the action/skill can be maintained. A bent knee version of the pose is not suggested, simply for the fact that it is difficult for many to develop tension across the anterior hip (Fig. A92).

Standing Marichi's Pose is harder than it looks. As previously established, suggested isometric hold time is 30–45 seconds, with multiple reps, inclusive of rest time between reps. Joint angle will vary considerably depending on the student. Action/skill can be practiced in both the standing leg and the target leg to prevent knee flexion in the standing leg or leaning the torso back to feign hip flexion (Fig. A93).

Extended Hand-to-Big-Toe Pose, as the name implies, uses the hand to increase hip flexion by pulling on the big toe. This variation is not incorrect but it is somewhat of an illusion in that it takes the emphasis off loading the anterior hip (Fig. A94). A popular variation, referenced by the letter "D," is to hover the leg without any support. If holding for 5–8 breaths, as is often instructed in yoga, it would approach, or even exceed the 30 second range, thereby making breath count a reasonable measure of time in a yoga class. A chair or wall might be available for those needing rest within a single rep as 30 seconds is challenging for those who have not trained in this position (Fig. A95).

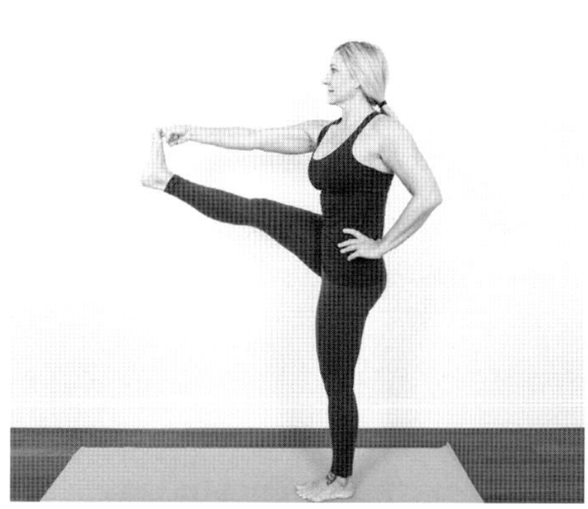

A94 Extended Hand-to-Big-Toe Pose, with external support.

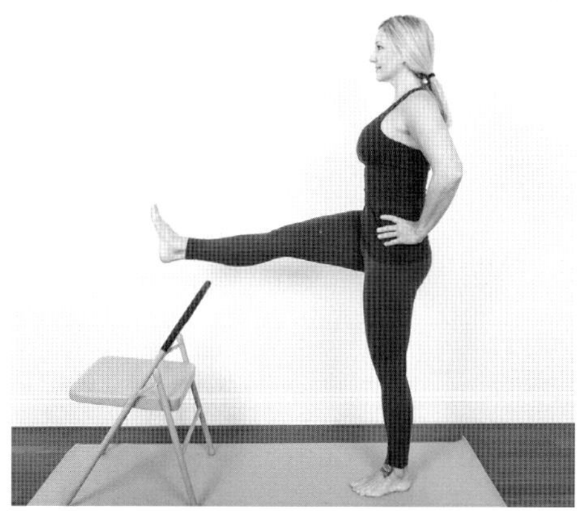

A95 Extended Hand-to-Big-Toe Pose, with emphasis on loading the anterior hip.

Finally, these poses can be progressed by providing external resistance (e.g. partner work, creative use of props, etc.), and varied by exploring combinations of joint angles while in flexion (e.g. external rotation).

Internal Rotation

It is often the case that an individual experiencing an aching or pinching anterior hip during deep flexion presents with limited internal rotation. While morphology determines end range, most people should have some degree of internal rotation if the hip is functioning well. I find that combining internal rotation training with flexion training can be quite effective, restoring ease with flexion almost immediately. Keep in mind that any adaptations that occur in real time are fleeting and that reinforcement via repetition over the long term is the only way to sustain persistent change.

Yoga poses do not generally emphasize internal rotation, so a simple Side Sitting position is a good place to start. To add an isometric load, the leg internally rotated at the hip (i.e. the leg bent behind) should be pressed down into the floor (Figs. A96-A98). The floor acts as a safety barrier, ensuring that range of motion is not pushed beyond the individual's natural range, while simultaneously providing an opposing, resistive force. If an individual has internal rotation to gain (i.e. her morphology will allow it), the isometric work should produce those gains in small increments over time. Some creativity with position, props, and cueing can provide endless variations and progressions.

As a bonus, similar work can be done on the leg that is externally rotated at the hip (i.e. the leg bent in front) while in this position.

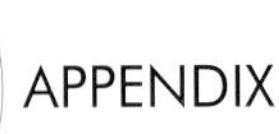

Internal Rotation

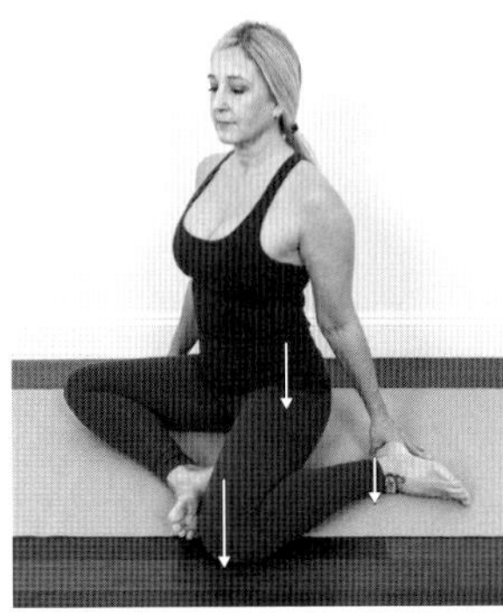

A96 Side Sitting, internal and external rotation with hip flexion.

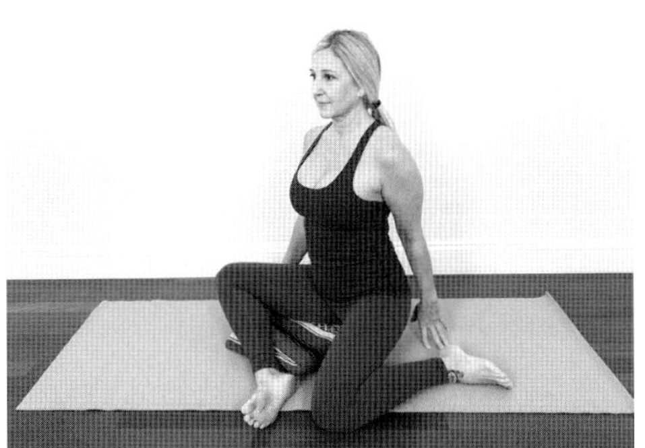

A97 Side Sitting with support under externally rotated hip if internal rotation is limited.

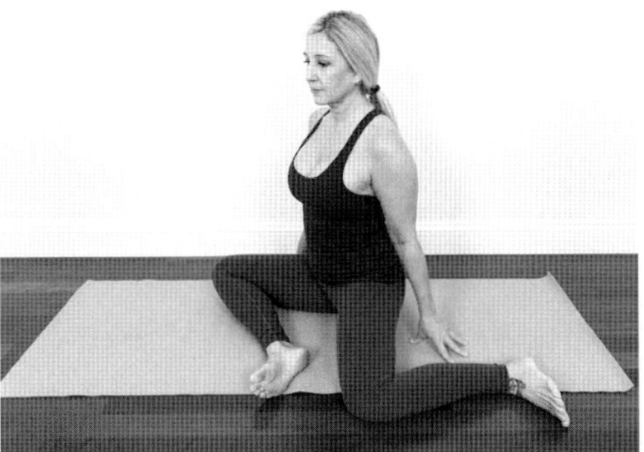

A98 Side Sitting with progressed abduction on internally rotated hip.

Long Range Postures

In addition to short range training, long range training and eccentric lengthening of the hip muscle group is beneficial. Once again, the suggestion here is not passive stretching, but rather introducing load during a stretch. Passive stretching is certainly not contraindicated, but the objective here is to increase load-bearing capacity.

Action/skill to bias the anterior hip

Lengthen from the hip crease toward the knee while simultaneously lengthening the hip crease up toward the shoulder, cultivating a *sense* of lifting, both of the thigh and of the chest (Fig. A99). Establish the action in a starting position and maintain during transition into and out of the pose, while holding the pose, and during any variations and progressions of the pose you may create. Relax during rest.

Kneeling Lunges for the anterior hip (Figs. A99-A101) are the equivalent of the Kneeling Lunges for the posterior hip. In fact, they can be combined to target both at

Long Range Postures

Kneeling Lunge

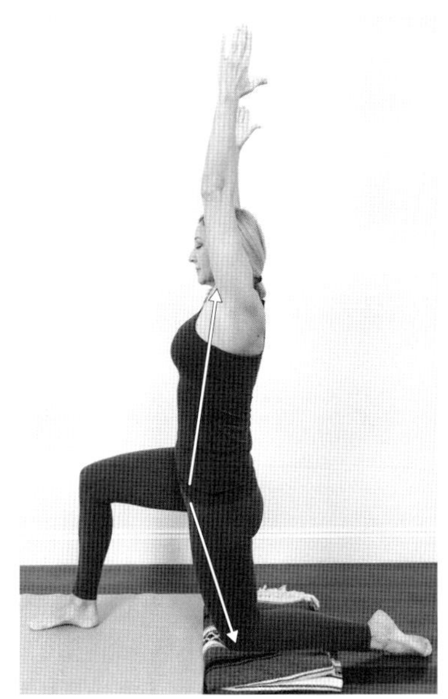

A99 Kneeling Lunge, isometric start position.

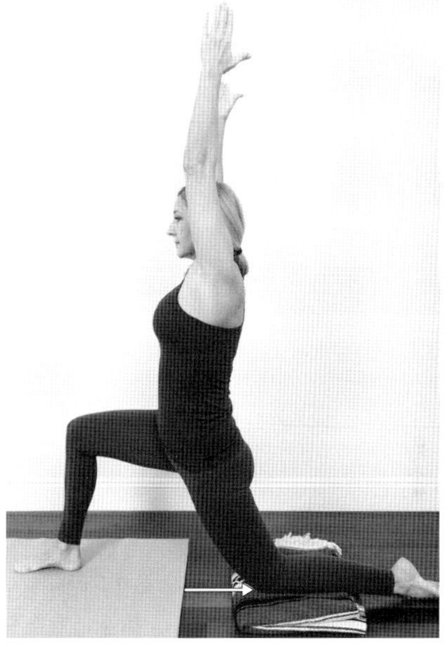

A100 Kneeling Lunge, eccentric variation.

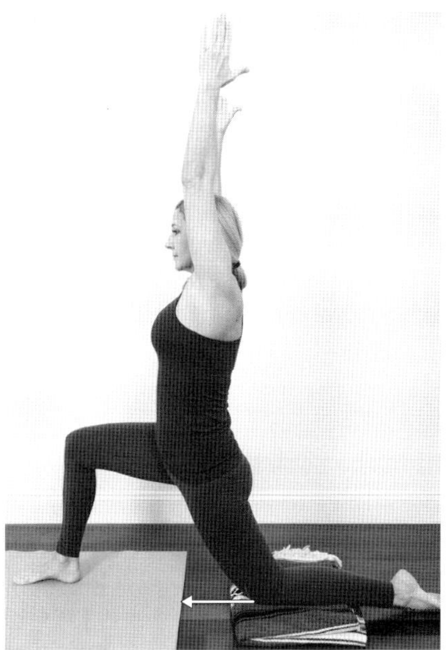

A101 Kneeling Lunge, concentric variation.

Eccentric Lunge

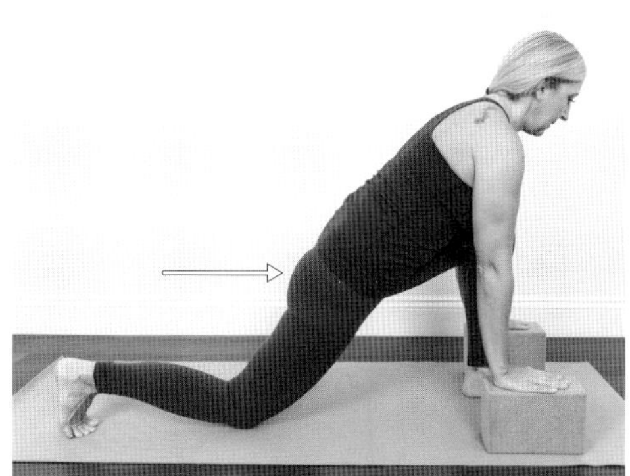

A102 Eccentric Lunge, start position.

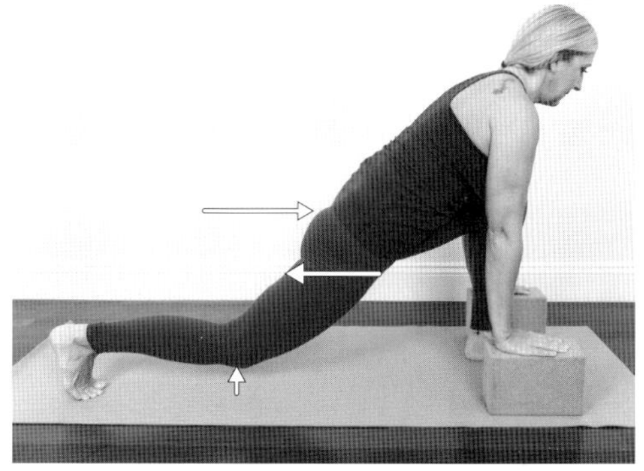

A103 Eccentric Lunge with internally created resistance.

once (i.e. the anterior hip of the back leg, and the posterior hip of the front leg).

In the Eccentric Lunge (Figs. A102-A103), the pelvis is secured in the start position and does not shift vertically, nor horizontally, while the back hip extends, and the knee starts to lift off the floor. The height of the knee is not the objective here, rather the resistance created across the anterior hip as the pelvis remains in position. This position can be held isometrically or performed as 3 sets of 10 reps.

Warrior I Pose demands quite a bit of hip extension in the back leg, more than most people anatomically have. In order to achieve the shape, some degree of lumbar extension is required. If an individual is unable to access the action/skill at the end range, the pose can be regressed by elevating the front foot to decrease the extension demanded by the back hip and lumbar spine (Figs. A104-A106).

These principles can eventually lead into bigger poses, such as Hanuman's Pose (forward splits) and One-Legged King Pigeon Pose, both of which will likely demand full end range hip and lumbar extension. By supporting the back hip (usually the limiting factor in these poses) prior to progressing, an appropriate height can be set where one can achieve the action/skill. The support might also be favorable for students with hypermobility. The front leg can eventually extend progress toward full splits, or the hip can externally rotate to progress toward Pigeon variation. A chair offers another way to add demand to the front hip while working the action/skill in the back hip. With a little creativity, both these poses could incorporate blanket slides to add eccentric and concentric contractions.

By bringing these long-range postures in a little bit (Figs. A107 and A108), the emphasis can be taken off pushing end range, and placed on increasing capacity. If range of motion improves as a side effect of these practices, then we know the individual was not limited by her morphology. If anatomical end range has already been reached, then ROM will not increase, and capacity remains the focus.

Warrior I Pose

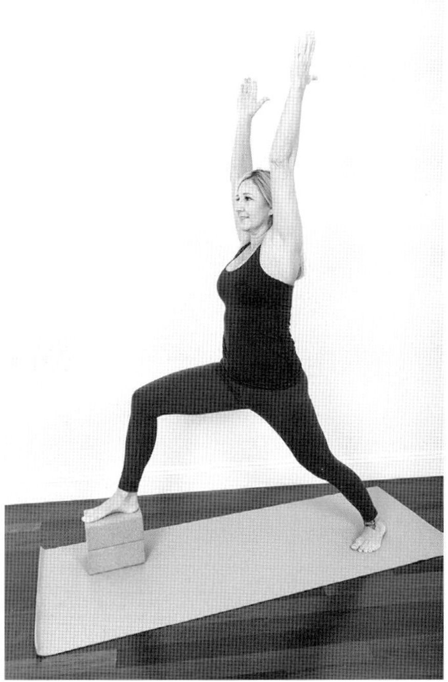

A104 Warrior I Pose with front foot on two blocks, minimizes hip extension.

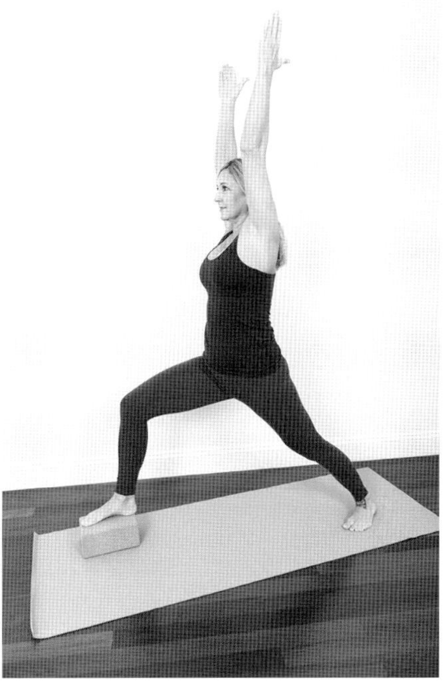

A105 Warrior I Pose with front foot on one block, moderate hip extension.

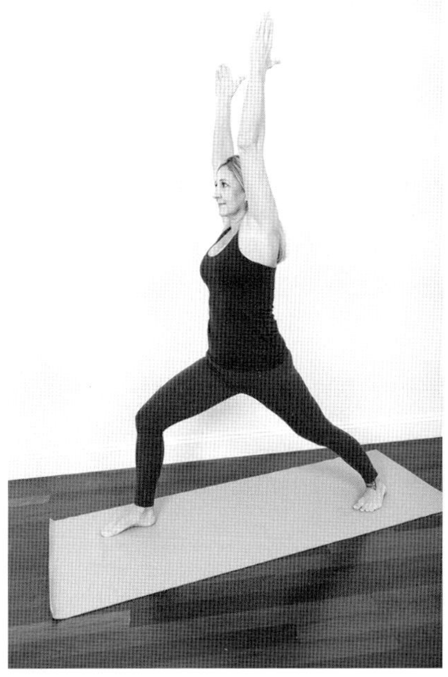

A106 Warrior I Pose with front foot on floor, maximizes hip extension.

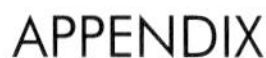

Bigger Pose Regressions

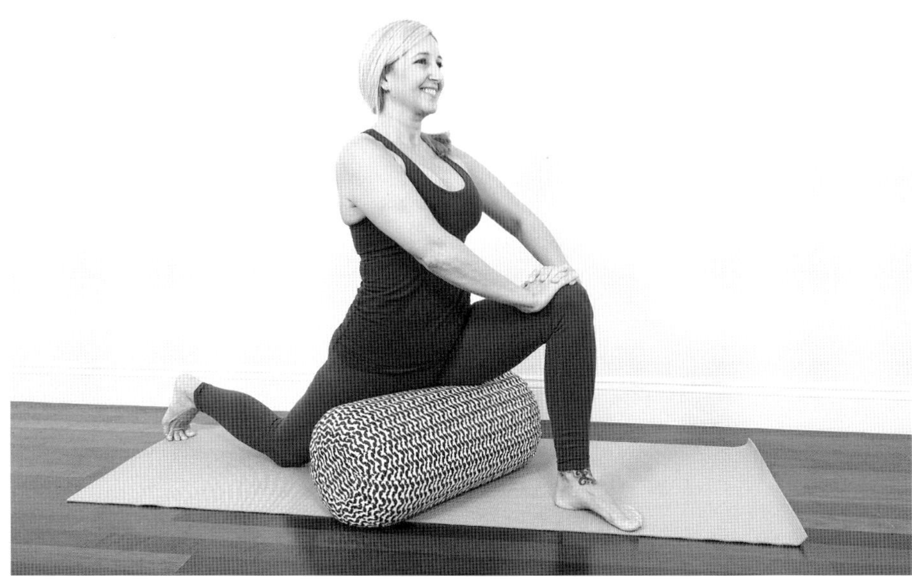

A107 Kneeling Lunge on a bolster (can be used for Pigeon, too).

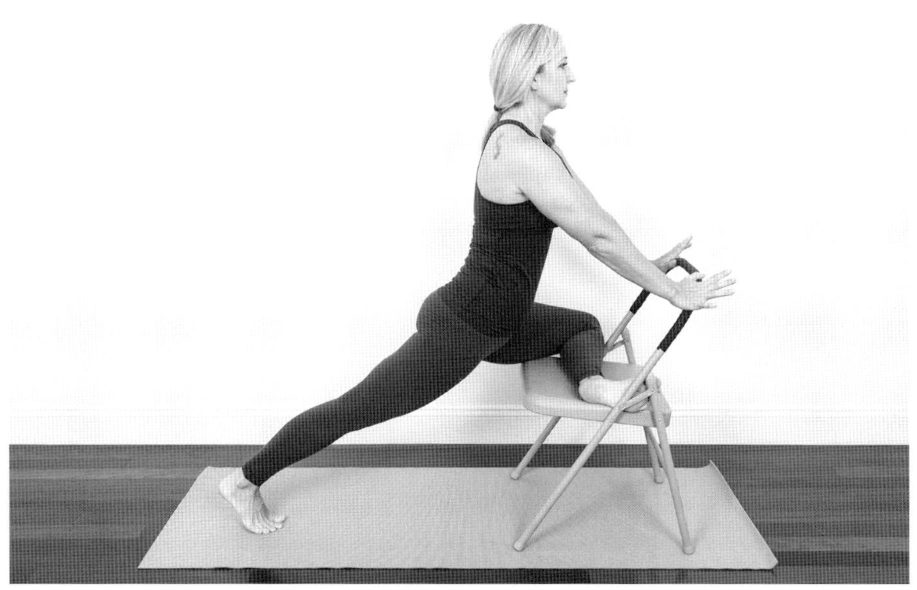

A108 One-Legged King Pigeon Pose on a chair.

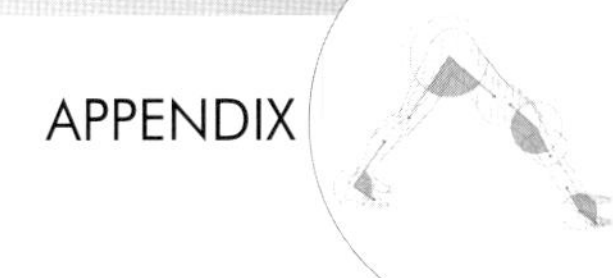

Modifying Loads for the Shoulder Complex

The following series targets the entire shoulder, increasing capacity wherever it may be needed in a certain individual. The emphasis in these upper body-focused postures is on balancing the contractions of the anterior and medial shoulder with those of the lateral and posterior shoulder, and all the neighboring structures as well. Alignment considerations should take a back seat to accessing the skill and avoiding aggravated sensations. As capacity increases, previously troublesome ranges should start to become more accessible.

Action/skill to bias the shoulder and scapular-thoracic region

Reach from the back of the shoulders, along the triceps, to the little fingers. Feel the entire length of the arm engage. Maintain that action while reaching from the thumbs, along the biceps, and to the inner shoulder where the arm meets the chest. Cultivating a *sense* of pushing and pulling simultaneously, maintain both actions during transition into and out of the pose, while holding the pose, and during all variations and progressions of the pose (Fig. A109). Relax during rest.

The degree of shoulder flexion should be determined by the ability to maintain the action/skill without bending the elbows or extending the spine (Figs. A110-A111). Students should work at this range until improvements are made. Note that students with hypermobility might need to grasp the block firmly while bending and straightening the elbow to discover how to maintain tension along the full length of the arms.

Planks

Once the action/skill has been established, it can be applied to weight-bearing postures. Plank Pose can be held for 30–45 seconds while maintaining the action/skill. Students may wish to maintain skill while slowly moving into Downward Facing Dog Pose, adding shoulder flexion. Again, the degree of shoulder flexion should be determined by the action/skill and not the final shape of the pose. Plank Pose (Fig. A112) can be regressed by elevating the hands on blocks, a chair, or even a wall (Fig. A113). It can be progressed by elevating the feet, or by adding single-leg variations, it can be varied, and sometimes further progressed, by creative hand placements (Figs. A114-A117). The same principles can be applied to Side Plank, keeping the action/skill central to the pose (Figs. A118-A120).

It is worth discussing the common cue to address elbow hyperextension here. While most often one is instructed to put a soft bend in the elbow, I will caution here that a soft bend absent of muscle tension transmitted across the joint may not be helpful for a student with hypermobility. Accessing the skill is more important than the micro-bend, and such is also the case with students who are *hypo*mobile.

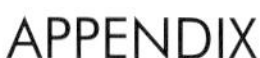

Finding the Skill/Action

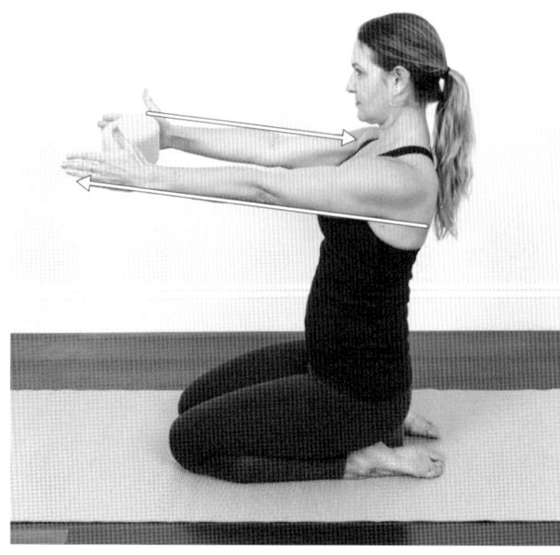

A109 Holding a block at 90° shoulder flexion, establish action/skill.

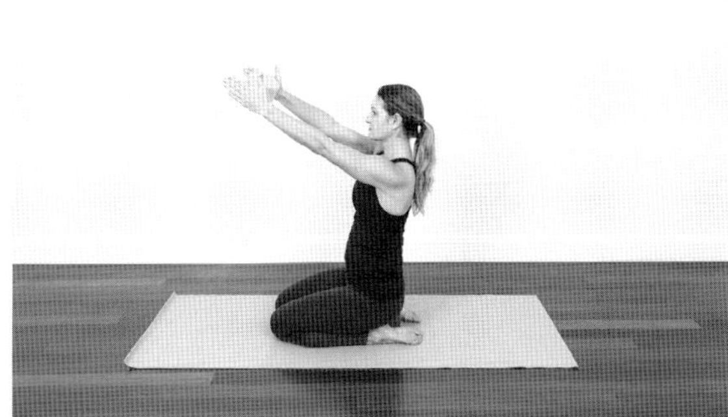

A110 Holding a block, increasing shoulder flexion while maintaining action/skill.

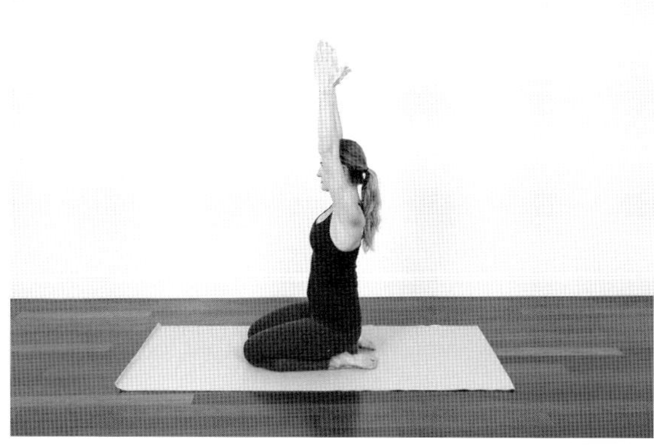

A111 Holding a block approaching 180° shoulder flexion while maintaining action/skill.

Planks

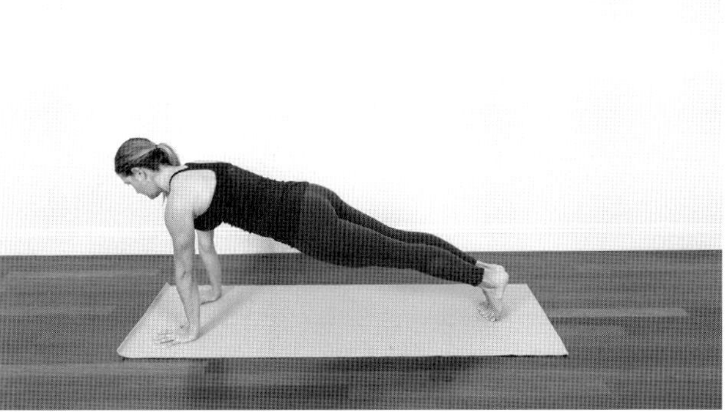

A112 Plank Pose, maintaining action/skill.

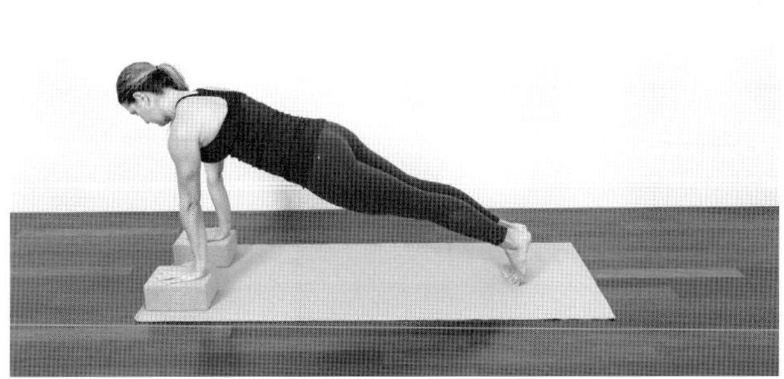

A113 Plank Pose regression, elevated hands.

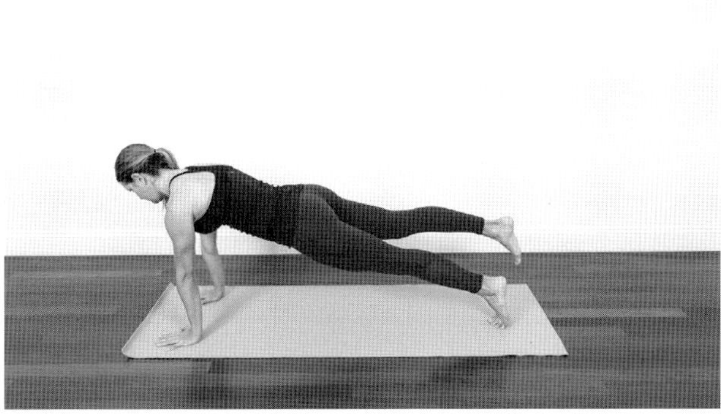

A114 Plank Pose progression, single leg.

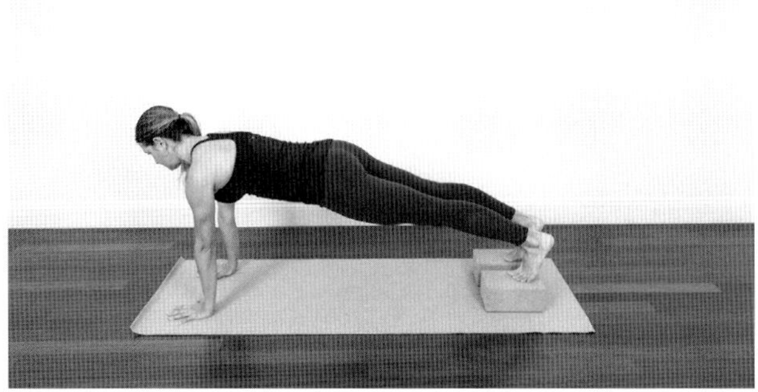

A115 Plank Pose progression, feet elevated.

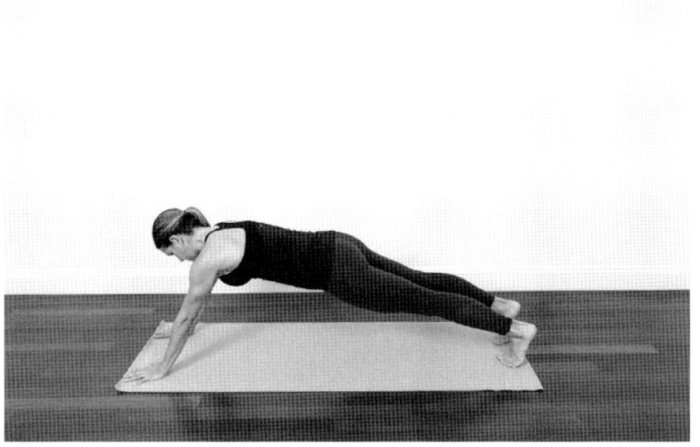

A116 Extended Plank, varied and progressive.

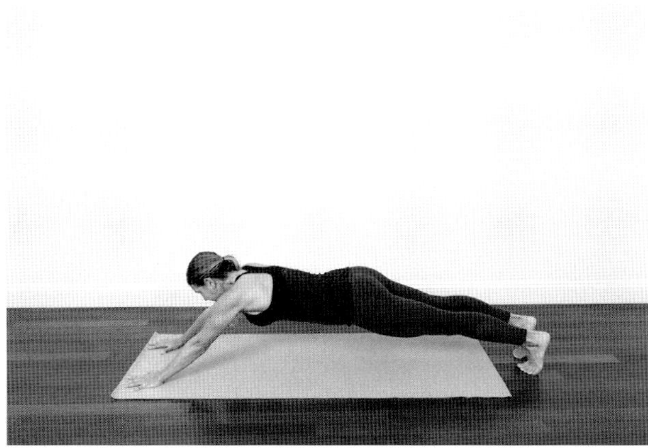

A117 Extended Plank, further varied and progressive.

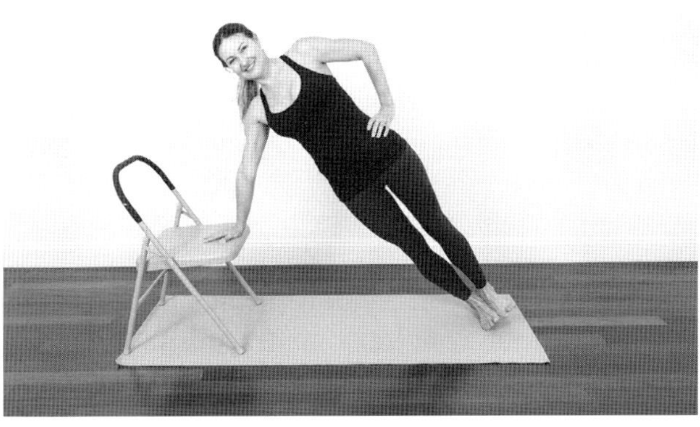

A118 Side Plank regression, hand on a chair.

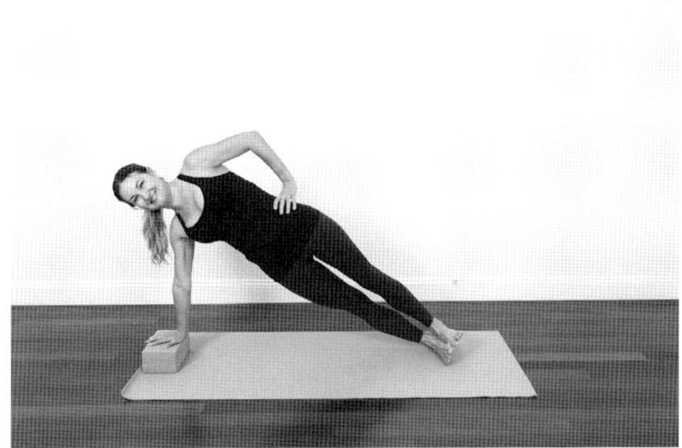

A119 Side Plank regression, hand on a block.

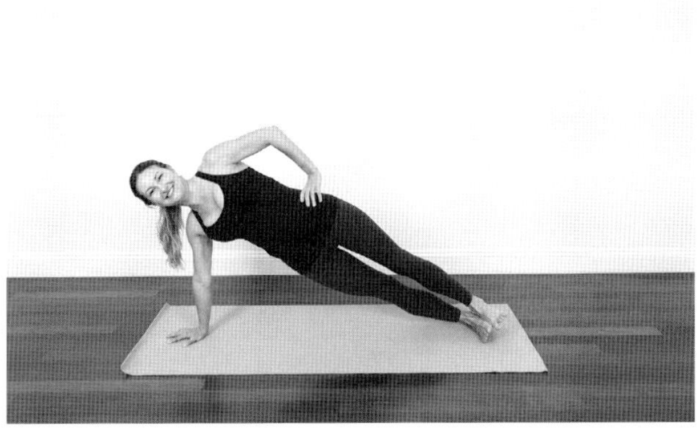

A120 Side Plank.

Push-Ups

The standard Push-Up might be one of the most overlooked skills in a typical yoga class where Low Tricep Plank (Chaturanga Dandasana) is often unattainable by many students. Even if a Low Plank can be executed with ease, one can still benefit from different Push-Up variations (Figs. A121-A134). The pose selection should focus on capacity, such that if only 1 rep can be achieved, the time under tension is not sufficient to promote adaptation. The student should build up to approximately 3 sets of 10 reps before moving on. Simply slowing the movement down is the easiest way to emphasize eccentric and concentric contractions. Varying hand placements can progress the pose, and can become increasingly complex and sophisticated, as with having the arms in different positions from each other, or with the use of sliders under the hands. Shown here is a basic series that should be mastered before attempting variations which may actually exceed capacity.

Because the elbows will bend and straighten during a Push-Up, the action/skill, which is generally instructed in straight arm positions, can be modified slightly to focus more on the chest and scapular muscles, as well as the latissimus dorsi. Some creative cueing should help achieve this.

Push-Ups

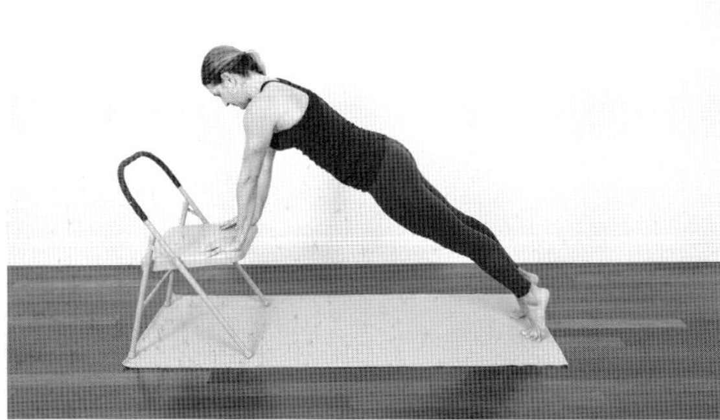

A121 Chair Push-Up, start position.

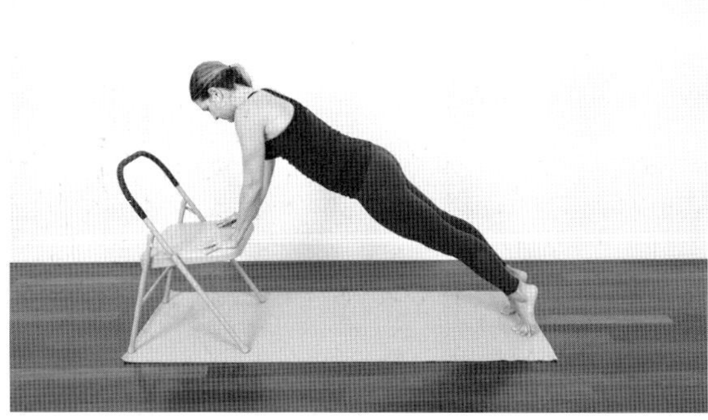

A122 Chair Push-Up, slowly lower.

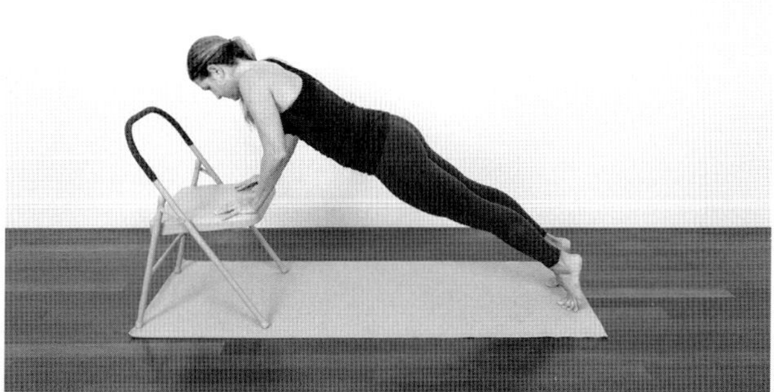

A123 Chair Push-Up, option to add isometric hold.

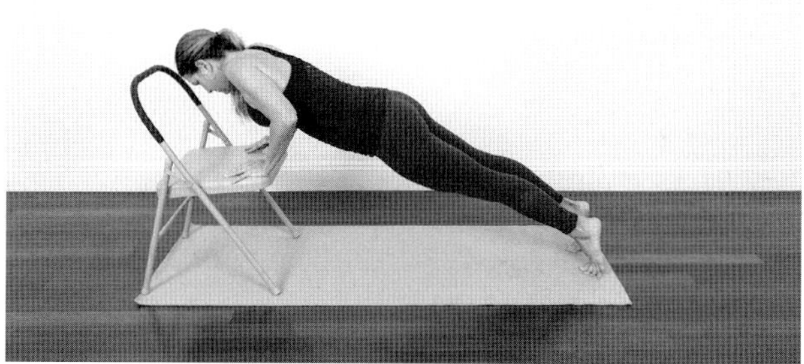

A124 Chair Push-Up, step up and reset to start position to lower again if control is lost.

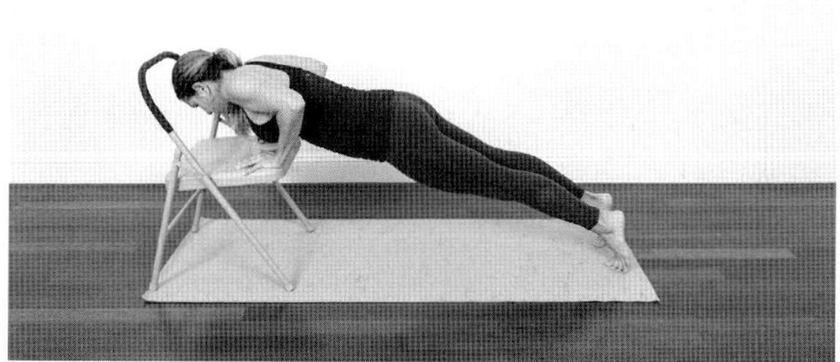

A125 Chair Push-Up, progress by pushing back up to start position when ready.

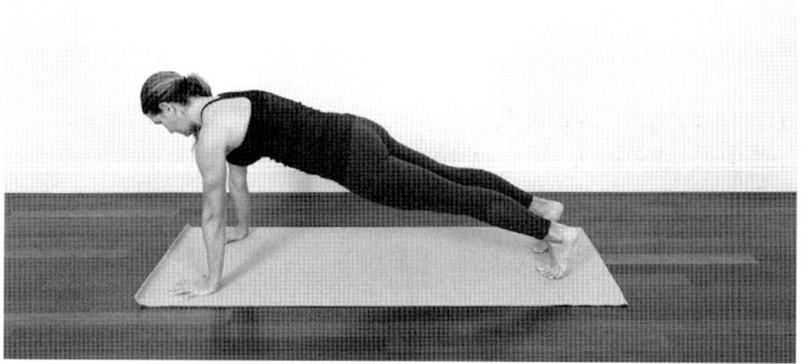

A126 Standard Push-Up, start position.

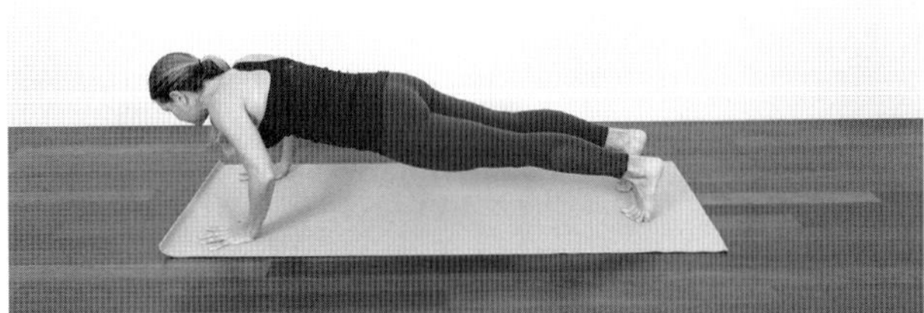

A127 Push-Up, elbows are approximately at 45°.

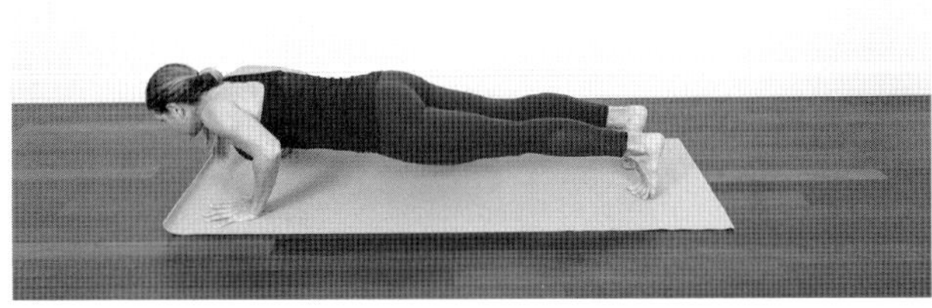

A128 Push-Up, with isometric hold option.

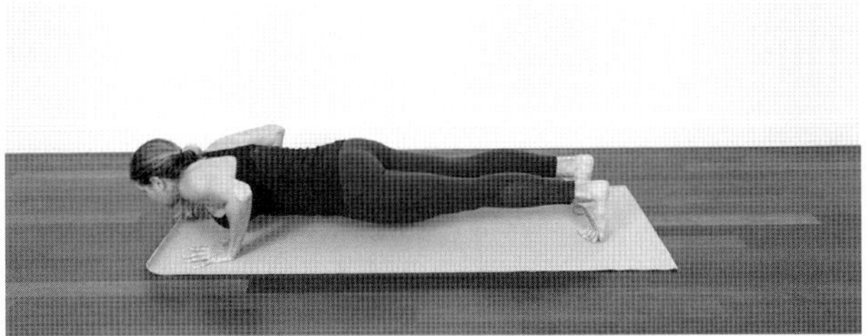

A129 Push-Up, can press back up to start position if floor feels too far.

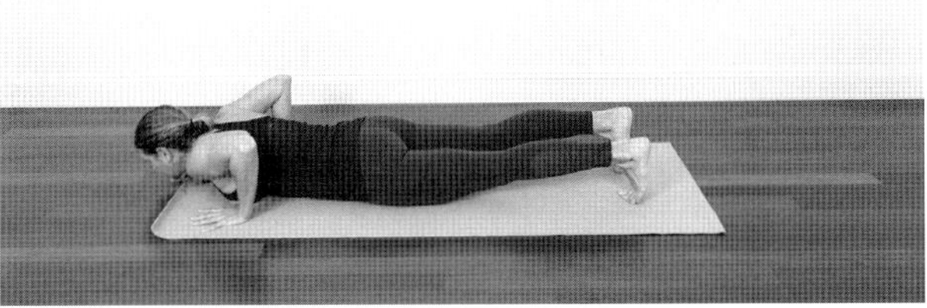

A130 Push-Up, full range down and back up.

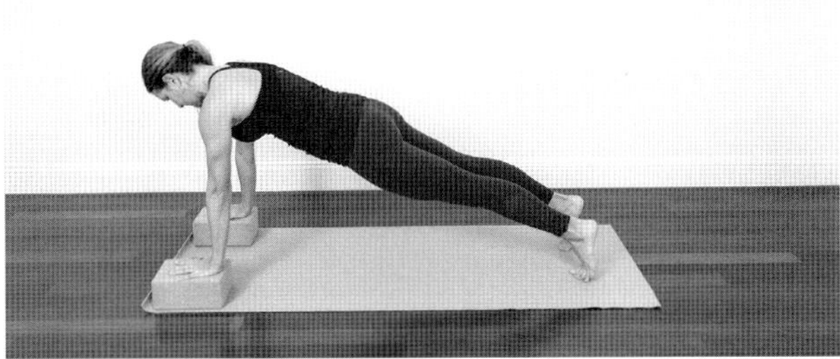

A131 Eccentric Push-Up, start position.

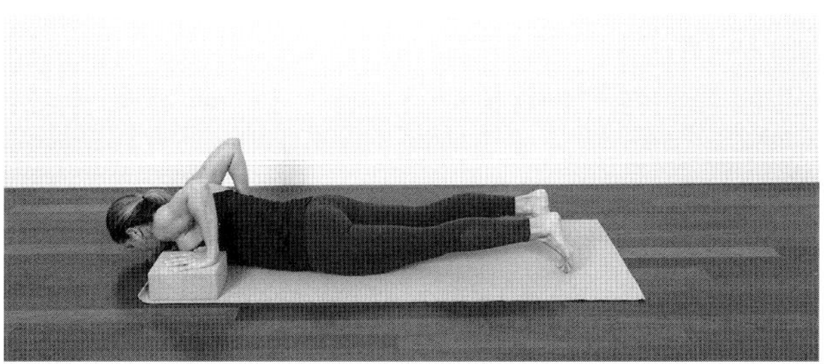

A132 Eccentric Push-Up, end position. Place knees down and reset.

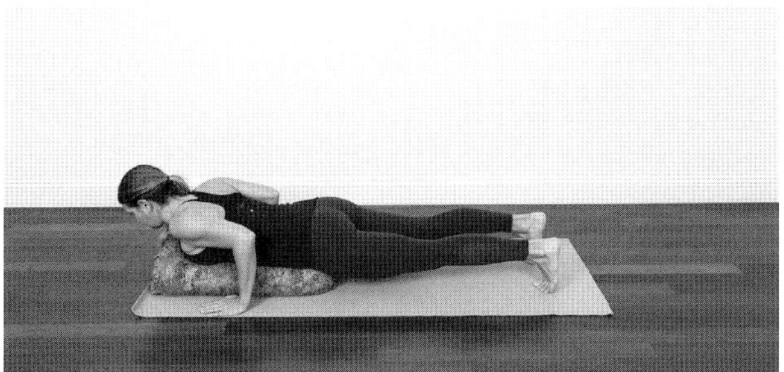

A133 Low Tricep Plank (known as Chaturanga Dandasana) with elbows closer to body, start position.

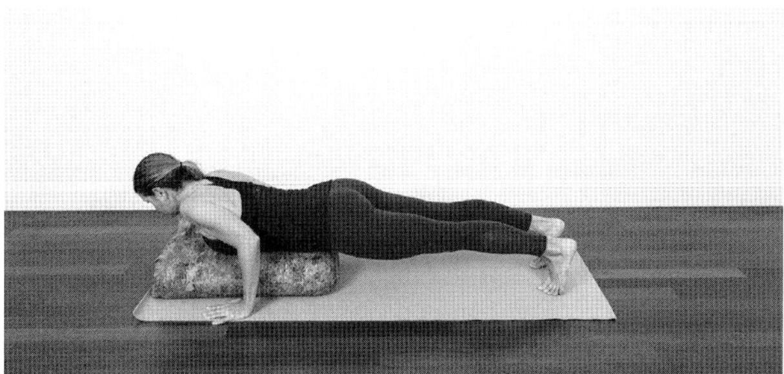

A134 Low Tricep Plank (known as Chaturanga Dandasana), hover above bolster, hold.

Inversions

One might say that yoga has a reputation for inversions. No doubt inversions are challenging and exhilarating, but they require substantial levels of strength, courage, and interest. If students are unable, fearful or simply uninterested, offering any of the previous poses in the series provides a fantastic option to develop shoulder capacity, rather than suggesting a passive stretch. Of course, a passive pose is an effective option if the student is too tired to continue.

The action/skill provided at the beginning of the shoulder section works well with most inversions and arm balances. Another option is to provide a prop that the student can press into, and pull away from, simultaneously (Figs. A135-A138). This will increase the isometric contraction as the opposing muscles co-contract.

Inversions

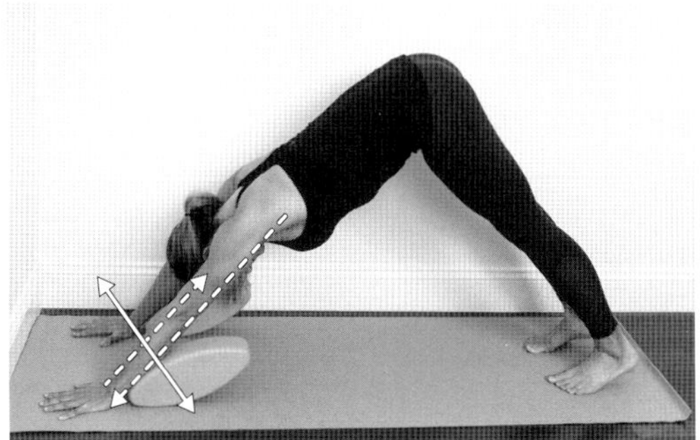

A135 Downward Facing Dog Pose with Three Minute Egg oval-shaped blocks or rolled-up blankets.

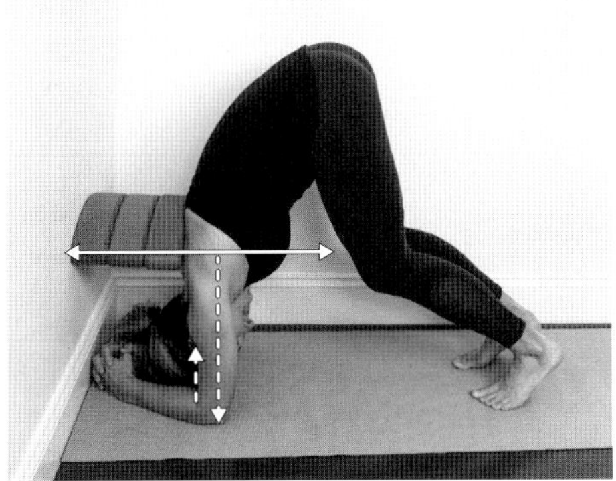

A136 Handstand at the wall with a bolster.

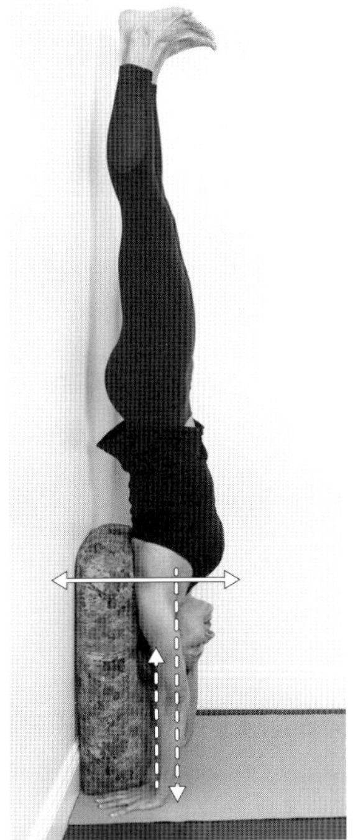

A137 Dolphin Pose at the wall with blocks.

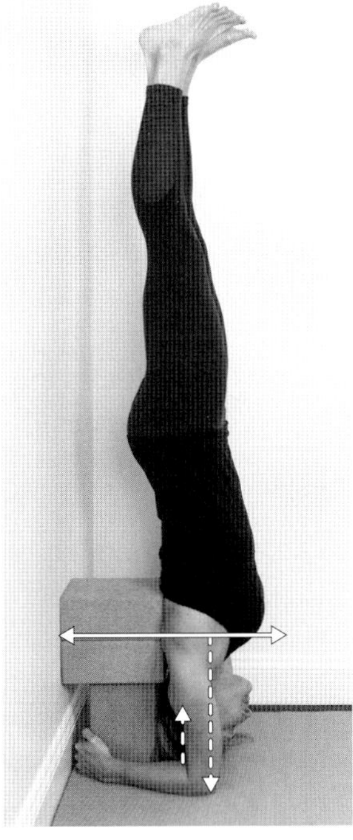

A138 Headstand at the wall with blocks.

Considerations and Contraindications

The narrative presented here is heavily biased toward increasing tolerance to load. It should be noted that there will always be a few exceptions. Osteoarthritis is one condition which might warrant reduced loading rather than progressive loading. Our current understanding of degenerative articular cartilage tells us that there is little to nothing we can do to promote adaptation. Teachers who work with students with osteoarthritis should understand that minimizing symptoms is central to their movement practice. Because symptoms vary from day to day, and among individuals, teachers should be prepared to adjust load parameters as needed.

It should go without saying that compound fractures should never be loaded until healed and cleared by a healthcare professional. Additionally, the discussion here in no way considers any medical condition, disease, or terminal illness and the effects these may have on musculoskeletal tissues. If capacity appears to diminish over the course of a loading program, it is suggested the student be referred to an appropriate healthcare professional, either in the field of physiotherapy or any other non-musculoskeletal focused area of healthcare (e.g. nutrition, psychology, internal medicine, etc.).

Finally, it is not appropriate for most yoga teachers to assess orthopedic conditions including, but not limited to, muscle imbalances, joint dysfunction and dyskinesis, compensatory patterns, inhibitions and facilitations, and minor injuries. Fortunately, the presence of any of these conditions should not preclude one from smart exposure to load. The information I have provided in this book is intended to empower a yoga teacher with the skills to make evidence-based decisions, determine optimal loading conditions, and ultimately, teach as safely as possible.

References

Abate M, Silbernagel KG, Siljeholm C, Di Iorio A, De Amicis D, Salini V, Werner S, Paganelli R (2009) Pathogenesis of tendinopathies: Inflammation or degeneration? Arthritis Research and Therapy 11(3): 235. doi: 10.1186/ar2723.

Adstrum S, Hedley G, Schleip R, Stecco C, Yucesoy CA (2017 [published online November 2016]) Defining the fascial system. Journal of Bodywork and Movement Therapies 21(1):173–177. doi: 10.1016/j.jbmt.2016.11.003.

American College of Sports Medicine (2017). Available: http://www.acsm.org/about-acsm/who-we-are [21 March 2017].

Arampatzis A, Karamanidis K and Albracht K (2007) Adaptational responses of the human Achilles tendon by modulation of the applied cyclic strain magnitude. Journal of Experimental Biology 210:2743–2753. doi: 10.1242/jeb.003814.

Askling C, Tengvar M and Thorstensson A (2013) Acute hamstring injuries in Swedish elite football: A prospective randomised controlled clinical trial comparing two rehabilitation protocols. British Journal of Sports Medicine 47(15):986–991. doi: 10.1136/bjsports-2013-092165.

Bahr R (2016) Why screening tests to predict injury do not work – and probably never will …: A critical review. British Journal of Sports Medicine 50:776–780. doi: 10.1136/bjsports-2016-096256.

Bartlett JL, Sumner B, Ellis RG, Kram R (2014) Activity and functions of the human gluteal muscles in walking, running, sprinting, and climbing. American Journal of Physical Anthropology 153(1):124–131. doi: 10.1002/ajpa.22419.

Battié MC, Videman T, Kaprio J, Gibbons LE, Gill K, Manninen H, Saarela J, Peltonen L (2009) The Twin Spine Study: Contributions to a changing view of disc degeneration. Spine Journal 9(1):47–59. doi: 10.1016/j.spinee.2008.11.011.

Beazley D, Patel S, Davis B, Vinson S, Bolgla L (2017) Trunk and hip muscle activation during yoga poses: Implications for physical therapy practice. Complementary Therapies in Clinical Practice 29:130–135. doi: 10.1016/j.ctcp.2017.09.009.

Behm D, Cavanaugh T, Quigley P, Reid JC, Nardi PS, Marchetti PH (2016a) Acute bouts of upper and lower body static and dynamic stretching increase non-local joint range of motion. European Journal of Applied Physiology 116(1): 241–249. doi: 10.1007/s00421-015-3270-1.

Behm D, Blazevich A, Kay AD, McHugh M (2016b) Acute effects of muscle stretching on physical performance, range of motion, and injury incidence in healthy active individuals: A systematic review. Applied Physiology, Nutrition, and Metabolism 41:1–11. doi: 10.1139/apnm-2015-0235.

Belavý DL, Quittner MJ, Ridgers N, Ling Y, Connell D, Rantalainen T (2017) Running exercise strengthens the intervertebral disc. Scientific Reports 7:45975. doi: 10.1038/srep45975.

Ben M, Harvey LA (2010) Regular stretch does not increase muscle extensibility: A randomized controlled trial. Scandinavian Journal of Medicine and Science in Sports 20(1):136–144. doi: 10.1111/j.1600-0838.2009.00926.x.

Bennett D, Hanratty B, Thompson N, Beverland DE (2009) The influence of pain on knee motion in patients with osteoarthritis undergoing total knee arthroplasty. Orthopedics 32(4):252.

Blazevich AJ, Cannavan D, Waugh CM, Miller SC, Thorlund JB, Aagaard P, Kay AD (2014) Range of motion, neuromechanical, and architectural adaptations to plantar flexor stretch training in humans. Journal of Applied Physiology 117(18):452–462. doi: 10.1152/japplphysiol.00204.2014.

Bogduk N, Aprill C, Derby R (2013) Lumbar discogenic pain: State-of-the-art review. Pain Medicine (United States) 14(6):813–836. doi: 10.1111/pme.12082.

Bohm S, Mersmann F, Arampatzis A (2015) Human tendon adaptation in response to mechanical loading: A systematic review and meta-analysis of exercise intervention studies on healthy adults. Sports Medicine – Open 1(1):7. doi: 10.1186/s40798-015-0009-9.

Borman NP, Trudelle-Jackson E, Smith SS (2011) Effect of stretch positions on hamstring muscle length, lumbar flexion range of motion, and lumbar curvature in healthy adults. Physiotherapy Theory and Practice 27(2):146–154. doi: 10.3109/09593981003703030.

Bourne MN, Duhig SJ, Timmins RG, Williams MD, Opar DA, Al Najjar A, Kerr GK, Shield AJ (2017) Impact of the Nordic hamstring and hip extension exercises on hamstring architecture and morphology: Implications for injury prevention. British Journal of Sports Medicine 51:469–477. doi: 10.1136/bjsports-2016-096130.

Brinjikji W, Diehn FE, Jarvik JG, Carr CM, Kallmes DF, Murad MH, Luetmer PH (2015) MRI findings of disc degeneration are more prevalent in adults with low back pain than in asymptomatic controls: A systematic review and meta-analysis. American Journal of Neuroradiology 36(12):2394–2399. doi: 10.3174/ajnr.A4498.

Brodsky BB, Persikov AV (2005) Molecular structure of the collagen triple helix. Advances in Protein Chemistry 70(4):301–339. doi: 10.1016/S0065-3233(04)70009-1.

Brughelli M, Cronin J (2007) Altering the length-tension relationship with eccentric exercise: Implications for performance and injury. Sports Medicine 37(9):807–826.

Brunelle J-F, Blais-Coutu S, Gouadec K, Bédard É, Fait P (2015) Influences of a yoga intervention on the postural skills of the Italian short track speed skating team. Open Access Journal of Sports Medicine 6:23–35. doi: 10.2147/OAJSM.S68337.

Butterfield TA, Leonard TR, Herzog W (2005) Differential serial sarcomere number adaptations in knee extensor muscles of rats is contraction type dependent. Journal of Applied Physiology 99(4):1352–1358. doi: 10.1152/japplphysiol.00481.2005.-Sarcomerogenesis.

Cao T, Hicks MR, Zein-Hammoud M, Standley PR (2015) Duration and magnitude of myofascial release in 3-dimensional bioengineered tendons: Effects on wound healing. Journal of the American Osteopathic Association 115(2):72–82. doi: 10.7556/jaoa.2015.018.

Cattalini M, Khubchandani R, Cimaz R (2015) When flexibility is not necessarily a virtue: A review of hypermobility syndromes and chronic or recurrent musculoskeletal pain in children. Pediatric Rheumatology 13(1):40. doi: 10.1186/s12969-015-0039-3.

Chaudhry H, Max R, Antonio S, Findley T (2012) Mathematical model of fiber orientation in anisotropic fascia layers at large displacements. Journal of Bodywork and Movement Therapies 16(2):158–164. doi: 10.1016/j.jbmt.2011.04.006.

Chiu CC, Chuang TY, Chang KH, Wu CH, Lin PW, Hsu WY (2015) The probability of spontaneous regression of lumbar herniated disc: A systematic review. Clinical Rehabilitation 29(2):184–195. doi: 10.1177/0269215514540919.

Cholewicki J, Panjabi MM, Khachatryan A (1997) Stabilizing function of trunk flexor-extensor muscles around a neutral spine posture. Spine 22(19):2207–2212. doi: 10.1097/00007632-199710010-00003.

Clemes SA, Haslam CO, Haslam RA (2009) What constitutes effective manual handling training? A systematic review. Occupational Medicine 60(2):101–107. doi: 10.1093/occmed/kqp127.

Cook JL, Rio E, Purdam CR, Docking SI (2016) Revisiting the continuum model of tendon pathology: What is its merit in clinical practice and research? British Journal of Sports Medicine 50:1187–1191. doi: 10.1136/bjsports-2015-095422.

Cook JL, Docking SI (2015) Rehabilitation will increase the – 'capacity' of your – insert musculoskeletal tissue here. Defining 'tissue capacity': A core concept for clinicians. British Journal of Sports Medicine 49(23):1484–1485. doi: 10.1136/bjsports-2015-094849.

Cook JL, Purdam CR (2009) Is tendon pathology a continuum? A pathology model to explain the clinical presentation of load-induced tendinopathy. British Journal of Sports Medicine 43:409–416. doi: 10.1136/bjsm.2008.051193.

Cramer H, Ward L, Saper R, Fishbein D, Dobos G, Lauche R (2015) The safety of yoga: A systematic review and meta-analysis of randomized controlled trials. American Journal of Epidemiology 182(4):281–293. doi: 10.1093/aje/kwv071.

Dickinson MH, Farley CT, Full RJ, Koehl MA, Kram R, Lehman S (2000) How animals move: An integrative view. Science 288(5463):100–106.

Docking SI, Cook J (2016) Pathological tendons maintain sufficient aligned fibrillar structure on ultrasound tissue characterization (UTC). Scandinavian Journal of Medicine and Science in Sports 26(6):675–683. doi: 10.1111/sms.12491.

Docking S, Samiric T, Scase E, Purdam C, Cook J (2013) Relationship between compressive loading and ECM changes in tendons. Muscles, Ligaments and Tendons Journal 3(1):7–11. doi: 10.11138/mltj/2013.3.1.007.

Endo K, Suzuki H, Nishimura H, Tanaka H, Shishido T, Yamamoto K (2014) Characteristics of sagittal spino-pelvic alignment in Japanese young adults. Asian Spine Journal 8(5):599–604. doi: 10.4184/asj.2014.8.5.599.

Farmer M, James SE (2001) Contractures in orthopaedic and neurological conditions: A review of causes and treatment. Disability and Rehabilitation 23(13):549–558. doi: 10.1080/09638280010029930.

Fergusson D, Hutton B, Drodge A (2007) The epidemiology of major joint contractures: A systematic review of the literature. Clinical Orthopaedics and Related Research 456(456):22–29. doi: 10.1097/BLO.0b013e3180308456.

Ferrer GA, Miller RM, Zlotnicki JP, Tashman S, Irrgang JJ, Musahl V, Debski RE (2018) Exercise therapy for treatment of supraspinatus tears does not alter glenohumeral kinematics during internal/external rotation with the arm at the side. Knee Surgery, Sports Traumatology, Arthroscopy 26(1):267–274. doi: 10.1007/s00167-017-4695-3.

Finan PH, Buenaver LF, Bounds SC, Hussain S, Park RJ, Haque UJ, Campbell CM, Haythornthwaite JA, Edwards RR, Smith MT (2013) Discordance between pain and radiographic severity in knee osteoarthritis: Findings from quantitative sensory testing of central sensitization. Arthritis and Rheumatism 65(2):363–372. doi: 10.1002/art.34646.

Flemons T (2006) Intension designs. Available: http://www.intensiondesigns.ca/ [15 June 2018]

Franchi MV, Reeves ND, Narici MV (2017) Skeletal muscle remodeling in response to eccentric vs. concentric loading: Morphological, molecular, and metabolic adaptations. Frontiers in Physiology 8:447. doi: 10.3389/fphys.2017.00447.

Freedman BR, Zuskov A, Sarver JJ, Buckley MR, Soslowsky LJ (2015) Evaluating changes in tendon crimp with fatigue loading as an ex vivo structural assessment of tendon damage. Journal of Orthopaedic Research 33(6):904–910. doi: 10.1002/jor.22875.

Freitas SR, Mendes B, Andrade RJ (2017) Can chronic stretching change the muscle-tendon mechanical properties? A review. Scandinavian Journal of Medicine and Science in Sports 28(3):794–806. doi: 10.1111/sms.12957.

Freitas SR, Mil-Homens P (2015) Effect of 8-week high-intensity stretching training on biceps femoris architecture. Journal of Strength and Conditioning Research 29(6):1737–1740.

Fritz ML, Grossman AM, Mukherjee A, Hunter SD, Tracy BL (2014) Acute metabolic, cardiovascular, and thermal responses to a single session of Bikram yoga. Medicine and Science in Sports and Exercise 46(5S):146–147. doi: 10.1249/01.mss.0000493613.83031.88.

Gabbett TJ (2016) The training-injury prevention paradox: Should athletes be training smarter and harder? British Journal of Sports Medicine 50(5):273–280. doi: 10.1136/bjsports-2015-095788.

Gallo RA, Silvis M, Smetana B, Mosher T, Stuck D, Lynch SA, Black KP (2013) Hip labral tears among asymptomatic professional hockey players identified on MRI: Four-year follow-up study. Orthopaedic Journal of Sports Medicine 1(4):2013. doi: 10.1177/2325967113S00057.

Garber CE, Blissmer B, Deschenes MR, Franklin BA, Lamonte MJ, Lee IM, Nieman DC, Swain DP, American College of Sports Medicine (2011) American College of Sports Medicine position stand. Quantity and quality of exercise for developing and maintaining cardiorespiratory, musculoskeletal, and neuromotor fitness in apparently healthy adults: Guidance for prescribing exercise. Medicine and Science in Sports and Exercise 43(7):1334–1359. doi: 10.1249/MSS.0b013e318213fefb.

Girish G, Lobo LG, Jacobson JA, Morag Y, Miller B, Jamadar DA (2011) Ultrasound of the shoulder: Asymptomatic findings in men. American Journal of Roentgenology 197(4):713–719. doi: 10.2214/AJR.11.6971.

Glasgow P, Phillips N, Bleakley C (2015) Optimal loading: Key variables and mechanisms. British Journal of Sports Medicine 49(5):278–279. doi: 10.1136/bjsports-2014-094443.

Goldring MB (2012) Articular cartilage degradation in osteoarthritis. HSS Journal 8(1):7–9. doi: 10.1007/s11420-011-9250-z.

Gracovetsky, Serge. (2007). Stability or controlled instability?. Movement, Stability & Lumbopelvic Pain. 279-294. 10.1016/B978-044310178-6.50021-9.

Gracovetsky S (2008) Is the lumbodorsal fascia necessary? Journal of Bodywork and Movement Therapies 12(3):194–197. doi: 10.1016/j.jbmt.2008.03.006.

Green D (2015) ACE Study examines effects of Bikram yoga on core body temps, www.acefitness.org. Available: https://www.acefitness.org/education-and-resources/professional/prosource/may-2015/5355/ace-study-examines-effects-of-bikram-yoga-on-core-body-temps [2 March 2018].

Greene GW, Banquy X, Lee DW, Lowrey DD, Yu J, Israelachvili JN (2011) Adaptive mechanically controlled lubrication mechanism found in articular joints. Proceedings of the National Academy of Sciences of the United States of America 108(13):5255–5259. doi: 10.1073/pnas.1101002108.

Guex K, Degache F, Morisod C, Sailly M, Millet GP (2016) Hamstring architectural and functional adaptations following long vs. short muscle length eccentric training. Frontiers in Physiology 7(August):340. doi: 10.3389/fphys.2016.00340.

Guimberteau JC (2005) The sliding mechanics of the subcutaneous structures in man. Illustration of a functional unit: The microvacuoles. Studies of the Académie Nationale de Chirurgie 4(4):35–42.

Halper J, Kjaer M (2014) Basic components of connective tissues and extracellular matrix: Elastin, fibrillin, fibulins, fibrinogen, fibronectin, laminin, tenascins and thrombospondins. Advances in Experimental Medicine and Biology, ed. J. Halper. Dordrecht: Springer Netherlands (Advances in Experimental Medicine and Biology), 802, pp. 31–47. doi: 10.1007/978-94-007-7893-1.

Hamilton AR, Beck KL, Kaulbach J, Kenny M, Basset FA, DiSanto MC, Behm DG (2015) Breathing techniques affect female but not male hip flexion range of motion. Journal of Strength and Conditioning Research 29(11):3197–3205. doi: 10.1519/JSC.0000000000000982.

Hanci E, Sekir U, Gur H, Akova B (2016) Eccentric training improves ankle evertor and dorsiflexor strength and proprioception in functionally unstable ankles. American Journal of Physical Medicine and Rehabilitation 95(6):448–458. doi: 10.1097/PHM.0000000000000421.

Harvey LA, Katalinic OM, Herbert RD, Moseley AM, Lannin NA, Schurr K (2017) Stretch for the treatment and prevention of contracture: An abridged republication of a Cochrane

Systematic Review. Journal of Physiotherapy. Korea Institute of Oriental Medicine 63(2):67–75. doi: 10.1016/j.jphys.2017.02.014.

Hauser R, Dolan EE, Phillips HJ, Newlin AC, Moore RE, Woldin BA (2013) Ligament injury and healing: A review of current clinical diagnostics and therapeutics. Open Rehabilitation Journal 6:1–20.

Hector R, Jensen JL (2015) Sirsasana (headstand) technique alters head/neck loading: Considerations for safety. Journal of Bodywork and Movement Therapies 19(3):434–441. doi: 10.1016/j.jbmt.2014.10.002.

Heinemeier KM, Schjerling P, Heinemeier J, Møller MB, Krogsgaard MR, Grum-Schwensen T, Petersen MM, Kjaer M (2016) Radiocarbon dating reveals minimal collagen turnover in both healthy and osteoarthritic human cartilage. Science Translational Medicine 8(346):346ra90. doi: 10.1126/scitranslmed.aad8335.

Herbert R (2005) How muscles respond to stretch, in K Refshauge, L Ada, E Ellis (eds) Science-Based Rehabilitation, Edinburgh: Elsevier Limited, pp. 107–130.

Herrington L (2011) Assessment of the degree of pelvic tilt within a normal asymptomatic population. Manual Therapy 16(6):646–648. doi: 10.1016/j.math.2011.04.006.

Herzog W, Schappacher G, DuVall M, Leonard TR, Herzog JA (2016) Residual force enhancement following eccentric contractions: A new mechanism involving titin. Physiology 31(4):300–312. doi: 10.1152/physiol.00049.2014.

Heslinga JW, te Kronnie G, Huijing PA (1995) Growth and immobilization effects on sarcomeres: A comparison between gastrocnemius and soleus muscles of the adult rat. European Journal of Applied Physiology and Occupational Physiology 70(1):49–57. Available: http://www.ncbi.nlm.nih.gov/pubmed/7729438.

Hodges PW, Richardson CA (1999) Altered trunk muscle recruitment in people with low back pain with upper limb movement at different speeds. Archives of Physical Medicine and Rehabilitation 80(9):1005–1012. doi: S0003-9993(99)90052-7 [pii].

Hogan DA, Greiner BA, O'Sullivan L (2014) The effect of manual handling training on achieving training transfer, employee's behaviour change and subsequent reduction of work-related musculoskeletal disorders: A systematic review. Ergonomics 57(1):93–107. doi: 10.1080/00140139.2013.862307.

Howarth SJ, Glisic D, Lee JG, Beach TA (2013) Does prolonged seated deskwork alter the lumbar flexion relaxation phenomenon? Journal of Electromyography and Kinesiology 23(3):587–593. doi: 10.1016/j.jelekin.2013.01.004.

Hrysomallis C (2010) Effects of stretching and strengthening exercises for postural correction of abducted scapulae: A review. Journal of Strength and Conditioning Research 24(2):567–574. doi 10.1519/JSC.0b013e3181c069d8.

Hrysomallis C, Goodman C (2001) A review of resistance exercise and posture realignment. Journal of Strength and Conditioning Research 15(3):385–390. doi: 10.1519/1533-4287(2001)015<0385:AROREA>2.0.CO;2.

Huijing PA (2009) Epimuscular myofascial force transmission: A historical review and implications for new research. International Society of Biomechanics Muybridge Award Lecture, Taipei, 2007. Journal of Biomechanics 42(1):9–21. doi: 10.1016/j.jbiomech.2008.09.027.

Ingber D, Wang N, Stamenović D (2014) Tensegrity, cellular biophysics, and the mechanics of living systems. Reports on Progress in Physics 77(4):46603. doi: 10.1088/0034-4885/77/4/046603.

Ipsos Public Affairs (2016) 2016 Yoga in America. Yoga Journal. Available: https://www.yogajournal.com/page/yogainamericastudy.

Iyengar B (1979) Light on Yoga. New York, NY: Schocken Books.

Junker D, Stöggl T (2015) The foam roll as a tool to improve hamstring flexibility. Journal of Strength and Conditioning Research 29(12):3480–3485. doi: 10.1519/JSC.0000000000001007.

Kadler KE, Baldock C, Bella J, Boot-Handford RP (2007) Collagens at a glance. Journal of Cell Science 120:1955–1958. doi: 10.1242/jcs.03453.

Kannus P, Jozsa L (1991) Histopathological changes preceding spontaneous rupture of a tendon. A controlled study of 891 patients. Journal of Bone and Joint Surgery 73(10):1507–1525.

Kawakami Y, Muraoka T, Ito S, Kanehisa H, Fukunaga T (2002) In vivo muscle fibre behaviour during counter-movement exercise in humans reveals a significant role for tendon elasticity. Journal of Physiology 540(2):635–646. doi: 10.1113/jphysiol.2001.013459.

Kelley K, Slattery K, Apollo K (2017) An electromyographic analysis of selected asana in experienced yogic practitioners. Journal of Bodywork and Movement Therapies 22(1):152–158. doi: 10.1016/j.jbmt.2017.05.018.

Kelly S, Beardsley C (2016) Specific and cross-over effects of foam rolling on ankle dorsiflexion range of motion. International Journal of Sports Physical Therapy 11(4):544–51. Available: https://www.ncbi.nlm.nih.gov/pubmed/27525179.

Khan KM, Scott A (2009) Mechanotherapy: How physical therapists' prescription of exercise promotes tissue repair. British Journal of Sports Medicine 43(4):247–252. doi: 10.1136/bjsm.2008.054239.

Konin JG, Wiksten DL, Isear JA, Brader H (2006) Special Tests for Orthopedic Examination, 3rd edn. Thorofare, NJ: Slack.

Konrad A, Tilp M (2014) Increased range of motion after static stretching is not due to changes in muscle and tendon structures. Clinical Biomechanics 29(6):636–642. doi: 10.1016/j.clinbiomech.2014.04.013.

Krabak BJ, Laskowski ER, Smith J, Stuart MJ, Wong GY (2001) Neurophysiologic influences on hamstring flexibility: A pilot study. Clinical Journal of Sport Medicine 11(4):241–246.

Kubo K, Kanehisa H, Kawakami Y, Fukunaga T (2001) Influence of static stretching on viscoelastic properties of human tendon structures in vivo. Journal of Applied Physiology 90(2):520–527.

Kubo K, Kanehisa H, Fukunaga T (2002) Effect of stretching training on the viscoelastic properties of human tendon structures in vivo. Journal of Applied Physiology 92(2):595–601. doi: 10.1152/japplphysiol.00658.2001.

Langevin HM, Huijing PA (2009) Communicating about fascia: History, pitfalls, and recommendations. International Journal of Therapeutic Massage and Bodywork 2(4):3–8.

Lauche R, Schumann D, Sibbritt D, Adams J, Cramer H (2017) Associations between yoga practice and joint problems: A cross-sectional survey among 9151 Australian women. Rheumatology International. Springer Berlin Heidelberg, 37(7):1145–1148. doi: 10.1007/s00296-017-3744-z.

Lavagnino M, Brooks AE, Oslapas AN, Gardner KL, Arnoczky SP (2017) Crimp length decreases in lax tendons due to cytoskeletal tension, but is restored with tensional homeostasis. Journal of Orthopaedic Research 35(3):573–579. doi: 10.1002/jor.23489.

Le Corroller T, Vertinsky AT, Hargunani R, Khashoggi K, Munk PL, Ouellette HA (2012) Musculoskeletal injuries related to yoga: Imaging observations. American Journal of Roentgenology 199(2):413–418. doi: 10.2214/AJR.11.7440.

Lederman E (2011) The fall of the postural-structural-biomechanical model in manual and physical therapies: Exemplified by lower back pain. Journal of Bodywork and Movement Therapies 15(2):131–138. doi: 10.1016/j.jbmt.2011.01.011.

Lu YH, Rosner B, Chang G, Fishman LM (2016) Twelve-minute daily yoga regimen reverses osteoporotic bone loss. Topics in Geriatric Rehabilitation 32(2):81–87. doi: 10.1097/TGR.0000000000000085.

Magnusson S, Heinemeier K, Kjaer M (2016) Collagen homeostasis and metabolism. Advances in Experimental Medicine and Biology 920:11–25. doi: 10.1007/978-3-319-33943-6_2.

Magnusson SP, Simonsen EB, Aagaard P, Sørensen H et al. (1996a) A mechanism for altered flexibility in human skeletal muscle. Journal of Physiology 497(1):291–298.

Magnusson SP, Simonsen EB, Aagaard P, Kjaer M (1996b) Biomechanical responses to repeated stretches in human hamstring muscle in vivo. American Journal of Sports Medicine 24(5):622–628.

Magnusson SP, Langberg H, Kjaer M (2010) The pathogenesis of tendinopathy: Balancing the response to loading. Nature Reviews. Rheumatology, 6(5):262–268. doi: 10.1088/nrrheurn.2010.43.

Malliaras P, Kamal B, Nowell A, Farley T, Dhamu H, Simpson V, Morrissey D, Langberg H, Maffulli N, Reeves ND (2013) Patellar tendon adaptation in relation to load-intensity and contraction type. Journal of Biomechanics 46(11):1893–1899. doi: 10.1016/j.jbiomech.2013.04.022.

Marshall PW, Cashman A, Cheema BS (2011) A randomized controlled trial for the effect of passive stretching on measures of hamstring extensibility, passive stiffness, strength, and stretch tolerance. Journal of Science and Medicine in Sport 14(6):535–540. doi: 10.1016/j.jsams.2011.05.003.

McNeill W, Jones S, Barton S (2018) The Pilates client on the hypermobility spectrum. Journal of Bodywork and Movement Therapies 22(1):209–216. doi: 10.1016/j.jbmt.2017.12.013.

Millett PJ, Giphart JE, Wilson KJ, Kagnes K, Greenspoon JA (2016) Alterations in glenohumeral kinematics in patients with rotator cuff tears measured with biplane fluoroscopy. Arthroscopy 32(3):446–451. doi: 10.1016/j.arthro.2015.08.031.

Mok NW, Hodges PW (2013) Movement of the lumbar spine is critical for maintenance of postural recovery following support surface perturbation. Experimental Brain Research 231(3):305–313. doi: 10.1007/s00221-013-3692-0.

Moonaz S, Jeter P, Schmalzl L (2017) The importance of research literacy for yoga therapists. International Journal of Yoga Therapy 27(1):131–133.

Moreside J, McGill S (2012) Hip joint range of motion improvements using three different interventions. Journal of Strength and Conditioning Research 26(5):1265–1273.

Moreside J, McGill S (2013) Improvements in hip flexibility do not transfer to mobility in functional movement patterns. Journal of Strength and Conditioning Research 27(10):2635–2643.

Morris ZS, Wooding S, Grant J (2011) The answer is 17 years, what is the question: Understanding time lags in translational research. Journal of the Royal Society of Medicine 104(12):510–520. doi: 10.1258/jrsm.2011.110180.

Mueller-Wohlfahrt HW, Haensel L, Mithoefer K, Ekstrand J, English B, McNally S, Orchard J, van Dijk CN, Kerkhoffs GM, Schamasch P, Blottner D, Swaerd L, Goedhart E, Ueblacker P (2013) Terminology and classification of muscle injuries in sport: The Munich consensus statement. British Journal of Sports Medicine 47(6):342–350. doi: 10.1136/bjsports-2012-091448.

Nakamura M, Ikezoe T, Takeno Y, Ichihashi N (2012) Effects of a 4-week static stretch training program on passive stiffness of human gastrocnemius muscle-tendon unit in vivo. European Journal of Applied Physiology 112(7):2749–2755. doi: 10.1007/s00421-011-2250-3.

Nakamura M, Ikezoe T, Takeno Y, Ichihashi N (2013) Time course of changes in passive properties of the gastrocnemius muscle-tendon unit during 5 min of static stretching. Manual Therapy 18(3):211–215. doi: 10.1016/j.math.2012.09.010.

Nakashima H, Yukawa Y, Suda K, Yamagata M, Ueta T, Kato F (2015) Abnormal findings on magnetic resonance images of the cervical spines in 1211 asymptomatic subjects. Spine 40(6):392–398. doi: 10.1097/BRS.0000000000000775.

Ni M, Mooney K, Balachandran A, Richards L, Harriell K, Signorile JF (2014) Muscle utilization patterns vary by skill levels of the practitioners across specific yoga poses (asanas). Complementary Therapies in Medicine 22(4):662–669. doi: 10.1016/j.ctim.2014.06.006.

Noorkõiv M, Nosaka K, Blazevich A (2014) Neuromuscular adaptations associated with knee joint angle-specific force change. Medicine and Science in Sports and Exercise 46(8):1525–1537. doi: 10.1249/MSS.0000000000000269.

O'Sullivan K, McAuliffe S, Deburca N (2012) The effects of eccentric training on lower limb flexibility: A systematic review. British Journal of Sports Medicine 46(12):838–845. doi: 10.1136/bjsports-2011-090835.

Orishimo K, McHugh MP (2015) Effect of an eccentrically biased hamstring strengthening home program on knee flexor strength and the length-tension relationship. Journal of Strength and Conditioning Research 29(3):772–778.

Pape JL, Brismée JM, Sizer PS, Matthijs OC, Browne KL, Dewan BM, Sobczak S (2018) Increased spinal height using propped slouched sitting postures: Innovative ways to rehydrate intervertebral discs. Applied Ergonomics 66:9–17. doi: 10.1016/j.apergo.2017.07.016.

Park CL, Riley KE, Braun TD (2016) Practitioners' perceptions of yoga's positive and negative effects: Results of a National United States survey. Journal of Bodywork and Movement Therapies 20(2):270–279. doi: 10.1016/j.jbmt.2015.11.005.

Petrofsky JS, Laymon M, Lee H (2013) Effect of heat and cold on tendon flexibility and force to flex the human knee. Medical Science Monitor 19:661–667. doi: 10.12659/MSM.889145.

Polsgrove MJ, Eggleston BM, Lockyer RJ (2016) Impact of 10-weeks of yoga practice on flexibility and balance of college athletes. International Journal of Yoga 9(1):27–34. doi: 10.4103/0973-6131.171710.

Pugh A (1976) An Introduction to Tensegrity. Berkeley: University of California Press.

Quandt E, Porcari J, Steffen J, Felix M, Foster C, Green DJ (2015) Heart rate and core temperature responses to Bikram yoga. ACE ProSource, May, pp. 1–5.

Reeves P, Narendra K, Cholewicki J (2007) Spine stability: the six blind men and the elephant. Clinical Biomechanics 22(3):266–274.

Riel H, Cotchett M, Delahunt E, Rathleff MS, Vicenzino B, Weir A, Landorf KB (2017) Is 'plantar heel pain' a more appropriate term than 'plantar fasciitis'? Time to move on. British Journal of Sports Medicine 51(22):1576–1577. doi: 10.1136/bjsports-2017-097519.

Rio E, Moseley L, Purdam C, Samiric T, Kidgell D, Pearce AJ, Jaberzadeh S, Cook J (2014) The pain of tendinopathy: Physiological or pathophysiological? Sports Medicine 44(1):9–23. doi: 10.1007/s40279-013-0096-z.

Ryan ED, Herda TJ, Costa PB, Walter AA, Hoge KM, Stout JR, Cramer JT (2010) Viscoelastic creep in the human skeletal muscle-tendon unit. European Journal of Applied Physiology 108(1):207–211. doi: 10.1007/s00421-009-1284-2.

Scarr G (2012) A consideration of the elbow as a tensegrity structure. International Journal of Osteopathic Medicine 15(2):53–65. doi: 10.1016/j.ijosm.2011.11.003.

Scarr G (2016) Comment on 'Defining the fascial system'. Journal of Bodywork and Movement Therapies 21(1):178. doi: 10.1016/j.jbmt.2016.11.004.

Scheper MC, de Vries JE, Verbunt J, Engelbert RH (2015) Chronic pain in hypermobility syndrome and Ehlers-Danlos syndrome (hypermobility type): It is a challenge. Journal of Pain Research 8:591–601. doi: 10.2147/JPR.S64251.

Schleip R, Findley TW, Chaitow L, Huijing PA (eds) (2012) Fascia: The Tensional Network of the Human Body. Edinburgh: Elsevier.

Schleip R, Müller DG (2013) Training principles for fascial connective tissues: Scientific foundation and suggested practical applications. Journal of Bodywork and Movement Therapies 17:103–115. doi: 10.1016/j.jbmt.2012.06.007.

Schwartzberg R, Reuss BL, Burkhart BG, Butterfield M, Wu JY, McLean KW (2016) High prevalence of superior labral tears diagnosed by MRI in middle-aged patients with asymptomatic shoulders. Orthopaedic Journal of Sports Medicine 4(1), p. 2325967115623212. doi: 10.1177/2325967115623212.

Scott A, Backman LJ, Speed C (2015) Tendinopathy: Update on pathophysiology. Journal of Orthopaedic and Sports Physical Therapy 45(11):833–841. doi: 10.2519/jospt.2015.5884.

Shin G, D'Souza C, Liu YH (2009) Creep and fatigue development in the low back in static flexion. Spine 34(17):1873–1878. doi: 10.1097/BRS.0b013e3181aa6a55.

Silvis ML, Mosher TJ, Smetana BS, Chinchilli VM, Flemming DJ, Walker EA, Black KP (2011) High prevalence of pelvic and hip magnetic resonance imaging findings in asymptomatic collegiate and professional hockey players. American Journal of Sports Medicine 39(4):715–721. doi: 10.1177/0363546510388931.

Sinaki M (2013) Yoga spinal flexion positions and vertebral compression fracture in osteopenia or osteoporosis of spine: Case series. Pain Practice 13(1):68–75. doi: 10.1111/j.1533-2500.2012.00545.x.

Smith BE, Hendrick P, Smith TO, Bateman M, Moffatt F, Rathleff MS, Selfe J, Logan P (2017) Should exercises be painful in the management of chronic musculoskeletal pain? A systematic review and meta-analysis. British Journal of Sports Medicine 51(23):1679–1687. doi: 10.1136/bjsports-2016-097383.

Smith BE, Littlewood C, May S (2014) An update of stabilisation exercises for low back pain: A systematic review with meta-analysis. BMC Musculoskeletal Disorders 15(1):416. doi: 10.1186/1471-2474-15-416.

Soligard T, Schwellnus M, Alonso JM, Bahr R, Clarsen B, Dijkstra HP, Gabbett T, Gleeson M, Hägglund M, Hutchinson MR, Janse van Rensburg C, Khan KM, Meeusen R, Orchard JW, Pluim BM, Raftery M, Budgett R, Engebretsen L (2016) How much is too much? (Part 1) International Olympic Committee consensus statement on load in sport and risk of illness. British Journal of Sports Medicine 50(17):1030–1041. doi: 10.1136/bjsports-2016-096572.

Stecco C, Adstrum S, Hedley G, Schleip R, Yucesoy CA (2018) Update on fascial nomenclature. Journal of Bodywork and Movement Therapies 22(2):354 doi: 10.1016/j.jbmt.2017.12.015.

Steele J, Bruce-Low S, Smith D, Osborne N, Thorkeldsen A (2015) Can specific loading through exercise impart healing or regeneration of the intervertebral disc? Spine Journal 15(10):2117–2121. doi: 10.1016/j.spinee.2014.08.446.

Stephens J, Davidson J, Derosa J, Kriz M, Saltzman N (2006) Lengthening the hamstring muscles without stretching using 'awareness through movement'. Physical Therapy 86(12):1641–1650. doi: 10.2522/ptj.20040208.

Straker LM (2002) A review of research on techniques for lifting low-lying objects: 1. Criteria for evaluation. Work 19(1):9–18.

Svensson RB, Hassenkam T, Hansen P, Peter Magnusson S (2010) Viscoelastic behavior of discrete human collagen fibrils. Journal of the Mechanical Behavior of Biomedical Materials 3(1):112–115. doi: 10.1016/j.jmbbm.2009.01.005.

Thornton GM, Hart DA (2011) The interface of mechanical loading and biological variables as they pertain to the development of tendinosis. Journal of Musculoskeletal and Neuronal Interactions 11(2):94–105.

van den Bekerom MP, Struijs PA, Blankevoort L, Welling L, van Dijk CN, Kerkhoffs GM (2012) What is the evidence for rest, ice, compression, and elevation therapy in the treatment of ankle sprains in adults? Journal of Athletic Training 47(4): 435–443. doi: 10.4085/1062-6050-47.4.14.

van der Wal J (2009) The architecture of the connective tissue in the musculoskeletal system – an often overlooked functional parameter as to proprioception in the locomotor apparatus. International Journal of Therapeutic Massage and Bodywork 2(4):9–23.

van Dyke JM, Bain JLW, Riley DA (2012) Preserving sarcomere number after tenotomy requires stretch and contraction. Muscle and Nerve 45(3):367–375. doi: 10.1002/mus.22286.

Vigotsky A, Halperin I, Lehman GJ, Trajano GS, Vieira TM (2017) Interpreting surface electromyography studies in sports and rehabilitation sciences. Frontiers in Physiology 8(January):985. doi: 10.17605/OSF.IO/FKBX8.

Vora AJ, Doerr KD, Wolfer LR (2010) Functional anatomy and pathophysiology of axial low back pain: disc, posterior elements, sacroiliac joint, and associated pain generators. Physical Medicine and Rehabilitation Clinics of North America 21(4):679–709. doi: 10.1016/j.pmr.2010.07.005.

Wallace IJ, Worthington S, Felson DT, Jurmain RD, Wren KT, Maijanen H, Woods RJ, Lieberman DE (2017) Knee osteoarthritis has doubled in prevalence since the mid-20th century. Proceedings of the National Academy of Sciences 114(35):9332–9336. doi: 10.1073/pnas.1703856114.

Wang N, Naruse K, Stamenović D, Fredberg JJ, Mijailovich SM, Tolić-Nørrelykke IM, Polte T, Mannix R, Ingber DE (2001) Mechanical behavior in living cells consistent with the tensegrity model. Proceedings of the National Academy of Sciences 98(14):7765–7770. doi: 10.1073/pnas.141199598.

Watson SL, Weeks BK, Weis LJ, Horan SA , Beck BR (2015) Heavy resistance training is safe and improves bone, function, and stature in postmenopausal women with low to very low bone mass: Novel early findings from the LIFTMOR trial. Osteoporosis International 26(12):2889–2894. doi: 10.1007/s00198-015-3263-2.

Wattanaprakornkul D, Cathers I, Halaki M, Ginn KA (2011) The rotator cuff muscles have a direction specific recruitment pattern during shoulder flexion and extension exercises. Journal of Science and Medicine in Sport 14(5):376–382. doi: 10.1016/j.jsams.2011.01.001.

Weppler CH, Magnusson SP (2010) Increasing muscle extensibility: A matter of increasing length or modifying sensation? Physical Therapy 90(3):438–449. doi: 10.2522/ptj.20090012.

Wilcox SJ, Hager R, Lockhart B, Seeley MK (2012) Ground reaction forces generated by twenty-eight Hatha yoga postures. International Journal of Exercise Science 5(2):114-126. Available: https://www.ncbi.nlm.nih.gov/pubmed/27182380

Willard FH, Vleeming A, Schuenke MD, Danneels L, Schleip R (2012) The thoracolumbar fascia: Anatomy, function and clinical considerations. Journal of Anatomy 221(6):507–536. doi: 10.1111/j.1469-7580.2012.01511.x.

Williams P, Catanese T (1988) The importance of stretch and contractile activity in the prevention of connective tissue accumulation in muscle. Journal of Anatomy 158:109–114.

Wolf JM, Cameron KL, Owens BD (2011) Impact of joint laxity and hypermobility on the musculoskeletal system. Journal of the American Academy of Orthopaedic Surgeons 19(8):463–471. Available: http://www.ncbi.nlm.nih.gov/pubmed/21807914.

Yosifon D, Stearns P (1998) The rise and fall of American posture. American Historical Review 103(4):1057–1095.

Yu SS, Wang MY, Samarawickrame S, Hashish R, Kazadi L, Greendale GA, Salem GJ (2012) The physical demands of the tree (vriksasana) and one-leg balance (utthita hasta padangusthasana) poses performed by seniors: A biomechanical examination. Evidence-based Complementary and Alternative Medicine: eCAM 2012:971896. doi: 10.1155/2012/971896.

Zhong M, Liu JT, Jiang H, Mo W, Yu PF, Li XC, Xue RR (2017) Incidence of spontaneous resorption of lumbar disc herniation: A meta-analysis. Pain Physician Journal 20(1):4E5–E52. Available: https://www.ncbi.nlm.nih.gov/pubmed/28072796.

Zöllner AM, Abilez OJ, Böl M, Kuhl E (2012) Stretching skeletal muscle: Chronic muscle lengthening through sarcomerogenesis. PloS one 7(10):e45661. doi: 10.1371/journal.pone.0045661.

Zorn A (2007) Physical thoughts about structure: The elasticity of fascia. Journal of the Rolf Institute. Available: https://www.rolf.org/docs/Journal_03-07_full.pdf.

Zwambag DP, Brown SHM (2015) Factors to consider in identifying critical points in lumbar spine flexion relaxation. Journal of Electromyography and Kinesiology 25(6):914–918. doi: 10.1016/j.jelekin.2015.10.017.

Index

A

B

C

D

E

F

G

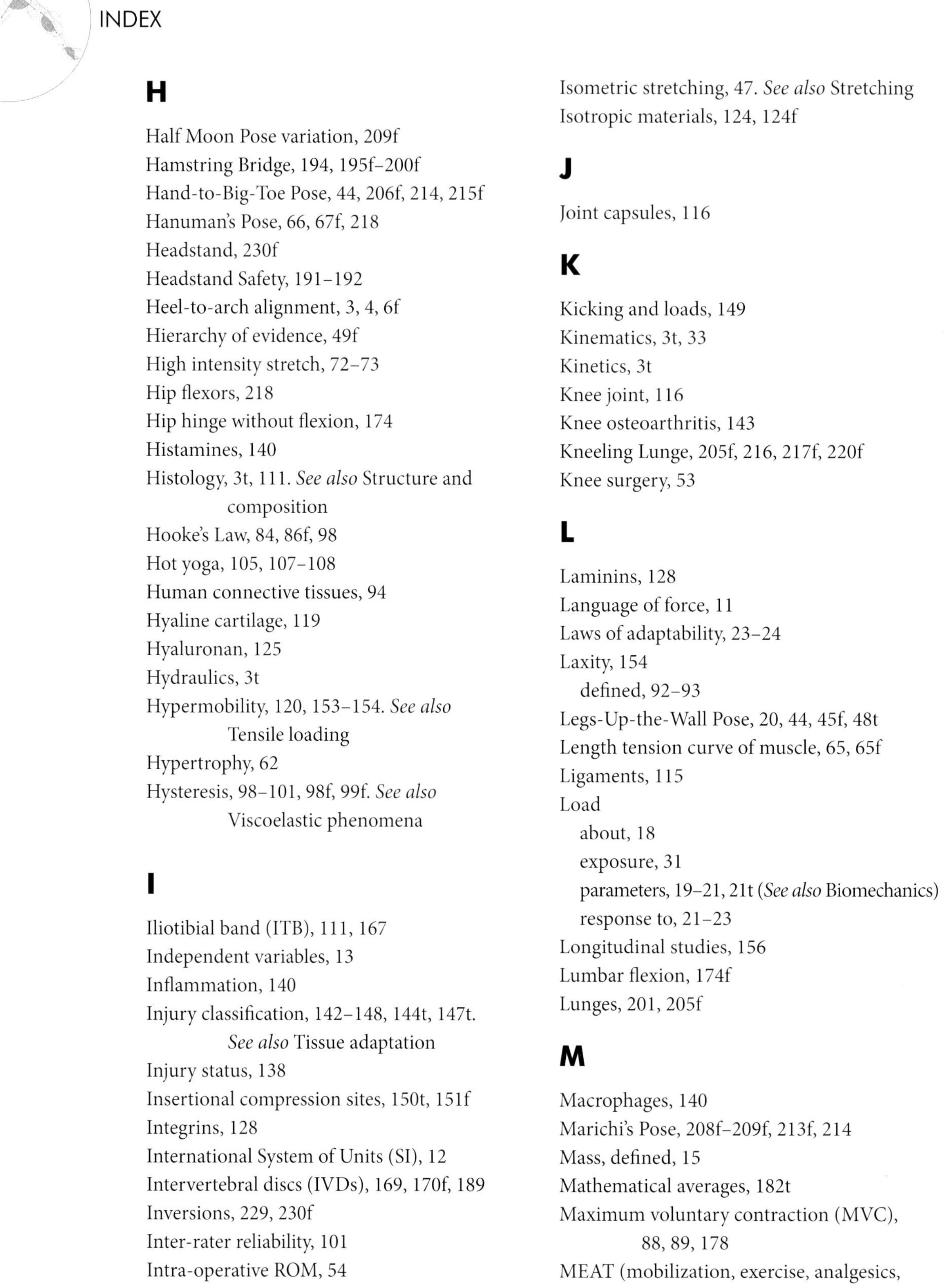

N

O

P

R

S

V

W

Y